"Across my career, I have enjoyed the privilege of reading literally thousands of books on psychoanalysis, but I cannot ever recall having encountered such a unique and stimulating publication as Dr. Todd Anderson's new text on *Unknowing as Truth: Epistemic Inversions and the Recursive Psyche*. This deeply original and profoundly scholarly tome provides us all with tremendous insights into the true complexity of listening to, speaking with, and understanding the rich minds of our patients. Anderson certainly thinks and writes with immense care and with deep detail about the very musicality of the psychoanalytical process. I strongly suspect that Sigmund Freud would be very proud of such a memorable book."

—**Prof. Brett Kahr**, *senior fellow, Tavistock Institute of Medical Psychology; honorary director of research, Freud Museum London; author of* Hidden Histories of British Psychoanalysis

"In this intelligent and erudite book, Todd Anderson proposes a novel approach to psychoanalytic treatment, one that privileges a transferential relationship grounded in empathy, affect, and the psychic margins—often difficult to grasp—rather than symbolic interpretation centered on the analysis of discourse. To accomplish this reconfiguration, he draws on post-Freudians such as Wilfred R. Bion and Hans Loewald, thereby reviving an interwar debate between Freud and Ferenczi, the former often considered too paternal, the latter too feminine. A major achievement."

—**Élisabeth Roudinesco, PhD**, *historian and psychoanalyst; author of* Freud: In His Time and Ours

"Dans ce livre intelligent et érudit, Todd Anderson propose une nouvelle approche de la cure psychanalytique, privilégiant une relation transférentielle fondée sur l'empathie, l'affect et les marges psychiques, souvent impossibles à saisir, plutôt que sur l'interprétation symbolique mettant en jeu l'analyse des discours. Pour effectuer cette refonte, il s'appuie sur les post-freudiens (Wilfred R. Bion et Hans Loewald) et renoue ainsi avec un débat de l'entre-deux-guerres qui avait opposé Freud et Ferenczi, l'un jugé trop paternaliste et l'autre trop féminin. Une réussite."

—**Élisabeth Roudinesco** (original French text)

Unknowing as Truth is a remarkable achievement — one of those rare works that doesn't just argue for a new way of thinking but enacts it on every page. The author's central move is as bold as it is clarifying: not-knowing is not the analyst's failure, but their most vital resource. What the author calls "epistemic inversion" — the recursive process by which every act of knowing generates new blind spots, every certainty its own shadow — reorients the entire analytic enterprise with elegant precision.

The writing itself is alive. Concepts return transformed, clinical moments breathe alongside theory, and the reader is genuinely surprised — which is, of course, exactly the point. This is a book that practices what it preaches, and the experience of reading it is inseparable from its argument.

What lingers most is the ethical vision: an analytic hospitality that refuses premature closure, that trusts the field, that treats surprise not as disruption but as evidence that something real is happening. This is psychoanalysis at its most honest and most generous.

Essential reading for clinicians, theorists, and anyone willing to discover that dwelling in uncertainty can be, sometimes, the most powerful form of presence.

Giuseppe Civitarese, MD, PhD, author of The Limits of Interpretation: Essays on Bion and Field Theory

"What if psychoanalysis were above all the practice of *docta ignorantia*? Learned ignorance as a key clinical tool: here is Todd Anderson's thesis when he proposes an 'ethics of unknowing' to rethink creatively psychoanalytic concepts like projection, aggression, and destruction, and stage exciting dialogues between thinkers like Bion and Levinas, Bollas and Derrida, Lacan and Loewald, Ferenczi and Laplanche. His numerous clinical vignettes, all imbued with a refreshingly Surrealist atmosphere, make the theoretical stakes very clear."

—**Jean-Michel Rabaté, PhD**, *University of Pennsylvania and American Academy of Arts and Sciences; author of* Lacan and Psychoanalytic Obsolescence

"*Unknowing as Truth: Epistemic Inversions and the Recursive Psyche* is an intellectually bold book that offers a provocative reading of the clinical practice of psychoanalysis. Eschewing the theoretical model of a system that would render all inconsistencies and difficulties transparent in light of a lucid totality, Todd Anderson opts for a mode of thinking that celebrates the opacity of the remainder—the residue of tensions, paradoxes, and asymmetries that cannot be assimilated into a coherent sense of the whole. Appreciating the epistemic centrality of unknowing to the process of human cognition sensitizes us to the truism that the fragment must always be subject to further fragmentation. Drawing upon the recursive form of the fugue, attested especially in the musical compositions of Bach, Anderson proffers an alternative to the conventional linear understanding of temporality that shapes the contours of consciousness. Just as the fugue doubles back on itself to reveal new dimensions, so the cadence of time—mirrored in the structure of the psyche—is informed by the paradoxical realization that each moment is the same because different and different because the same. The future, accordingly, is such that we are continually returning in the present to a past where we have never been. I am confident that this monograph will contribute significantly to the shifting yet continuous pursuit of the ethics of unknowing that is at the heart of analytic truth, and to the aesthetic temperament necessary to engage the complex structures of human subjectivity."

—**Elliot R. Wolfson, PhD**, *distinguished professor emeritus of religious studies, University of California, Santa Barbara; author of* Heidegger and Kabbalah *and* a Dream Interpreted within a Dream

"What Todd Anderson accomplishes in *Unknowing as Truth* is utterly revelatory. By reframing psychoanalysis as recursive topology and epistemic inversion, he draws the reader into a genuinely psychoanalytic odyssey: what is deeply familiar is rendered strange, what is strange or faintly perceived rendered articulate, even obvious, and what emerges is nothing less than uncanny. The content, the book's recursive structure, and the writing itself work synergistically to create these effects. Anderson reminds us that psychoanalysis's true potential lies in the creative, unresolved potential of what surprises, exceeds epistemic capture, and risks new symbolic form. This is a reawakened psychoanalysis—not only relevant, but necessary for a new era of human consciousness."

—**Jill Gentile, PhD**, *NYU Postdoctoral Program; author of* Feminine Law: Freud, Free Speech, and the Voice of Desire

"This book is, in its own words, 'an invitation to risk surprise at the edge of the sayable.' Its premise is that psychoanalytic ideas are recursive, always folding back on themselves and opening out again in new ways. This pushes creatively at the boundaries of theory, and brings a specific, very valuable kind of openness ('hospitality' is Todd Anderson's apt word) into the clinical situation. There is a remarkable range of reference, including music, art, literature, and even Tibetan mysticism. Without question, a book that will enrich its readers."

—**Michael Parsons**, *distinguished fellow of the British Psychoanalytical Society; author of* The Dove That Returns, the Dove That Vanishes

"With this powerful text, Todd Anderson draws us into the complex textures and challenges of the opaque and fluid emotional dimensions of analytic interaction. He uses contributions from major theorists to weave a convincing sense of the significance of recursiveness as it manifests to open up possibilities, or not, for any analytic encounter. With his emphasis on recursiveness, Anderson helps the analyst tolerate limits that haunt the ideals of any attempt to understand and represent self experience, analytically or otherwise."

—**Steven H. Knoblauch, PhD,** *New York University Postdoctoral Program in Psychotherapy & Psychoanalysis; Institute for the Psychoanalytic Study of Subjectivity*

"In this scholarly, sophisticated volume, Todd Anderson pushes beyond the expected and challenges us to interrogate the clinical and theoretical value of *inversion.* Turning our ordinary assumptions about the value of paradox, Anderson invites us to consider how 'unknowing' deepens our clinical work and the way we conceptualize it."

—**Joyce Slochower, PhD, ABPP**, *NYU Postdoctoral Program; author of* Psychoanalysis and the Unspoken

"Psychoanalysis is often said to lack innovation. Be aware, dear reader: with this book you'll encounter highly intelligent clinical wisdom and a fresh way of theorizing what can be 'seen' and 'heard'—and made available to us and our patients. Among its most important contributions is 'recursion,' including a temporal dimension that Anderson calls 'recursive scaffolding.' What better way to restore the analytic building, a hundred years on, than a scaffold that holds while we look deeper? Throughout, Anderson honors contemporary clinical authors and brings their insights to new heights so we may see further."

—**Prof. Dr. Dr. Michael B. Buchholz,** *International Psychoanalytic University (IPU) Berlin*

"Todd Anderson's proposal to replace paradox with epistemic inversion is as innovative as it is timely. By focusing on affect, atmosphere, and surprise, he shows that psychoanalysis remains a vital method for understanding our current moment and orienting ourselves within it. To celebrate open-endedness rather than fixed certainty is both an epistemological and an ethical opportunity."

—**Prof. Dr. Dr. Elisabeth Bronfen**, *University of Zürich; global distinguished professor, New York University*

"*Unknowing as Truth* is a groundbreaking, highly sophisticated, and wholly original work that will inspire and enrich psychoanalytic theory and practice for a long time to come. It sets new standards for recognizing what eludes knowledge and integration—and opens a space in which surprise, atmosphere, and remainder can be productively lived and thought."

—**Prof. Dr. Hans-Jürgen Wirth**, *professor of psychoanalytic social psychology, University of Frankfurt am Main; psychoanalyst and publisher, Psychosozial-Verlag, Gießen*

"Anderson knows that even the most abstract psychoanalytic and philosophical chains of concepts matter for their music. He invites us to read this text of his as a series of toccatas and fugues in the manner of Baroque music. In the shimmering of meanings, the reader will savor the dynamic geometry of ideas."

—**Sergio Benvenuto**, *Institute for Advanced Studies in Psychoanalysis (ISAP), Rome; editor,* European Journal of Psychoanalysis

Unknowing as Truth

Unknowing as Truth reframes psychoanalysis as a discipline of recursive hospitality through the lens of epistemic inversion—treating unknowing not as a deficit but as the living medium of analytic truth.

This book invites clinicians to work at the rim of symbolization—where refusals, reversals, and surprises preserve vitality—and cultivate an ethic of presence that lets meaning arrive without force. It shifts the axis from paradox to inversion, toward a recursive, "curved" epistemology that privileges atmosphere over linear mastery and recasts the analytic field as a participatory climate. Chapters map the grammar of *inversion*, articulate *ethical refusal* as protection of *remainder*, and show how *recursive return* keeps analysis alive when language thins. It integrates classical theory, contemporary relational work, and post-structural thought drawing on cross-disciplinary strands of poetry, music, and visual art as models of open form. Anderson establishes a coherent clinical method for working with not-knowing—moving beyond "tolerance of ambiguity."

With a rich blend of clinical vignettes, teaching pathways, study prompts, and a lexicon for supervision, this book offers a teachable, clinically resonant architecture for psychoanalysts.

Todd Anderson, PhD, PsyD, is a New York–based psychoanalyst. His work explores how dissociation, desire, and symbolic remainder shape psychic survival, drawing together object relations, relational psychoanalysis, and contemporary philosophy in a vivid, practice-centered prose.

PSYCHOANALYSIS IN A NEW KEY

DONNEL STERN

When music is played in a new key, the melody does not change, but the notes that make up the composition do: change in the context of continuity, continuity that perseveres through change. Psychoanalysis in a New Key publishes books that share the aims psychoanalysts have always had, but that approach them differently. The books in the series are not expected to advance any particular theoretical agenda, although to this date most have been written by analysts from the Interpersonal and Relational orientations.

The most important contribution of a psychoanalytic book is the communication of something that nudges the reader's grasp of clinical theory and practice in an unexpected direction. Psychoanalysis in a New Key creates a deliberate focus on innovative and unsettling clinical thinking. Because that kind of thinking is encouraged by exploration of the sometimes surprising contributions to psychoanalysis of ideas and findings from other fields, Psychoanalysis in a New Key particularly encourages interdisciplinary studies. Books in the series have married psychoanalysis with dissociation, trauma theory, sociology, and criminology. The series is open to the consideration of studies examining the relationship between psychoanalysis and any other field—for instance, biology, literary and art criticism, philosophy, systems theory, anthropology, and political theory.

But innovation also takes place within the boundaries of psychoanalysis, and Psychoanalysis in a New Key therefore also presents work that reformulates thought and practice without leaving the precincts of the field. Books in the series focus, for example, on the significance of personal values in psychoanalytic practice, on the complex interrelationship between the analyst's clinical work and personal life, on the consequences for the clinical situation when patient and analyst are from different cultures, and on the need for psychoanalysts to accept the degree to which they knowingly satisfy their own wishes during treatment hours, often to the patient's detriment.

A full list of all titles in this series is available at:
https://www.routledge.com/Psychoanalysis-in-a-New-Key-Book-Series/book-series/LEAPNKBS

Unknowing as Truth

Epistemic Inversions and the Recursive Psyche

Todd Anderson

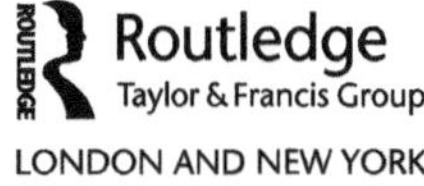

LONDON AND NEW YORK

Designed cover image: Getty Images

First published 2026
by Routledge
4 Park Square, Milton Park, Abingdon, Oxon OX14 4RN

and by Routledge
605 Third Avenue, New York, NY 10158

Routledge is an imprint of the Taylor & Francis Group, an informa business

British Library Cataloguing-in-Publication Data
A catalogue record for this book is available from the British Library

Library of Congress Cataloging-in-Publication Data
A catalog record has been requested for this book

ISBN: 9781041255208 (hbk)
ISBN: 9781041250845 (pbk)
ISBN: 9781003747109 (ebk)

DOI: 10.4324/9781003747109

Typeset in Times New Roman
by codeMantra

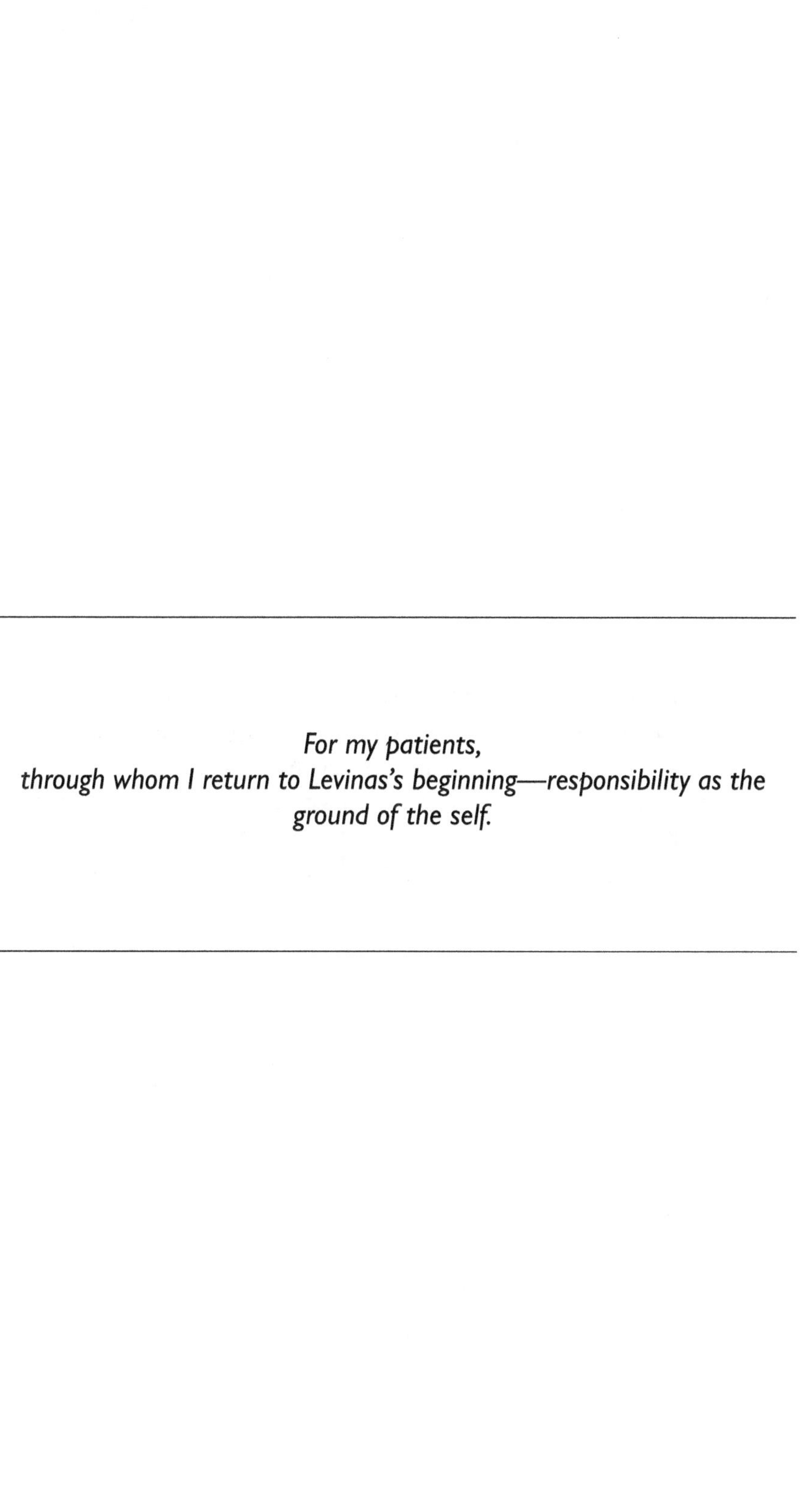

For my patients,
through whom I return to Levinas's beginning—responsibility as the ground of the self.

**Power arises from the desire for closure.
Only afterward does it enter the discursive forms
Foucault described.
Openness overwhelms; the mind totalizes to feel secure.
Hospitality is the steadiness that holds the infinite
responsibility Levinas saw in the face of the other.**

Contents

About the Cover

The cover image presents a spiral interior organized around a central opening of light. What appears initially as a single aperture becomes, upon closer attention, a kind of structured emptiness—an interior void that the architecture turns around without ever resolving. As the spiral descends, each rotation repeats the last with a slight temporal shift, creating a sense of recursive movement rather than linear direction. This echoes the experience of moving through self-states—returning again and again to familiar shapes of feeling, but altered, displaced, or newly illuminated.

Near the base, a reflective surface bends the light into iridescent color, introducing a subtle distortion that unsettles any stable point of view. The image invites the reader into this book's central concerns—how psychic life is shaped by what cannot be fully known, how time folds back on itself in the spaces between self-states, and how a generative emptiness at the center of experience becomes the quiet source of transformation.

Acknowledgments

This book, like any analytic process, emerged through the slow reciprocity of influence, listening, and care. Its pages are shaped by the voices that have accompanied my thinking—teachers, colleagues, patients, and friends—each of whom left traces in the work even where their names are absent.

I am deeply grateful to Donnel Stern, whose trust and editorial stewardship gave this project a home in *Psychoanalysis in a New Key*. His belief in the work's trajectory lent it both courage and continuity.

To Nancy McWilliams, I extend profound thanks for steady encouragement, generative conversations, and enduring faith in the work.

Sergio Benvenuto, Elisabeth Bronfen, Michael B. Buchholz, Giovanni Foresti, Brett Kahr, Steven H. Knoblauch, Michael Parsons, Jean-Michel Rabaté, Élisabeth Roudinesco, Joyce Slochower, Hans-Jürgen Wirth, and Elliot R. Wolfson—your generosity of thought and presence has helped clear space for this work. Each of you models a hospitality of mind that this book strives to reciprocate.

I am indebted as well to those whose ideas have shaped the contours of my thought—Thomas Ogden, Christopher Bollas, André Green, Jean Laplanche, Michael Eigen, Emmanuel Levinas, and Maurice Merleau-Ponty—figures who taught me that theory is not explanation but transmission.

Warm thanks to Kate Hawes and Aakriti Aggarwal, the editorial team at Routledge, and to the readers whose presence, sometimes named and sometimes anonymous, sustains the living dialogue that makes writing possible.

To Tim, I extend deep appreciation for love, patience, and the quiet forms of sustenance without which none of this would have been written.

Finally, I thank my patients, whose courage and honesty are the true source of every idea in these pages. The analytic hour remains where thought becomes experience, and experience becomes truth.

This book, like all analysis, belongs to no one. It is an offering—an attempt to listen back into the field that first called it forth.

Preface

On Form and Temperament

This book appears in *Psychoanalysis in a New Key*—a metaphor I owe to Donnel Stern, whose invitation to "a new key" makes this work possible. I write not only in a different key, but also in a different **temperament**. A key organizes tones around a center; a temperament sets how those intervals are tuned, and how consonance and dissonance are distributed across the system. To change temperament is to change how a key itself is heard—what it can mean. My work, then, composes in new keys but also in another temperament: one that **preserves remainder and opacity** rather than smoothing them away.

In J. S. Bach's time, **well temperament** was a genuine innovation. Earlier systems (like meantone) made some keys glorious and others nearly unplayable. Well temperament smoothed remainder just enough to make all keys usable on a single clavier, yet it preserved unequal intervals so each key kept its own atmosphere—its shimmer and strain. In such tunings, a C–E major third can ring near the pure 5:4, while the "same" third in a distant key (say G♭–B♭) carries more tension. Bach did not neutralize those differences; he composed **with** them. The *Well-Tempered Clavier* is a tour of key-characters inside a specific tuning world; the pieces were written for those keys in that temperament and lose real color when transposed or played under a different system.

By contrast, **equal temperament** spreads discrepancies evenly across the octave, making every semitone the same size. That uniformity gives modern instruments their effortless transposability—but at the cost of key-character. In well temperament, intervals often sound "perfectly out of tune"—perplexing at first—and yet, in the hands of a master like Bach, that **remainder** becomes a medium of beauty itself.

By **remainder**, I mean the residue that resists smoothing: the tensions, paradoxes, and asymmetries coherence cannot fully absorb. In music, remainder is the difference that makes one key radiant and another shadowed, even when the "same" interval is played. In psychoanalysis, remainder is the unformulated affect, the paradox, the fragment that cannot be assimilated without loss. **Opacity** names the refusal to flatten that remainder into transparency: the part of experience that must remain resistant to full recognition, not because it fails symbolization but because it is constitutive of truth itself. Where equal temperament seeks clarity through erasure, well temperament composes with remainder and sustains opacity as a form of fidelity.

And if temperament is the tuning, the **fugue** is the recursive form. A fugue begins with a subject that re-enters again and again—through inversion, augmentation, diminution, and stretto. It is the same and not the same: recognizable, yet altered by each return, each context, each crossing of voices. The theme doubles back on itself until it reveals new dimensions, carrying both continuity and transformation. This recursive unfolding mirrors the psyche as I present it here—layered, repetitive, self-referential, and never exhausted by a single statement. **Clinically, each "entry" is a return to a problem the field can now bear differently.** Just as Bach composed fugues to let one theme disclose its variations, I write to follow the psyche's themes as they recur across time—shifting yet continuous, unresolved yet luminous.

This is how I want my writing to be heard—not only in a different key, but also in a different temperament. Not equalized, not flattened into a single register, but composed with **paradox, remainder, opacity, and dissonance** as materials. Each chapter belongs to its register; its uneven consonances and resistances are part of its truth. I am not seeking premature resolution. Like Bach, I want to preserve the distinct weather of each key—the shine and the grit—so the psyche can be heard in its opacity and remainder.

Listening note: If you may be curious, listen to a prelude and fugue from the *Well-Tempered Clavier* in equal temperament and then in a historical well temperament (e.g., Werckmeister, Kirnberger, Vallotti); the difference in "shimmer" is the remainder I mean.

On Perception and Subjectivity

We call the world "reality," but what we mean by that is always already bounded by human perception. We never meet the thing-in-itself; we meet what our senses and symbols can register, and then we call that the real. Our sciences, our philosophies, and even our most ordinary talk about "what is" have been constructed within this constraint. What shows up is not neutral—it appears through structures of subjectivity.

This is why I speak of structures of subjectivity across music, analysis, physics, and philosophy. Subjectivity does not simply impose itself on the world, nor does it passively receive what lies outside. Rather, it perceives its own form mirrored back. In this sense, perception itself is **recursive**: the psyche recognizes itself in what it apprehends. Dzogchen's *tögal* makes this vivid—appearance as self-display, the world as the psyche's own light, remainder, shimmer.

So the tradition sounds its theme and answer, one after another: Klein reveals part-objects—split and remainder before wholeness; Jung names archetypes—forms psyche meets as world; Winnicott opens transitional space—reality played-into-being; Bion transforms beta-elements—container and contained; Loewald retunes integration—tempered rather than smoothed; Lacan maps RSI—the Real as what resists symbolization; Laplanche preserves the enigma—opacity at the origin; Bollas and Stern keep what organizes before it is said; Green insists on the negative as real; Ogden writes reverie as a fugue of subjects. I gather these lines into one ethic: **preserve opacity, protect remainder, and listen for recursive return.**

Reality does not divide into the ordinary and the beyond; the given is always more than it gives. To miss that is to reduce the world to a flat register where nothing ever exceeds itself. To affirm it is to allow each key, each encounter, and each subject to preserve its remainder and opacity—the excess by which things are most themselves.

Listening to music is practice in this kind of perception. To hear temperament is to hear how consonance and dissonance are distributed; to hear a fugue is to hear repetition with difference—opacity preserved in return. In learning to hear music structurally, we are also learning to hear the psyche. And in analysis, this listening becomes the capacity to hear the patient not as a single melody, but as a layered, recursive form whose truth lies in its remainder.

Listening to music, then, is not just an art but an ethic: to hear how form carries remainder, and how perception reveals its own opacity. Psychoanalysis extends this same listening to the human subject. What I seek in these pages is not resolution but **resonance**—the way a cadence can settle without erasing its dissonance, the way a phrase can end while leaving something still sounding.

What follows turns this musical figure into a clinical one: how analysts work with remainder, opacity, and return in the hour.

Introduction

The Ethics of Epistemic Inversion

This introduction lays the conceptual foundation for *Unknowing as Truth*, presenting the book's core movement: a shift from paradox to inversion as the lens for rethinking psychoanalytic concepts, technique, and ethics. It traces how "epistemic inversion"—the reversal of knowing and unknowing, defense and revelation, subject and object—emerges as both a clinical method and an ethical stance. Distinguishing this volume as recursive, bottom-up, and "curved" in its epistemological structure, the introduction draws on classical and contemporary psychoanalytic theorists while weaving throughlines from earlier works. By foregrounding atmosphere over linear mastery, the introduction recasts unknowing not as failure but as a resource—a mode of analytic hospitality to difference. The introduction orients the reader to the book's recursive structure and invites participation in its climate of surprise, opacity, and generative ambiguity.

Inversion as Method—The Turn from Paradox to Epistemic Reversal

Psychoanalysis has long circled the paradoxical. Its most enduring insights, from the double logic of repression to the tension between drive and defense, have flourished in the in-between: the neither-nor, the both-and, the unresolvable edge where desire and impossibility meet. Paradox, in its many guises, has given psychoanalytic thought its distinctive power to hold together what cannot be synthesized, to witness divisions that refuse neat repair. But this book marks a departure—not a renunciation of paradox, but an inversion of the very axis along which knowledge and unknowing have traditionally been arrayed.

DOI: 10.4324/9781003747109-1

Here, “inversion” names a methodological wager: not a simple swap of terms, but a destabilization of the frame that makes such binaries feel self-evident. In this sense, epistemic inversion is both a clinical strategy and an ethical stance: it refuses to take the given categories of knowing and not-knowing as fixed, instead rendering them contingent, permeable, and recursively entangled.

The history of psychoanalysis is, at a certain level, a history of inversion. Freud’s earliest insights emerged from reversals: the symptom as both expression and disguise, the dream as wish-fulfillment and censorship, the analyst as a knowing subject and a not-knowing witness. Klein’s work on projective and introjective processes further complicated these boundaries, suggesting that what is “inside” is always already shaped by what is “outside,” and vice versa. Later theorists, drawing on these traditions, have pushed the dialectic even further, exploring how subject and object, self and other, reality and fantasy, are constituted through recursive processes of transmission, containment, and transformation.

Yet, in most psychoanalytic discourse, these inversions have often been subsumed under the umbrella of paradox—a holding of opposites, a suspension of resolution, a fidelity to tension. Paradox has been indispensable, allowing analysts to resist the premature closure of the unknown, to dwell in the ambiguity that analytic life demands. Still, the language of paradox tends to preserve the symmetry of the opposed terms. The subject and the object, the analyst and the patient, the known and the unknown: these are placed in balance, each incomplete without the other, but each retaining its essential identity.

The epistemic inversion proposed here is subtler, and more destabilizing. It is not merely a matter of tolerating contradiction, but of reversing the direction of inquiry: asking not, “How do we move from unknowing to knowing?” but, “How does the act of knowing create new sites of unknowing? How does the wish to know generate its own blind spots, resistances, and refusals?” In this sense, inversion is not a static pose but a movement, a recursive process by which every claim to knowledge is haunted by its shadow, every certainty by its excess, every revelation by the residue it cannot absorb. This movement is felt most acutely in the clinical encounter. The analyst’s traditional task—to interpret, to reveal, to make the unconscious conscious—is inverted here. Interpretation becomes less mastery than opening—an invitation to risk surprise at the edge of the sayable. The "success" of analysis becomes not the achievement of clarity, but the cultivation of a discipline of staying-with ambiguity, opacity, and reversal.

The shift from paradox to inversion is thus not simply conceptual, but experiential. It shapes the analyst's presence in the room, their tolerance for uncertainty, their hospitality to the not-yet-formulated. It informs an ethics of restraint—an unwillingness to foreclose the unknown with hasty interpretation, a discipline of waiting for the field to speak in its own time. In the recursive structure of analytic life, what is most alive is not what is finally known, but what returns, loops, and surprises. Inversion is the signature of this return: the refusal to allow knowledge to calcify, the commitment to remain open to the reversals that animate the symbolic field.

This inversion also reorients the analytic gaze. Rather than viewing the psyche as a puzzle to be solved or a landscape to be mapped, the analytic field is imagined as a curved, recursive space—one in which every act of knowing folds back on itself, creating new openings, blind spots, and forms of hospitality. This approach resonates with diverse subjectivities, where bottom-up attention and recursive engagement can reveal the limits of fixed epistemic frames, including in autistic ways of knowing.

What emerges, then, is not a prescription for technique, but a methodological atmosphere—a climate in which inversion becomes a mode of attention, a willingness to let knowledge bend, recur, and open onto its own limits. The following chapters pursue this inversion across the terrain of psychoanalytic concepts: from Oedipal law to fantasy, projection to introjection, destruction to the uncanny, and beyond. In each, the analytic stakes are not only theoretical but ethical: how do we remain hospitable to the surprises of the field? How do we accompany our patients—and ourselves—through the recursive inversions that sustain analytic life?

The turn from paradox to inversion, then, is a call to practice: to risk not-knowing as a source of analytic presence, to welcome reversal as the birthplace of new symbolic forms, and to inhabit the recursive, curved atmosphere that is the true home of psychoanalytic thought.

Epistemic Stakes—Atmosphere, Affect, and the Limits of Knowing

What is at stake when psychoanalysis turns from paradox to inversion, from the mastery of meaning to the recursive climate of not-knowing? The answer is not merely theoretical. It is lived as atmosphere, as the felt sense of possibility and risk in every analytic hour. Psychoanalytic work is saturated with the atmospheres of epistemic life: moods of urgency or indeterminacy, climates of hope, dread, or surprise, and those subtle shifts in weather that mark the difference between interpretation and genuine presence. Epistemic inversion, in this sense, is not only a change in thought but a reorientation of the entire psychic field—one in which affect, mood, and symbolic excess come to the fore.

For Freud, knowing was never a purely cognitive act. The moment of insight was always accompanied by a discharge of affect, a relief or intensification of tension. The "aha" of interpretation is, at heart, an affective event—a release, a shift, a reorganization of psychic energy. Yet, Freud also understood that interpretation is never final. Each revelation brings with it new resistances, new sites of uncertainty, and a lingering aftertaste of the unknown. The limit of knowing is always inscribed within the act of knowing itself, a reminder that the drive to understand is never free of its own defenses, blind spots, and inversions.

Melanie Klein radicalized this insight by showing that affective atmospheres precede the formation of meaning. For Klein, the infant's earliest experience is one of undifferentiated mood—of good and bad, comfort and threat, all fused in a swirling atmosphere of feeling. These affective climates are not the byproduct of cognition but its very ground. The mind comes into being in an atmosphere; it is curved and colored by the moods that animate the internal and external world. Phantasy, for Klein, is never simply a thought or an image; it is a lived mood, a climate, a recursive return to the feelings that cannot be fully contained or symbolized.

The analytic hour, viewed through this lens, becomes a field experiment in atmosphere. Analyst and patient co-inhabit a symbolic climate—one that is always shifting, recursive, and alive with the excesses of affect and meaning. The "weather" of the session may turn with a word, a silence, a sigh, or a passing glance. Some days, the air is thick with anxiety or longing; on others, a surprising lightness enters, making new forms of thought and play possible. The analytic field is not a backdrop to knowledge, but its very medium—the curved space in which knowing and unknowing loop, fold, and surprise.

This attention to atmosphere and affect finds echoes in the work of later theorists. Hans Loewald envisioned the analytic encounter as a symbolic climate in which old meanings are dissolved and new ones can emerge.

He spoke of the presence of absence, the affective residue that lingers after an interpretation, the unformulated mood that shapes what can and cannot be thought. Thomas Ogden developed the idea of the "analytic third"—a shared, emergent field generated by the interplay of analyst and patient, neither reducible to either party's subjectivity nor to the sum of their separate minds. This analytic third is not a static thing but a living atmosphere, one that is recursive, affective, and surprising.

Crucially, the field is not only composed of content—thoughts, images, associations—but of mood, weather, and affective resonance. Christopher Bollas describes the "unthought known"—those elements of psychic life that can only be sensed, not yet symbolized, that circulate as atmospheres, moods, or resonant patterns. Michael Eigen writes of the field of the between, the affective and symbolic climate that is always more than either participant can own or contain. The analytic hour, in this sense, is a climate for surprise: a recursive environment in which knowledge is always being revised, unsettled, and renewed by the movement of affect through the field.

The affective climate of analytic work is also marked by its limits. No matter how much is said, something remains unsaid; no matter how thoroughly an experience is interpreted, a residue of the unknown persists. André Green's "dead mother" complex offers one vision of this: a psychic field saturated not by the presence of affect, but by its withdrawal, its deadness, its refusal to be metabolized. The atmosphere here is not one of play or surprise, but of suspension, absence, or numbness. Even these climates have their recursive logics: the repetition of absence, the looping of a mood that cannot be shifted by insight alone.

This affective and atmospheric dimension becomes especially pronounced in those whose epistemic stance resists linearity—those for whom knowing is always provisional, recursive, or bottom-up. Here, I am thinking not only of neurotypical or "well-integrated" subjectivities, but of the many for whom knowledge is a matter of assembling, layering, or revisiting the field from below, rather than grasping it from above. For some on the autism spectrum, for example, knowing is less about synthesis and more about recursive assembly, the building up of experience from detail, mood, or resonance. This approach to knowing—neither hierarchical nor linear—reveals the artificiality of the very boundaries psychoanalysis often presumes.

Thus, epistemic inversion is not simply a theoretical move, but an atmospheric one. It invites the analyst to attend to the moods and climates that shape analytic life—the recursive "weather" that moves through the room, bringing with it both surprise and risk. The ethic here is one of hospitality: a willingness to remain with uncertainty, to let the atmosphere do its work, to resist the premature foreclosure of the unknown. The discipline is not only intellectual but affective: it is the practice of staying-with, of witnessing the recursive play of mood and meaning, of letting the limits of knowing become the very ground of analytic presence.

In sum, the stakes of epistemic inversion are existential as much as theoretical. To turn from mastery to atmosphere, from paradox to recursive unknowing, is to risk a new kind of analytic hospitality—one that honors the generativity of the field, the surprise of affect, and the ethical demands of presence in the face of the unknown. The climate of the analytic hour becomes the laboratory for this practice, and the challenge is not to master the field, but to remain open to the recursive atmospheres that sustain it.

From Paradox to Inversion—Methodology and Conceptual Innovations

Psychoanalytic thought has long been enchanted by paradox: the simultaneous holding of incompatible truths, the oscillation between presence and absence, and the endless doubling-back of psychic life upon itself. Yet, paradox—so generative in its day—can become a resting place, a horizon beyond which the field is hesitant to venture. The conceptual move at the heart of this book is the leap from paradox to inversion: not the simple coexistence of opposites, but the turning-inside-out of epistemic, affective, and clinical assumptions. Inversion is not simply the negative of a prior term; it is the recursive transformation of the entire field, a reorientation of structure and atmosphere that yields new forms of symbolic life.

What, then, does it mean to move from paradox to inversion? Paradox, in its classical psychoanalytic register, is the acknowledgment that the psyche is split, that every assertion of truth is shadowed by its negation, that the mind is always already double. Winnicott's "capacity to be alone in the presence of another," Freud's dream logic, or Klein's simultaneous love and hate for the same object—each of these embodies paradox as both insight and predicament. The paradoxical attitude values holding, waiting, and the refusal to resolve contradiction too quickly. It is the ethic of the "not yet," of patience with what cannot be integrated.

But inversion introduces something further: a reversal in which what was formerly foreground becomes background, and vice versa; where the "unknown" is no longer a lack to be filled but the atmosphere in which knowledge is formed. Inversion is not the same as opposition. It is a folding, a recursive turning of form and content, subject and object, inside and outside. When analytic knowing is inverted, interpretation does not simply uncover what is hidden; it becomes an act of participating in the field's ongoing reformation. The interpretive act is no longer final or unidirectional; it loops back, alters the field, and opens further layers of unknowing.

This methodological shift is both conceptual and clinical. Methodologically, inversion means that psychoanalytic concepts are continually subjected to their own reversal—not to destroy them, but to discover their recursive generativity. A defense becomes a resource; a symptom, a creative reply; the unknown, a form of hospitality rather than a danger. Each analytic category is read not for its binary logic, but for its curved, atmospheric, recursive possibilities. The focus is not on resolving oppositions, but on living at the edge of their inversion, allowing meaning to be continually folded and reassembled.

Clinically, the ethic of inversion transforms the stance of the analyst. The analyst is not only the interpreter of paradox but also the participant in the recursive atmosphere of the field. Presence is not merely the backdrop for interpretation; it is the active condition that allows surprise, reversal, and unknowing to become generative. The analyst practices a discipline of "recursive hospitality"—remaining open to the unpredictable ways in which the field inverts, recurs, and surprises both participants. This demands a form of humility and presence attuned to what cannot be anticipated, a willingness to let the field lead rather than seeking to control its direction.

The logic of inversion becomes especially vivid in the way the book treats core psychoanalytic concepts. Each is examined not only in terms of its classical function but also for how it inverts under recursive conditions. Take introjection, for example: traditionally seen as a means of incorporating or metabolizing aspects of the other, it is reframed here as a practice of hospitality—one that is always haunted by the limits of what can be welcomed, metabolized, or refused. Destruction, rather than simply the breakdown of integration, is read as a necessary counter-force, an ethic that exposes the creative limits of containment and the generativity that may arise from ruin or refusal.

Even the most foundational narratives—such as the Oedipal myth—are subject to inversion. The law of linearity, the demand to know and integrate, is refused in favor of recursive, looping, and nonlinear alternatives. The myth becomes not a script to be reenacted but a field to be inverted, allowing the "riddle" of Oedipus to point beyond its own impasses toward new forms of psychic and analytic life. Similarly, the concept of the uncanny, so often approached as a symptom of failed repression or return of the repressed, is reconfigured as a marker of curved structure and affective surprise—a signal not merely of unresolved conflict, but of new forms of recursive knowing and being.

Inversion also shapes the book's approach to epistemology itself. Traditional psychoanalytic knowing has often been framed as an ascent to truth: a movement from symptom to meaning, from surface to depth, from ignorance to knowledge. But epistemic inversion suggests a different trajectory: knowledge is not the endpoint but the product of recursive, atmospheric process; unknowing is not simply ignorance but the condition for surprise, emergence, and ethical engagement. The analyst's discipline becomes the capacity to remain with the unknown, to let it shape the field, to trust that what cannot be known may, in time, become the very site of new symbolic forms.

This recursive, inverted methodology requires a "bottom-up" sensitivity. Rather than imposing structure from above, the analytic process assembles, layers, and revisits the field from below—from the level of affect, detail, and atmosphere. For subjectivities marked by autistic modes of knowing, for instance, the epistemology is not linear or hierarchical, but recursive, assembling knowledge through repeated contact with detail, mood, and symbolic resonance. The analyst's task is to honor these bottom-up processes, to resist the seductions of mastery, and to recognize the curved, recursive assembly of meaning as a generative force.

The conceptual innovation, then, is not simply a new theory but a practice—a recursive discipline of unknowing, an openness to inversion, and a commitment to accompanying the patient and the field wherever the curved path may lead. Each chapter of the book enacts this logic: concepts are inverted, atmospheres traced, clinical vignettes woven in as living illustrations of how the recursive field operates. The method is recursive not only in argument but also in form; the structure of the book itself folds back on earlier themes, returns to prior concepts, and allows meaning to emerge in unexpected ways.

To move from paradox to inversion is, ultimately, to risk a new form of psychoanalytic life—one that values atmosphere over mastery, surprise over certainty, and the recursive play of the field over the finality of explanation. The challenge is not simply to understand this logic, but to practice it: to become attuned to the moments when meaning inverts, when knowledge gives way to surprise, and when the analytic field itself becomes the most vital participant in the work.

Recursive Structure and the Curved Field—Atmosphere, Surprise, and Clinical Presence

To speak of "recursive structure" in psychoanalysis is to depart from the image of theory and technique as a ladder to be ascended or a code to be cracked. Instead, recursive structure imagines the analytic field as a space of continual looping, return, and atmospheric reformation. It is a structure whose very law is that of surprise: a movement not toward resolution, but toward repeated opening—a folding and unfolding of meaning in which neither patient nor analyst can anticipate the final form.

This "curved field" is not merely a metaphor for psychic complexity; it is an experiential reality, palpable in both clinical process and lived subjectivity. In a curved field, the boundaries between inside and outside, past and present, self and other, are never linear or absolute. Instead, they are always in the process of being negotiated, bent, and reconstituted by recursive contact. The analytic hour itself becomes curved—less a sequence of steps toward insight than a climate in which affect, mood, and symbol loop back, refract, and return in altered form.

Atmosphere is the essential medium of this curved field. Traditional psychoanalytic technique privileges content: dreams, memories, associations, interpretations. But the recursive model foregrounds atmosphere as the principal register of analytic life. Atmosphere is both the "weather" of the session and the substrate in which new forms become possible. It is the felt sense of presence, mood, and possibility—an implicit, often unspoken climate that saturates the analytic encounter and sets the conditions for surprise.

Clinical vignettes repeatedly demonstrate that transformation does not unfold through the linear accretion of knowledge or the stepwise integration of insight. Rather, it is in the recursive looping—returning to the same affect, the same impasse, the same unformulated tension—that the field becomes charged, and something unexpected may emerge. The patient may find themselves repeating a theme, not as a symptom but as a search for the new inflection, the yet-unspoken angle that the curved field alone can generate.

Atmosphere also determines the timing of surprise. There are moments in the analytic process when the field thickens—when silences, shared affect, or unexpected reveries descend, creating a sense of suspension. The old analytic impulse is to interpret, to fill the silence with meaning. But in the recursive model, the analyst learns to accompany, to wait, to trust that the field's atmosphere is itself the precondition for emergence. When surprise comes—a new association, a shift in affect, a sudden recognition—it arises not from mastery, but from the atmosphere's capacity to support reversal, return, and creative rupture.

The logic of the curved field also reframes resistance and deadness. What classical technique may regard as "resistance"—the patient's refusal to move forward, to remember, to know—becomes, in the curved field, a signal that the atmosphere has entered a recursive phase. Deadness is not simply defense; it may be a necessary part of the cycle, a pause before the next surprise. The analyst's task is not always to disrupt or interpret but sometimes to bear witness, to stay present in the climate of not-knowing, and to model a discipline of patience and humility.

Curved structure is particularly salient for analytic work with neurodivergent subjectivities, especially those on the autism spectrum. In these encounters, meaning is often assembled "bottom-up"—through repeated contact with detail, affect, and pattern, rather than through top-down synthesis. The recursive field allows the analyst to honor this mode of knowing, to resist the imposition of premature narrative, and to discover, with the patient, new forms of coherence that emerge only through looping, atmospheric return. This attunement to curved assembly not only deepens the clinical work but also challenges the field's own habits of mastery and linearity.

Surprise, in this context, is not a disruption but a marker of field vitality. In recursive structure, surprise is both the goal and the byproduct: a sudden shift in atmosphere, a new affective weather front, a recognition that emerges where neither analyst nor patient expected it. These surprises may be small—an unexpected laughter, a new word, a silent look that changes the tone of the session. Or they may be large—a moment of reversal, a collapse of old certainties, the birth of a new subjectivity. What matters is not the content, but the recursive process that allowed the field to generate the new.

The recursive and curved model also has implications for analytic presence. The analyst is no longer positioned as the outside interpreter, the master of the field. Instead, presence becomes recursive: the analyst is both participant and witness, both affected by and affecting the atmosphere. The challenge is to remain porous but not engulfed, receptive but not dissolved, able to bear the field's surprises without retreating into premature knowing. Analytic presence is thus not only a stance but also a discipline—a willingness to be implicated in the recursive life of the field, to be changed by it, and to risk one's own unknowing.

This recursive stance is echoed in the very architecture of the book. Chapters loop back to prior themes, ideas are inverted and revisited, and clinical material is woven throughout not as illustration but as active ingredient. The aim is to enact, in both argument and form, the recursive, atmospheric, and curved logic that the book advocates. Each chapter becomes a site for surprise, each clinical moment an invitation to participate in the field's ongoing transformation.

Finally, atmosphere, surprise, and clinical presence are not only methodological commitments but also ethical imperatives. To stay with the recursive field is to honor the unknowable, to refuse the violence of forced closure, and to model a hospitality to difference that psychoanalysis must reclaim. The curved field is not a resting place, but a discipline—a practice of holding open the space for surprise, for emergence, for the new forms that only recursive, atmospheric contact can bring.

Conclusion and Orientation for the Reader

This book opens with a paradox: that psychoanalysis finds its greatest vitality not in what it knows, but in what it is able to un-know, to reverse, and to hold open. The preceding sections have charted a shift from mastery and interpretation to epistemic inversion, recursive structure, and the ethics of curved hospitality. The chapters to come will return, again and again, to these themes—not as fixed doctrine, but as invitations to linger, question, and participate in the generative atmosphere of the analytic field.

What does it mean, then, to read this book? The orientation is both simple and subtle: the reader is invited to approach each chapter not merely as an argument or a series of clinical techniques, but as a recursive climate. The structure is intentionally circular and refractive. Concepts introduced in the opening chapters—unknowing, projection, fantasy, introjection, destruction—will reappear, reversed and transformed, as the book unfolds. The field itself becomes the curriculum: the repeated returns, the atmospheric thickening, the surprise and reversal that animate both clinical practice and the analytic imagination.

To read recursively is to allow the chapters to echo across one another, to hold insights provisionally, and to trust that meaning will accumulate not only through explanation but through atmosphere, resonance, and return. The clinical vignettes are not simply illustrative; they are sites of emergence—places where the reader, too, may find their own affect, uncertainty, and curiosity engaged. Theoretical arguments loop and refract; technical claims are offered as invitations to risk surprise, rather than as recipes to be mastered.

As Knoblauch (2000, 2020) has shown, the analytic field is as much rhythmic and embodied as it is verbal. His attention to micro-movements of tone, breath, and timing clarifies how contact occurs through the body's rhythms as much as through language. This work underlies my own sense of recursiveness as an affective rhythm—a return through which the psyche gathers time and form.

This approach also honors the diversity of analytic subjectivities, including those for whom bottom-up, detail-driven, or atmospheric modes of knowing are primary. The recursive, curved structure resists closure and welcomes what cannot yet be integrated. In this sense, the book is less a manual than a field—a climate in which both analyst and reader may discover new forms of relation to knowledge, to not-knowing, and to the surprises that emerge in the act of sustained encounter.

Crucially, the introduction also frames the book's stance toward its own discipline. By declining to name earlier works by title, the book gestures toward a psychoanalytic lineage without reifying its own authority or fixity. Instead, the aim is to keep the analytic project alive—open to the reversals, refusals, and recursive re-entrances that mark both the field and the analytic hour. The text itself participates in the recursive ethics it describes, circling its own themes, staging the very atmosphere and surprise it advocates.

For the reader—clinician, theorist, or simply one who cares about the fate of unknowing in human life—this orientation asks for patience and a willingness to dwell in ambiguity. Surprise is not a problem to be solved but a sign that the field is alive. The analytic future, the book suggests, lies not in the triumph of knowledge, but in the hospitality to difference, opacity, and reversal. Each chapter will contribute a facet to this unfolding climate, and each will invite the reader to risk staying present with what resists integration.

As you move forward, let yourself be accompanied by the book's central commitment: that the richest psychic and analytic realities are not those that can be finally mastered, but those that remain generative, recursive, and atmospherically alive. The task is not to know everything but to participate in the field—to risk, to reverse, to be surprised, and to let new forms arise from the climate of unknowing. With this, the introduction cedes its authority to the recursive movement of the book itself. Let the field guide you; let surprise find you; and let the curved, recursive discipline of psychoanalytic hospitality open the way for what remains to be discovered.

Part I

The Inverted Frame

Turn the picture and the room rearranges.
Inside becomes edge; background begins to speak.
Perception loosens its grip and a truer outline appears.
We learn by letting the frame be moved by what it holds.

DOI: 10.4324/9781003747109-2

Chapter 1

Unknowing at the Threshold—From Interpretation to Epistemic Refusal

This chapter traces the evolution of psychoanalytic interpretation from its classical foundations in the quest for hidden knowledge to its contemporary inversion: the embrace of unknowing as the core of analytic truth. Beginning with the mythic authority of the interpreter in Freud and the classical tradition, this chapter unfolds the logic of inversion as a structural and affective principle—one that recasts the analytic hour as a recursive encounter with what resists sense. Through clinical vignette and theoretical reflection, the affective atmosphere of not-knowing is explored as an essential feature of the analytic field, demanding from the analyst not mastery, but presence and ethical hospitality. This chapter culminates in a meditation on epistemic refusal: the practice of honoring opacity, bearing witness to what cannot be named, and cultivating recursive structures in which new experience becomes possible. In doing so, it reframes psychoanalysis not as a method for mastering the unknown, but as an art of dwelling with it—a field where unknowing is not a deficit, but the very ground of transformation.

The Classical Frame of Interpretation

Psychoanalysis has always been shadowed by the myth of the interpreter—the analyst as a figure who, by virtue of theoretical training and patient listening, is able to peer beneath the manifest surface of a patient's words and actions to discover latent truths. This frame, foundational to the classical tradition, structures the analytic encounter as an epistemological drama: the analyst possesses a "method," a technique that slices through the overgrowth of defenses and misdirection, drawing forth the kernel of meaning supposedly hidden in the unconscious. The clinical setting is thus cast as a space of unmasking, and the analyst's interpretation as a tool for revelation (Freud, 1900/1953, 1901/1960).

DOI: 10.4324/9781003747109-3

We inherit from Freud a vision of analysis in which the work is, above all, a work of knowing. The patient arrives with symptoms whose origins are obscure; the analyst, by way of free association, dream interpretation, and the deciphering of slips and parapraxes, reveals the hidden logic beneath suffering (Freud, 1900/1953, 1901/1960). The therapeutic action—so goes the narrative—lies in the making-conscious of what has been repressed. The patient is cured, or at least relieved, by gaining knowledge of the true sources of their distress.

To revisit *The Interpretation of Dreams* (Freud, 1900/1953) or *The Psychopathology of Everyday Life* (Freud, 1901/1960) is to be struck by the confidence with which the classical analyst approaches the field of meaning. Each symptom, each mistake, or each fragment of narrative is presumed to bear significance, albeit in displaced, condensed, or symbolic form. The work of the analyst is to restore these fragments to the continuous, rational narrative from which they have become estranged. Knowledge is the instrument of cure, and interpretation is the privileged site at which knowledge becomes transformative.

But this classical frame is more than a set of techniques or even a theory of mind. It is a *scene*—a theatrical and ethical arrangement in which the analyst assumes a particular stance: the interpreter as decipherer, the patient as the one who brings material to be decoded. This scene is steeped in the language of unveiling, of discovery, of illumination. There is an implicit hierarchy of knowledge, even as the analytic ideal claims neutrality or abstinence. The analyst's role is to *know*, or at least to occupy the place of knowing, and to offer this knowledge as an intervention (Laplanche & Pontalis, 1973/1974).

The gravity of interpretation—its moral and epistemic weight—is nowhere more evident than in the ritual of the analytic hour. The patient speaks, sometimes circling the same themes with obsessive regularity, sometimes veering into silence, sometimes dazzling with associative leaps. The analyst listens, waiting for the opportune moment when an interpretation may be offered: "It seems to me that you are speaking about your father when you talk about your boss," or "Perhaps your fear of illness is connected to your early experiences of abandonment." In these moments, interpretation functions as a vector of meaning, a bid for coherence, an invitation to remember what has been split or forgotten (Loewald, 1960).

If there is an ethos to the classical frame, it is one of epistemic optimism. The world of the mind, however shadowed and conflicted, can be brought into the light of understanding. The past, even if fragmented, can be recollected. Trauma, even if unspeakable, can be rendered in language. The analyst's task is to guide the patient through this process of unveiling—not only to provide interpretations, but to foster a form of psychic integration that is equated, implicitly or explicitly, with the attainment of knowledge (Freud, 1912/1958).

Yet this classical frame also bears within it the seeds of its own destabilization. The very gesture of interpretation, so central to psychoanalysis, is haunted by questions: whose knowledge is being privileged? What is lost in the act of naming? How does the analyst's own unconscious structure the field of possible meanings? Even in Freud, the dream of a "science of the unconscious" is shadowed by a persistent anxiety about the limits of knowing—about the resistance of the psyche to full illumination (Freud, 1937/1964).

The subsequent history of psychoanalysis, especially in the post-Freudian and relational traditions, can be read as a progressive complication of the classical frame. Melanie Klein and her followers emphasize the symbolic function of interpretation but also the violence implicit in the act of naming the patient's experience (Klein, 1932/1975). Winnicott, with his emphasis on play and the transitional space, subtly shifts the locus of analytic action from interpretation to holding (Winnicott, 1971). Loewald re-envisions interpretation as a form of making present rather than simply uncovering the past (Loewald, 1960). And the relational turn, with figures like Mitchell and Aron, foregrounds the mutuality—and therefore the instability—of meaning in the analytic dyad (Benjamin, 1990; Mitchell & Aron, 1999).

Nevertheless, the classical frame remains a gravitational center. Even when we reject or problematize the stance of the all-knowing interpreter, we orbit around its absent presence. The analytic hour is still organized, however tacitly, around the fantasy that meaning is to be found, that there is a truth to be unveiled. The patient's suffering demands sense; the analyst is called, in one way or another, to respond to this demand with an offering of knowledge.

But what if interpretation is not only a tool for revealing truth but also, inevitably, a site of error, projection, and misrecognition? What if knowing itself, as enacted in the analytic frame, is sometimes a defense—against uncertainty, against unformulated experience, against the otherness of the patient? The remainder of this chapter, and indeed this book, will circle these questions. We begin, however, by situating ourselves within the classical frame, not in order to dismiss it, but to recognize its lingering hold on our clinical imagination—and to prepare the ground for its inversion.

The Logic of Inversion

To question the classical frame of interpretation is not merely to resist tradition or to critique from outside, but rather to inhabit the very core of psychoanalysis—its capacity to turn itself inside out. Psychoanalysis is unique among theories of mind for its insistence on the recursive; the idea that what appears as surface is always already the effect of something hidden, and yet that the act of looking for what is hidden can itself become the latest surface. This is the paradoxical inheritance of our field: an endless movement of reversal, a logic of inversion at the heart of our most cherished concepts (Freud, 1925/1961; Laplanche, 1999).

What does it mean to approach the analytic situation through the lens of inversion? On one level, it is to recognize that psychoanalytic knowledge is never simply additive—that is, we do not simply accumulate truths, one upon another, until we arrive at the whole. Rather, we encounter a series of epistemic reversals: symptoms that resist meaning, interpretations that generate new confusions, and insights that dissolve upon contact. Freud himself was attuned to this, noting that the path to the unconscious is not linear but labyrinthine, a "navel of the dream" that resists final understanding (Freud, 1900/1953, p. 525).

Inversion is present from the very origins of psychoanalytic theory. Consider repression, the foundational mechanism by which the psyche refuses certain knowledge, only to return it in disguised or inverted form. The repressed is both absent and omnipresent, silent and noisy, known and unknown (Freud, 1915/1957). In this way, repression is not simply a wall but a portal, a hinge between meaning and unmeaning—a perpetual oscillation. In Kleinian theory, splitting operates similarly, dividing the object into good and bad, only for these attributes to recombine and reverse, each always haunted by its shadow (Klein, 1946/1975). In both models, the mind operates not through the stable acquisition of knowledge, but through the restless exchange and inversion of positions.

Psychoanalytic thinking is thus structurally recursive: each claim to knowledge is shadowed by its own undoing. To interpret is to risk being interpreted in turn; to offer meaning is to expose oneself to the counter-interpretation of the patient's unconscious, or to the resistance of the analytic situation itself (Bollas, 1987; Ogden, 1994). There is no final ground, no fixed vantage point outside of transferential entanglement. As Loewald (1960) reminds us, the analyst is not a neutral observer, but a participant whose subjectivity is always implicated in the field of meaning—subject to the very inversions they seek to elucidate.

But what is the *logic* of inversion, if not simply contradiction? Inversion is not the negation of knowledge, but its recursive doubling. It is the recognition that every act of knowing produces a new field of unknowing; every revelation is a concealment; every interpretation, an evasion. The more fervently we pursue the kernel of truth, the more intricately we wrap it in the textures of language, desire, and defense (Derrida, 1978; Laplanche, 1999).

This logic is evident in the clinic, often in the very moments that unsettle our theoretical certainties. A patient, for example, arrives insisting that nothing is wrong, that analysis is unnecessary—yet week after week, their presence in the room testifies to a different kind of knowledge, one that cannot be directly owned. Here, negation is not mere denial, but a form of inverted affirmation: "I am not anxious," spoken with the tremor of anxiety; "I don't care about you," uttered with the eyes fixed on the analyst's face. The analytic task, in these moments, is not to pierce the surface with a more powerful interpretation, but to witness the inversion itself as a mode of truth (Freud, 1925/1961; Bollas, 1987).

Inversion is also at play in the structure of the analytic relationship. Transference itself is an epistemic inversion: the past returns as the present, the analyst is made to stand in for forgotten figures, and the analytic hour becomes a scene of both repetition and reversal (Freud, 1912/1958; Loewald, 1960). The countertransference, likewise, turns the analyst's own subjectivity inside out, so that the boundaries between knowing and being known, interpreting and being interpreted, are constantly in flux (Benjamin, 1990; Ogden, 1994).

Such inversions are not pathologies to be corrected, but evidence of the depth at which psychoanalytic truth operates. The patient's symptom is not simply a coded message to be deciphered, but a living paradox—an action that both conceals and reveals, an expression that protects by distorting what is most vital (Bollas, 1987; Eigen, 1999). The analyst's own theories, too, are subject to inversion: what once seemed clarifying becomes occluding; the drive for meaning is itself unmasked as a defense against not-knowing (Bion, 1962; Ogden, 1994).

Epistemic inversion is also a mode of ethical responsibility. To interpret is always to risk violence—the violence of premature knowing, of collapsing ambiguity, of failing to honor the patient's right to opacity (Benjamin, 1990; Glissant, 1997). In this light, unknowing is not a deficit but a stance: a willingness to let meaning hover, to tolerate paradox, to dwell in the curved space between knowing and not-knowing (Eigen, 1999). The analyst's humility is not the opposite of expertise, but its recursive deepening—a form of knowledge that contains within itself the capacity to be undone.

The logic of inversion also invites us to rethink the temporal structure of analytic work. In classical accounts, analysis moves from past to present, symptom to meaning, unknowing to knowing. In the logic of inversion, time folds upon itself: the past returns in the present, the future is anticipated in every act of listening, and the very desire to know becomes a repeating motif, itself subject to reversal. The analyst's interpretations may become, over time, not answers but openers—thresholds to further uncertainty, invitations to a recursive mode of engagement (Loewald, 1960; Bollas, 1987; Ogden, 1994).

This mode of thinking is not alien to psychoanalysis but embedded in its most radical traditions. Bion's (1962) notion of "negative capability" (after Keats [1817/1958]), the capacity to suspend the drive for premature understanding, is itself an embrace of inversion—a movement from meaning to the generative field of not-knowing. Eigen (1999) writes of the analyst's capacity to be undone, a recursive openness to the unknown that is as much affective as intellectual. Laplanche (1999) insists that the enigma of the other is never finally deciphered, and that all interpretation is provisional—a translation that leaves the original text forever in reserve.

In the logic of inversion, we find not only a critique of classical knowing but a resource for new forms of clinical and theoretical life. To inhabit the curved stance is to recognize that knowledge, in psychoanalysis, is never settled. It is always at risk of becoming its opposite: certainty shading into blindness, interpretation into enactment, truth into concealment. The analytic process is thus not a linear movement from ignorance to knowledge, but a recursive orbit around the impossibility of full understanding—a dance of inversion, a poetics of unknowing (Derrida, 1978; Ogden, 1994).

To close, the logic of inversion is not a detour or aberration, but the very engine of psychoanalytic thought. It is what allows us to continually renew the field of inquiry, to listen for what escapes our own formulations, to remain receptive to the surprises of the analytic encounter. As we move forward in this chapter and this book, we will explore how inversion serves not only as a method but also as an ethic, a way of holding space for truths that cannot be assimilated without loss. The analyst, in this frame, becomes not only an interpreter but also a witness to inversion itself—a presence attuned to the recursive play of knowing and unknowing at the heart of analytic life.

The Affective Atmosphere of Not-Knowing

If the classical frame rests on the assumption that knowledge is curative, and the logic of inversion exposes the instability of knowledge, then we must now attend to the lived affective atmosphere of not-knowing itself. For within the analytic encounter, unknowing is never a purely intellectual state. It is experienced—by analyst and patient alike—as mood, tension, charge, and atmosphere. It shapes the psychic field as palpably as words or interpretations, permeating the room with its particular climate.

This affective texture is more than a background condition. To enter not-knowing in the analytic sense is to cross a threshold: from certainty to ambiguity, from narrative to silence, from the comfort of explanation to the unease of the unformulated. The analyst may feel it as a subtle anxiety, a sense of vertigo, a gravitational pull toward meanings that remain just out of reach. The patient, too, often oscillates between relief and terror in the presence of uncertainty. Together, they inhabit a space charged with potential but stripped of guarantee (Bion, 1962; Ogden, 1994; Eigen, 1999).

In the early years of analysis, Freud's method was steeped in the faith that hidden meaning could be uncovered with enough interpretive effort. Yet, as the analytic hour unfolds in lived time, both participants are confronted with the presence of absence (Loewald, 1960)—the feeling that something important is in the room, though unnamed, and perhaps unnamable. The analyst's own unknowing is not a deficit, but a stance, a kind of ethical hospitality to what exceeds comprehension.

Bion (1962) famously urged analysts to suspend "memory and desire"—to bracket not only their preconceived theories, but also the urge for premature sense-making. For Bion, the capacity to sit with not-knowing, to dwell in what he called "negative capability" (after Keats), is not only a technique but also a psychological achievement. The analytic attitude he advocates is a receptive openness, a trust in the field of the unknown, and a willingness to let meaning emerge in its own time and form. This stance is itself affectively saturated: the analyst's patience is tinged with longing and loss, curiosity and dread.

Yet not-knowing is not a void; it is a dynamic field. In the analytic hour, the atmosphere of uncertainty is shaped by subtle cues—hesitations, associations, bodily tensions, glances, even the tempo of breath. These are the ways in which the analytic couple marks the territory of what cannot be said or known directly. Unknowing, in this sense, is felt in the body: the heart quickens at a certain silence, a shiver runs through the chest at a moment of hesitation, a heaviness gathers in the air when both analyst and patient approach the unspeakable (Ogden, 1994; Eigen, 1999).

Clinically, this field of not-knowing often reveals itself in the form of "analytic impasses." An impasse is not simply a failure of technique, but an affective state—a shared sense that something is stuck, ungraspable, or on the brink of collapse. Yet such impasses are also moments of greatest potential, precisely because they disrupt the momentum of ordinary understanding. The patient may express this by saying, "I don't know what I'm feeling," or "Nothing comes to mind." The analyst, too, may feel lost, blank, uncertain what to say. In these moments, the atmosphere of not-knowing is thick and tangible, a psychic weather front moving through the room (Bollas, 1987; D. B. Stern, 2010).

What is demanded of the analyst in these moments is a particular kind of presence—a willingness to dwell in, rather than flee from, the discomfort of not-knowing. This is a relational stance, one that privileges affective attunement over interpretive mastery. The analyst's task is not to dissolve the tension with a quick interpretation, but to bear witness to it, to hold it with the patient, to lend it a form of psychic hospitality. This hospitality is not passive; it is an active, embodied practice of "containing" (Bion, 1962; Ogden, 2005). The analyst becomes a vessel for the atmosphere of uncertainty, so that the patient may begin to tolerate and symbolize it themselves.

Michael Eigen (1999) describes the analyst's capacity to be undone—to allow their own sense of certainty, and even their identity as the one-who-knows, to be suspended. This capacity is not a mere technique but a fundamental aspect of analytic presence. The analyst does not merely model uncertainty; they risk it, they feel it, they enter it. In doing so, they enact an ethic of co-experiencing—the willingness to join the patient at the edge of what can be known, to be present at the threshold of articulation.

The atmosphere of not-knowing is also, crucially, affectively creative. When the analyst can remain present in this field, the patient often begins to experiment—playing with words, images, silences, even contradictions. Paradox is not resolved but inhabited. Meanings emerge not as fixed answers, but as living questions, constellated around the gap. New psychic forms are possible precisely because the field of not-knowing has not been prematurely foreclosed (Winnicott, 1971; D. B. Stern, 2010).

It is here, in the affective atmosphere of not-knowing, that the ethical stakes of psychoanalytic work come most fully into view. To refuse premature knowing is not to abdicate responsibility, but to take up a different kind of care—one that values ambiguity, risk, and the creative potential of unformulated experience. The analyst's presence in this atmosphere is not neutral; it is marked by the willingness to witness what cannot be possessed, to let what is unknown remain unknown for as long as necessary (Benjamin, 2018).

Yet this stance is always unstable, always at risk of collapse. The urge to resolve, to name, to impose meaning is powerful, for both analyst and patient. It is precisely here that the discipline of not-knowing must be cultivated: not as a withdrawal from engagement, but as an ongoing, affectively charged commitment to what Eigen (1999) calls the life in waiting. The analytic room becomes a site where knowledge and unknowing interpenetrate, generating an atmosphere thick with the charge of possibility.

The recursive structure of analytic experience—the doubling, echoing, and mirroring of uncertainty—creates a symbolic atmosphere, a shared space in which both participants feel the gravitational pull of what cannot yet be known. This is not a deficit, but a resource. For in the presence of unknowing, both analyst and patient become available to new forms of experience, new symbolic articulations, new ways of being together. This atmosphere is the invisible infrastructure of psychoanalytic transformation.

As this book argues, unknowing is not simply the backdrop for interpretation, but a primary mode of analytic truth. The capacity to dwell in not-knowing, to contain and transmit its affective charge, is itself a therapeutic action. It is the generative tension from which symbolization, recognition, and psychic movement arise (Loewald, 1960; D. B. Stern, 2010). The analyst's willingness to sustain the atmosphere of uncertainty creates the conditions for something genuinely new to appear.

In summary, the affective atmosphere of not-knowing is both the ground and the horizon of psychoanalytic work. It is a charged field—at once anxious and creative, destabilizing and opening. It requires from the analyst a discipline of presence and an ethic of containment. To practice within this field is to take unknowing as a form of truth: not a lack to be corrected, but a potential to be lived. This is the atmosphere in which all true analytic discovery takes place—and it is to this field that the work of inversion and epistemic refusal perpetually returns.

Clinical Vignette—Holding the Unformulated

A winter morning. My office is dimly lit, the city muffled behind drawn shades. I sit with Sam, a patient I have seen for almost a year. He arrives as always: precise, even courteous, yet his presence is ringed by a subtle atmospheric unease—a sense that something hovers just outside our shared space, unspoken but urgently alive.

Sam begins to speak about his week, describing a conflict at work with his supervisor. His words are measured, slightly abstracted, circling the facts rather than entering them. I listen and notice my own response: a faint impatience rising, a restlessness, the sense that I am waiting for something that has not yet arrived. This, I have learned, is often the first signal of unformulated experience—a subtle affective pressure at the edge of sense (D. B. Stern, 2010).

As the session progresses, Sam's narrative falters. He pauses, glances at the window, and then looks at me and shrugs. "I don't know why I'm telling you this," he says, voice thin. "It's not important. I feel like I'm wasting your time." I sense an old recursive pattern: the patient anxious about disappointing the analyst, both of us suspended in the gravity of expectation. For a moment, I am tempted to interpret—to suggest that his self-effacement mirrors childhood experiences of being unseen or dismissed. But I notice, too, a deeper current in the room: the presence of not-knowing, thickening between us.

I recall Bion's admonition to be "without memory and desire" (Bion, 1970b)—to bracket my habitual search for meaning and attend instead to what is unfolding in the present. I let myself rest in the uncertainty, resisting the pull to fill the silence with knowledge. The air between us grows dense, charged with feeling yet without clear narrative. I reflect on Ogden's (1994) concept of the analytic third—the emergent field shaped by both subjectivities, neither wholly mine nor his, but something that arises in the interstice, shaped by the affective atmosphere of not-knowing.

Sam breaks the silence first. "Sometimes I just feel… blank," he says. "Like I'm not really here. Or like I should have something to say, but there's nothing." He looks embarrassed, his voice fading. My own anxiety quickens in response—the analyst's ancient urge to rescue, to supply meaning, to relieve the discomfort. But instead, I say quietly, "I wonder what it's like, right now, to be with that blankness here with me." The words feel risky, almost insubstantial, but they open a small space.

Sam's eyes flicker. "I don't know," he says again, but something shifts: his posture softens, his breathing slows. We sit together, not in the absence of experience but in the presence of something unformulated—affect without name, sense without content. The mood is fragile, but in this moment, I sense a subtle intimacy: the shared endurance of uncertainty. My attention is not on what is missing, but on what is alive in the gap.

Time stretches. I remember Winnicott's (1971) insistence that play—and thus psychic growth—emerges only in the potential space between certainty and chaos, between what is already known and what cannot yet be known. In this analytic hour, the play is not overt: it is the play of presence, of mutual endurance, of risking contact without the shield of explanation. The analytic space becomes, for a moment, a field of aliveness in waiting (Eigen, 1999).

Sam speaks again, this time hesitantly: "Sometimes I feel like if I don't say the right thing, it'll all just… stop. Like you'll get bored, or leave, or just give up on me." He glances away. I notice the urge to reassure him, to protest that I am here, that I am not leaving. But instead I hold the feeling with him, noticing its quality—anxiety and yearning intertwined. The atmosphere is saturated with the tension of not-knowing, and in this field, Sam's longing for recognition becomes palpable, even as it cannot be spoken directly.

What occurs next is small but unmistakable. Sam sighs, slumps a little in the chair, then looks at me. "I guess I'm always afraid I'm too much. Or not enough. Or both." The paradox is out in the open—not resolved, but registered. I nod, letting his words settle between us. I do not interpret further, nor do I seek to clarify. The hour ends with a feeling of incompletion, a lingering uncertainty. Yet as Sam leaves, he looks back and meets my gaze. "See you next week," he says, voice steadier. There is, for the first time in many sessions, a trace of warmth.

Later, I reflect on the session. The work, I realize, was not in finding a new narrative or supplying insight, but in holding the affective atmosphere of not-knowing. The analytic field, for that hour, became a space where unformulated experience could be borne without collapse. The recursive tension—the oscillation between anxiety and contact, between blankness and recognition—was not a problem to be solved, but a ground to be inhabited. In this, the session became an enactment of epistemic refusal: a choice not to force sense, but to hold open the possibility of emergence.

Clinically, such moments are easily missed or dismissed. The pressure to "do" something, to interpret, to heal, is immense. Yet the most transformative shifts often occur in the patient's (and analyst's) capacity to stay with the unformulated—to bear the feeling of not-knowing together, and thus to create the conditions for something new to arise (Ogden, 2005; D. B. Stern, 2010). This is not passive; it is an active, even courageous form of presence. It is an ethical stance as much as a technical one.

It is also a recursive process. The next week, Sam returns, mentioning nothing of the previous session's tension. He speaks about work, about a friend's new relationship, about plans for the holidays. But something is different: he seems a little less defended, a little more present in his body. The atmosphere is lighter, as if the field of not-knowing has subtly shifted, making more room for play. Midway through the session, he pauses and says, "It's weird, but I feel okay not having anything big to talk about." I smile, recognizing the quiet revolution underway.

As I write this vignette, I am aware that the affective texture of not-knowing is not easily captured in narrative. It is something that happens in the in-between: a quality of the air, a resonance between bodies, a vibration in the analytic field. Yet it is precisely here that the heart of analytic work unfolds. The refusal to resolve too quickly, the willingness to dwell in uncertainty, the capacity to contain affect that has no name—these are not failures of technique, but the work itself. They are the soil from which psychic transformation grows.

In sum, the clinical encounter is not simply a site for the delivery of knowledge, but a field for the cultivation of unknowing as a form of truth. The analytic hour, at its most alive, is saturated with the recursive tension of what cannot be named. To hold the unformulated is to trust in the potential of the psyche, to honor the unknown not as a void but as a generative horizon. This, perhaps, is the deepest ethic of psychoanalysis: to become a companion in the field of not-knowing, and to witness what may emerge when nothing is forced, and nothing is foreclosed.

Epistemic Refusal and the Ethics of Unknowing

The analytic hour is saturated with the impulse to know—to decipher, interpret, illuminate. The patient's suffering demands meaning; the analyst's calling is, in some way, to respond with knowledge. Yet the most radical aspect of psychoanalysis may not be its drive toward sense, but its capacity for epistemic refusal: the ethical stance of not-knowing, not as abdication, but as a form of fidelity to what is irreducible in the analytic field.

To practice epistemic refusal is to recognize the shadow side of interpretation—the violence of premature naming, the foreclosure of ambiguity, the tendency to grasp for coherence where none yet exists (Glissant, 1997; Benjamin, 2018). Even careful interpretations can recast the patient in the analyst's terms, translating the enigma of the other into the grammar of the self. Epistemic refusal interrupts this movement: it is the willingness to bear the anxiety of ambiguity, to hold the question open rather than rush toward resolution.

This refusal is neither passive nor nihilistic. It is, as Foucault (1997) might have said, an ethic of discomfort—a practice of remaining with the tension that arises when the limits of one's own knowing become visible. In the analytic relationship, this often means attending to what remains unsymbolized, unspoken, or affectively charged but as yet unformulated. It is a discipline of listening for the silence beneath the story, the excess that does not fit established categories (Eigen, 1999; Ogden, 2005).

What is at stake in epistemic refusal is not merely a technique, but a radical form of care. To refuse the comfort of knowledge is to honor the patient's right to opacity, to protect the psychic space where new forms of experience may gestate without the pressure of immediate sense-making (Bollas, 1987; Glissant, 1997). This is the paradoxical ethic of psychoanalysis: a commitment to the patient's freedom from the analyst's certainties, even from the analyst's desire to heal through understanding.

At times, epistemic refusal is enacted through silence. The analyst resists the urge to interpret, allowing affect to circulate in the analytic field without immediate capture by language. At other times, refusal takes the form of a gentle questioning: "I wonder if we can stay with not knowing, for now?" Such interventions do not close down meaning; rather, they open space for the emergence of the unexpected, for the recursive play of sense and nonsense, presence and absence.

This ethic of not-knowing is especially vital in encounters with trauma, dissociation, and states of psychic fragmentation. Here, the analyst's rush to coherence can be retraumatizing, imposing narrative where the psyche has been ruptured by the impossibility of symbolization (Ferenczi, 1988/1932;

Laub & Auerhahn, 1993). Epistemic refusal becomes a holding action—a containment of the affective fragments until, or unless, the patient is ready to risk symbolization. It is a stance of waiting-with, rather than pushing-for, the emergence of meaning.

The psychoanalytic literature is replete with warnings about the dangers of omniscience and interpretive excess. Winnicott (1971) famously cautioned against premature object usage—the analyst who insists on being the one-who-knows forecloses the patient's experience of creative relating. Loewald (1960) insisted that the analyst's interpretations should be invitations, not impositions—offerings that may or may not be taken up by the patient, and always provisional. Laplanche (1999) went further, arguing that all translation leaves something untranslated; the residue of the enigmatic is the site of ongoing psychic work.

To practice epistemic refusal is to trust the analytic field: to allow that meaning may arise unpredictably, to tolerate the analyst's own anxiety about not-knowing, to bear witness to what cannot yet be spoken. It is, in Eigen's (1999) language, a discipline of being "undone" by the encounter with the other—an ethic of humility, openness, and affective risk.

Epistemic refusal is not only about the analyst's stance but also about the structure of the analytic situation itself. The analytic frame becomes a laboratory for living with the limits of knowledge: both analyst and patient are invited to risk the discomfort of unknowing, to let meaning emerge from the recursive interplay of desire, fear, language, and silence (Ogden, 2005; D. B. Stern, 2010). The analytic hour is not a space of mastery, but a field of potential—an atmosphere charged with the possibility of transformation, precisely because it is not foreclosed by certainty.

There is also an important social and political dimension to epistemic refusal. As Glissant (1997) argues in the context of colonial and postcolonial experience, the demand to be known is often a demand for transparency, a form of domination masquerading as care. Psychoanalysis, at its most radical, sides with opacity—with the right of the subject to remain ungraspable, unfinalizable, resistant to capture by another's schema. The ethics of unknowing thus echoes far beyond the analytic hour, resonating with questions of difference, recognition, and freedom.

In practice, this ethic demands a particular discipline of the analyst's own mind. It is easy to believe that our training and experience grant us privileged access to truth; it is far harder to risk the humility of not-knowing, to recognize that every interpretation is a wager, not a fact. The analyst's authority is reconfigured, not as mastery, but as presence: a willingness to remain alongside, to companion the patient through the shifting fields of sense and nonsense, emergence and retreat.

Perhaps the most difficult moments are those when unknowing feels unbearable—when the urge to interpret, to "do something," reaches its peak. Here, the ethic of epistemic refusal is most tested, and most needed. To hold the tension without collapsing into action is to enact a different kind of care, one that honors both the patient's and the analyst's vulnerability to the unknown. This is a care that is recursive, affectively saturated, and ethically alive.

To close, epistemic refusal is not a detour from the analytic task, but its ethical heart. It is the willingness to suspend the drive for mastery, to welcome the atmosphere of not-knowing, to recognize that the deepest transformations occur not through knowledge imposed, but through unknowing inhabited. The analyst's fidelity is to this recursive field: a commitment to the ongoing, unfinished work of being-with what cannot be fully known.

Recursive Structures and the Symbolic Atmosphere of Unknowing

Unknowing in psychoanalysis is not simply a momentary lapse or a tolerable blank—it is a structural principle, shaping the very field in which analyst and patient move. The recursive quality of the analytic situation means that unknowing is never a one-time event, but an ongoing, self-referential process: a structure that re-echoes, refracts, and folds back upon itself, constantly reconfiguring what counts as meaning, presence, and truth.

This recursive structure is most palpable in the way analytic themes return, not as repetitions of the same, but as variations on a theme, orbiting around the unsymbolized core. The patient's stories, dreams, and symptoms often circle unresolved affective knots, approaching from new angles, shifting in emotional coloration, sometimes dissolving into ambiguity, sometimes crystallizing into new insight. The analytic conversation, too, is recursive: we return to familiar words or images, only to find their meaning altered by the context, the mood, or the passage of time (Ogden, 1994; D. B. Stern, 2010). This looping quality is not a failure of progress, but a sign of psychic work: the psyche moving around what cannot yet be formulated, playing at the edges of knowing.

Recursive structure is also mirrored in the analyst's own experience. As the hour unfolds, the analyst may feel caught in a cycle—wondering if they are simply "doing the same thing again," or if something new is emerging within the repetition. This is particularly acute in work with patients for whom knowing and not-knowing are bound up with trauma or early relational uncertainty. Here, the recursive structure is not merely conceptual but affective, alive in the analyst's body and mind: anxiety, boredom, frustration, hope, and uncertainty looping in the countertransference, echoing the patient's own recursive affective patterns (Bollas, 1987; Eigen, 1999).

It is in this looping, recursive movement that the symbolic atmosphere of unknowing is generated. Symbolic atmosphere refers to the subtle, often pre-reflective field of meaning that permeates the analytic room—a field shaped by words, gestures, affects, and silences, but not reducible to any one element. It is the mood, the gravity, the charge of possibility and constraint that envelops analyst and patient alike. This atmosphere is not static; it shifts as meanings are risked, resisted, deferred, or left open. Unknowing is its signature: the sense that something is in play, alive, but not yet owned or defined (D. B. Stern, 2010).

Consider a patient who returns, session after session, to an unfinished story—a lost childhood object, a mysterious bodily symptom, a recurring dream with shifting details. Each return is both a repetition and a new creation: the meaning is never fully captured, and yet something changes. The patient senses the pattern but cannot quite articulate it. The analyst, too, feels the pull—the urge to name, to synthesize, but also the gravity of what remains unformulated. In this recursive atmosphere, new possibilities for symbolization open, precisely because the field is not closed by premature knowing.

Recursive structure is thus both a clinical and a symbolic principle. It is enacted in the rhythm of sessions, the pacing of speech, the timing of silences. It is present in the way language is used not only to clarify but also to gesture, to question, to hover. Ogden (1994) describes this as the analytic third: the emergent, co-created field that is neither wholly the analyst's nor the patient's, but a product of their recursive engagement. The analytic third is saturated with the symbolic atmosphere of unknowing; it is the space in which not-knowing is not a lack, but an active process of creative waiting.

This atmosphere is fragile and easily foreclosed. The pressure to resolve, to interpret, to escape the discomfort of uncertainty is ever-present. It is the analyst's task to protect the recursive structure: to notice when the field is closing, when premature coherence is being imposed, and to gently reopen the space of potential. This may involve naming the pressure to know ("I notice we're both searching for an answer here") or simply holding the silence a moment longer, allowing the symbolic atmosphere to thicken and deepen.

The recursive quality of analytic unknowing also shapes the analyst's self-reflection. Each session is not only a meeting with the patient but also a return to one's own limits—the edges of understanding, the recurrence of familiar anxieties, the looping of interpretive patterns. The analyst is continually returned to their own not-knowing, and it is this recursive humility that underwrites the ethic of the work. As Eigen (1999) suggests, the analyst's capacity to be repeatedly undone, to re-enter the atmosphere of unknowing without retreating into certainty, is what allows genuine transformation to occur.

This symbolic atmosphere of recursive unknowing is not unique to the analytic hour. It reverberates through the broader culture: in literature, myth, ritual, and spiritual practice, where unformulated truths are carried in symbol and gesture, in silence and song. Psychoanalysis joins this lineage by making the recursive structure of not-knowing central, not peripheral. The analytic hour becomes a small laboratory for living with uncertainty—a symbolic field in which the recursive movement of knowing and unknowing can be studied, endured, and, sometimes, celebrated.

In some cases, this recursive atmosphere is the very substance of change. The patient, learning to tolerate uncertainty, begins to relate differently to their own experience—to see patterns without forcing them into premature sense, to notice repetitions as invitations rather than indictments. The analyst, too, becomes attuned to the creative potential of the loop: the way an old theme returns with a new resonance, the way absence itself becomes generative. In these moments, the analytic hour is more than a site for the delivery of insight; it is a crucible for the symbolic transformation of affect, meaning, and selfhood.

Finally, recursive structure challenges the very notion of analytic "progress." Change is not a linear ascent from ignorance to knowledge, but an ongoing movement through cycles of openness, closure, and renewed uncertainty. This is not to say that analysis is futile, or that all is repetition without difference. Rather, it is to affirm that the deepest changes may be recursive: old patterns returned to with new feeling, new symbolic possibility, new forms of unknowing. The analyst's stance is thus one of faith—not in mastery, but in the generative power of returning, of dwelling, of letting the symbolic atmosphere of unknowing do its work.

As we prepare to conclude this chapter, it is worth underscoring that the recursive structures and symbolic atmospheres of unknowing are not failures to be overcome, but achievements to be cultivated. They are the conditions of possibility for all genuine analytic transformation: the field in which new experience can arise, where the old can be returned to without foreclosure, and where the mystery at the heart of the psyche can be respected, even loved.

Closing Reflection—Unknowing as the Heart of Analytic Truth

To arrive at the end of this opening chapter is, in a sense, to return to its beginning. The promise of psychoanalysis has always been entangled with knowing: to illuminate, to decipher, to name what was hidden and thereby relieve suffering. Yet, as we have followed the recursive pathways of the analytic hour, the atmosphere of not-knowing has gathered force—not as a deficit, but as the core condition of psychic life and analytic transformation. If there is a center to psychoanalytic truth, it is not the secure possession of knowledge, but the willingness to circle its impossibility.

What distinguishes psychoanalysis among the healing arts is not simply its theory of the unconscious, but its radical hospitality to what cannot be assimilated. The analytic situation is structured around the recurrent, looping encounter with what escapes understanding—symptoms that resist interpretation, affects that cannot be named, repetitions that refuse closure. This is not a flaw in the method, but its essential ground. The analytic frame itself is built to contain the unformulated, to hold open the space of potential, to value unknowing as a form of care.

In the classical frame, the analyst's power rests on their capacity to know: to see beneath the surface, to reveal the truth, to cure by making conscious. Yet every act of interpretation also risks foreclosure, an inadvertent violence done to the patient's right to remain opaque, ambiguous, irreducible. The logic of inversion, as we have traced it here, exposes the ambivalence at the heart of interpretation: every knowing is shadowed by unknowing; every revelation by loss; every act of care by the possibility of erasure.

It is in the affective atmosphere of not-knowing—those charged, uncertain, and creative fields of experience—that psychoanalysis most fully realizes its potential. Here, the analyst's discipline is not mastery, but presence: the capacity to remain with the patient in the field of the unsymbolized, to lend their own nervous system as a container for the patient's unformulated affects. The analyst's capacity to be undone (Eigen, 1999) becomes, paradoxically, the very source of their authority: an authority rooted in humility, responsiveness, and the ongoing risk of being changed.

To hold unknowing in the analytic hour is to risk everything that feels safe about the clinical encounter. The analyst is asked to relinquish their scripts, their desire to cure, even their identity as "the one who knows." The patient, too, is invited to enter the atmosphere of uncertainty, to discover new forms of subjectivity in the absence of a fixed narrative. The analytic dyad becomes, in these moments, a laboratory for the transformation of experience: not by making sense of the unknown, but by dwelling with it, giving it symbolic body, and allowing it to become the ground for something new.

This is not a call for analytic quietism or passivity. On the contrary, the discipline of unknowing is a fiercely active stance—a refusal to foreclose meaning, an openness to the recursive play of sense and nonsense, an ethical commitment to the other's right to remain ungrasped. The analyst's refusal to rush toward coherence is not a withdrawal from care, but its highest form: a witness who does not abandon the field of ambiguity, who trusts in the patient's capacity for emergence, who honors the unknown as a site of possibility rather than a problem to be solved.

The recursive structures and symbolic atmospheres we have described are not exclusive to the analytic hour; they reverberate throughout the broader field of human life. Every relationship, every encounter with art, every act of creation, is shaped by the tension between what can be known and what must remain unknown. Psychoanalysis, in this sense, offers not only a clinical method but also a philosophy of living—a way of being present to the world's irreducible complexity, its endless loops, its capacity for surprise.

At the edge of unknowing, a new ethic emerges. This is the ethic of epistemic refusal: a commitment to resist the violence of explanation, to cultivate the patience required by emergence, to love what is unfinished and unfinishable. The analyst, in this frame, becomes a kind of cosmic companion—bearing witness to the recursive pulse of the psyche, protecting the creative potential of the gap, and honoring the singularity of every analytic encounter.

To conclude is, inevitably, to begin again. The work of psychoanalysis is recursive in the deepest sense: each hour a return to the threshold, each insight an invitation to unknowing, each transformation a beginning anew. The chapters that follow will unfold this central paradox—exploring how classical concepts are inverted, how epistemic refusals generate truth, and how the recursive structure of the psyche is both a wound and a source of vitality.

To practice psychoanalysis, then, is not to master the unknown, but to dwell with it, to let it shape us, to become—again and again—anew in its presence. Unknowing is not an absence at the heart of analytic truth, but its deepest ground. It is here that analysis becomes not only a science of the mind but also an art of living at the edge of what can be known.

Chapter 2

Oedipus as Myth of Knowing—Refusing the Law of Linearity

This chapter reinterprets the Oedipal complex not as the emblem of linear psychic development or inevitable submission to law, but as a recursive myth of unknowing, detour, and creative refusal. Moving from Freud's classical narrative through Lacanian, feminist, and queer critiques, this chapter tracks how the figure of Oedipus becomes a site of paradox, where the pursuit of knowledge produces catastrophe and mastery is always shadowed by loss. Inverting the traditional frame, the unconscious is conceptualized as a recursive field—a curved psychic space in which riddles, desire, and the law circulate endlessly, opening possibilities for transformation through repetition and return. Through clinical vignette and symbolic exploration, this chapter develops an ethics of not-knowing: the analyst's task shifts from solving riddles to sustaining an atmosphere of ambiguity, recursive play, and emergent meaning. Refusing linearity, analysis is reframed as a discipline of accompaniment and creative wandering, where the detours and excesses of Oedipal desire become resources for psychic renewal and new forms of subjectivity.

The Oedipal Complex—The Law of Linearity in Classical Psychoanalysis

The Oedipal complex, perhaps the most enduring and contentious mythic figure in psychoanalysis, stands at the origin of the field's grand narrative about knowing. Its arc is inseparable from the very notion of the unconscious as a site of forbidden knowledge, hidden desire, and the impossible longing to resolve what cannot be named. The story of Oedipus—he who answers the riddle and brings ruin by knowing—has served as the emblem of psychic development, of the crossing from confusion to truth, from incestuous desire to the acceptance of law and limitation. It is here that

DOI: 10.4324/9781003747109-4

psychoanalysis enshrined the law of linearity: the presumption that psychic life unfolds as a progression from ignorance to knowledge, from chaos to order, from fusion to separation (Freud, 1900/1953, 1923/1961).

Freud's discovery of the Oedipal complex was as much an epistemological breakthrough as a clinical one. In the late 19th and early 20th centuries, as the boundaries of the self and the unconscious were first being mapped, the Oedipus myth provided a narrative skeleton for the new science of the mind. For Freud, the child's passage through the Oedipal stage—his or her forbidden longing for the parent of the opposite sex, rivalry with the same-sex parent, and eventual submission to the law—became the central drama of psychosexual development. In this frame, psychic maturation depended on a successful traversal of the Oedipal terrain: the renunciation of impossible desire, the internalization of the father's law, the assumption of a knowable and bounded identity (Freud, 1905/1953, 1923/1961).

This is the founding linear fantasy of psychoanalysis: that development is a story with a beginning, middle, and end, a passage from not-knowing to knowing, from immersion in affect to the formation of symbolic order. The Oedipal narrative is teleological, aiming always toward the resolution of conflict and the restoration of law. Its logic mirrors the structure of classical interpretation itself: there is something hidden, an enigma to be unraveled, and the analyst's task is to guide the patient from the darkness of confusion into the light of understanding.

The riddle of the Sphinx—central to the Oedipus myth—becomes, in this reading, a metaphor for the analytic enterprise. The child (and later, the analysand) is cast as the one who must solve the puzzle of desire, decode the hidden messages of the unconscious, and accept the authority of the law. The Oedipal narrative, then, is not merely a story about sexual development or family romance; it is a foundational myth about the nature of knowledge itself: what can be known, what must be renounced, and what it costs to solve the riddle (Freud, 1900/1953; Lacan, 1977).

Yet this linear structure has always been shadowed by ambivalence and loss. The law of the father, the supposed endpoint of development, is never fully internalized; desire, though renamed, is never fully relinquished. The knowledge that Oedipus wins is catastrophic; the truth he uncovers destroys the very frame of meaning that made the quest intelligible. In this sense, the Oedipal myth is haunted by its own refusal: knowledge is both cure and curse, and the drive to solve the riddle is never simply progressive, but recursive—always circling the unspeakable, the impossible, the traumatic kernel at the heart of psychic life (Laplanche, 1999).

Still, the classical tradition clings to its linearity. The analytic process, in its most traditional telling, is structured as a passage through and beyond the Oedipal impasse. The child must accept separation and difference, symbolized by the law; the adult must come to terms with the limits of knowledge, desire, and identity. Interpretation, in this frame, is an act of progress—a means of moving forward, resolving conflict, and achieving integration (Loewald, 1960; Chodorow, 1994).

This narrative has proven both powerful and constraining. On the one hand, it offers an intelligible path through the chaos of the drives, a story in which meaning can be found and suffering transformed. On the other hand, it risks reducing the multiplicity of psychic experience to a singular, normative arc. Linearity becomes not only a structure of narrative but also a law unto itself—a demand for coherence, resolution, and mastery. Those aspects of psychic life that resist integration—regression, repetition, the uncanny, the non-linear logic of trauma—are either pathologized or rendered invisible (Benjamin, 1990; Bersani, 2010).

The Oedipal complex, then, is not just a developmental stage or mythic event; it is an epistemic structure that orders the field of psychoanalysis. It shapes our sense of what counts as knowledge, what is valued or excluded, and what it means to be a subject at all. Even as later generations of analysts have critiqued and revised Freud's original formulations, the gravitational pull of Oedipal linearity continues to organize much analytic thought and practice. The child's journey through the labyrinth of desire remains, for many, the model of psychic progress—a template against which all deviations are measured.

Yet, as the following sections will explore, the myth of Oedipus is more complex than the classical frame allows. Beneath its apparent linearity lie loops, reversals, refusals—recursive structures that destabilize the very law they are said to enact. The law of linearity, far from resolving the enigma of desire, may itself be the riddle: a demand for knowledge that is haunted by the impossibility of ever fully knowing. To open the Oedipal narrative to recursive, affective, and symbolic inversion is to reimagine the very foundations of psychoanalytic thought—not as a march toward knowledge, but as a field of unknowing, return, and creative ambiguity.

Oedipus and the Paradox of Knowing—Psychoanalytic Readings and Their Limits

From its inception, psychoanalysis has been marked by the ambition to make sense of the enigmatic, to trace the hidden origins of psychic life. Nowhere is this more apparent than in the readings of the Oedipus myth that have shaped the field's understanding of subjectivity, desire, and the law. Yet, at the very heart of these readings lies a paradox: the more vigorously psychoanalysis has pursued the meaning of Oedipus, the more the myth resists closure, splintering into contradictions, ambiguities, and recursive enigmas.

Freud's own engagement with the myth of Oedipus reveals this paradox in its earliest form. For Freud, Oedipus stands as the figure who both knows and does not know—the solver of the Sphinx's riddle, yet ignorant of the more catastrophic riddle of his own existence (Freud, 1900/1953). The Oedipal narrative is thus double-edged: it promises that knowledge can resolve the threat of the unknown, but it also demonstrates the disastrous consequences of attaining forbidden knowledge. The analyst, much like Oedipus, is tempted by the allure of knowing, even as every revelation is shadowed by the risk of loss, guilt, and ruin.

Subsequent psychoanalytic readings have returned to this paradox, each in their own register. Lacan's (1977) engagement with Oedipus foregrounds the centrality of lack and the impossibility of complete knowledge. For Lacan, the Oedipal law is not simply a developmental milestone, but an encounter with the limits of symbolization itself—the "Name-of-the-Father" marking the place of prohibition, impossibility, and desire's perpetual displacement. The Sphinx's riddle, in Lacan's hands, is not so much solved as suspended: it becomes a signifier of absence, a wound around which subjectivity organizes itself in endless loops. The analyst's own knowledge is destabilized, revealed as contingent and partial, always haunted by the real that exceeds representation (Lacan, 1977).

Feminist and queer critiques have further complicated the Oedipal narrative, exposing the limitations of its linear, heteronormative, and patriarchal assumptions. Juliet Mitchell (1974), for example, highlights the ways in which the Oedipal frame has marginalized maternal desire, rendering the mother a mere obstacle in the child's psychic journey rather than a subject in her own right. Others, such as Jessica Benjamin (1990), have argued that the law of the father is only one possible outcome of

Oedipal struggle, and that mutual recognition, ambivalence, and nonlinearity are equally intrinsic to the psychic field. These readings fracture the unity of the myth, opening the analytic situation to other forms of desire, identification, and knowledge—forms that may be cyclical, ambiguous, or resistant to closure.

What these alternative readings reveal is that the Oedipal myth, far from being a single key to psychic life, is a generative site of paradox. Every effort to extract a univocal meaning from the story generates new contradictions: Oedipus is at once the seeker of truth and the agent of disaster, the solver of riddles and the embodiment of what cannot be solved. The Sphinx's riddle is never exhausted; the trauma at the heart of the myth is never wholly symbolized. In this sense, the analytic hour recapitulates the Oedipal drama—not as a linear passage from ignorance to knowledge, but as a recursive movement between enigma and meaning, law and desire, knowing and unknowing (Laplanche, 1999).

Even the most conceptually ambitious efforts to stabilize the Oedipal myth are undone by its internal excesses. Laplanche's (1999) reading foregrounds the enigmatic signifier—the messages from the other that the subject cannot fully translate. For Laplanche, the unconscious is constituted by these enigmatic demands, by the residue of the other's desire that remains unformulated. The Oedipal field is thus marked by the impossibility of closure: every act of interpretation is haunted by what is left unsaid, unsymbolized, or ungraspable. The analyst's fidelity, in this view, is not to the revelation of hidden truth, but to the recursive movement of translation and untranslation, knowing and misrecognition.

Leo Bersani (2010), writing in a different register, contends that psychoanalysis too often reduces the Oedipal myth to the law of structure and meaning, at the expense of its unruly, excessive, and queer dimensions. The true radicalism of Oedipus, for Bersani, lies in his refusal—or inability—to submit to the law, to resolve the paradox of his own desire. The analyst, faced with the recurrence of Oedipal themes in the clinic, must be attuned to these points of rupture: the moments when linear explanation fails, when desire undoes the law, when the riddle reasserts itself against every effort to solve it.

The clinical implications of these readings are profound. If the Oedipal situation is not a developmental stage to be traversed and left behind, but an ever-present paradox, then the analyst's task shifts. Rather than leading the patient toward a final, integrative knowing, the work becomes a recursive engagement with the limits of sense: circling the sites of enigma, bearing witness to what cannot be assimilated, honoring the affective intensity of what resists closure (Loewald, 1960; Ogden, 1994). The analytic hour is revealed as a field of oscillation, not resolution—a place where the paradox of knowing is lived, not overcome.

This is not to say that psychoanalysis abandons interpretation, or that knowledge is irrelevant to psychic transformation. Rather, it is to insist that all knowledge in the analytic field is provisional, partial, and recursively structured. The Oedipal myth, in its very resistance to closure, offers a model for an analysis that is always in motion: looping back, doubling, fragmenting, and returning again to the question of what cannot be known. The analyst is drawn, like Oedipus, to the lure of truth but is called also to remain faithful to the riddle—the recursive play of knowledge and its undoing.

In sum, psychoanalytic readings of Oedipus do not exhaust its enigma; rather, they multiply its paradoxes. The myth persists not as a static law, but as a recursive site of engagement—a field in which knowing and unknowing, law and desire, continually invert and transform one another. The limits of these readings, far from being failures, are the ground upon which new forms of analytic presence can emerge. The task, as we will see in the sections that follow, is not to solve the Oedipal riddle once and for all, but to dwell within its paradox: to let the law of knowing be unsettled by the ethics of unknowing, and to find in the recursive atmosphere of the analytic hour the possibility of transformation.

Inverting the Oedipal Logic—The Unconscious as Recursive Field

To invert the Oedipal logic is not simply to reverse the valences of desire or transgression, but to challenge the very temporality and topology that the Oedipus myth installs at the heart of psychoanalysis. The linear sequence—unknowing to knowing, forbidden desire to law, question to answer—has become so foundational that its frame is often invisible. Yet the clinical realities of analytic work, as well as the ambiguities of the myth itself, constantly strain against this presumption of linearity. What if, instead, we apprehend the unconscious as a recursive field—a space of looping, folding, and curved return, where knowledge and unknowing generate each other in perpetual motion?

This alternative topology can be glimpsed in the moments of analytic encounter where neither patient nor analyst can claim stable ground. The Oedipal "resolution" that classical theory posits is rarely so clean in lived experience. Patients return, session after session, to childhood scenes that are not stories but gravitational wells: fragments of feeling, flashes of fear, traces of erotic longing that resist narrative progression. The analytic hour becomes less a straight line and more a spiral, orbiting around unsymbolized centers—what Loewald (1960) describes as a generative lack at the heart of experience, and what Ogden (1994) later frames as the analytic third.

The myth of Oedipus, reread through this lens, reveals its recursive structure. The riddle is not solved and discarded; rather, it mutates, recurs, returns as trauma and dream, repetition and symptom. Oedipus' journey is not a single crossing from ignorance to knowledge, but a circling of the unspeakable—the very "navel" of the unconscious that Freud (1900/1953) recognized as forever resisting full interpretation. Each act of knowing begets new unknowing; every revelation is shadowed by further questions, each solution a new riddle.

Laplanche (1999), with his theory of the enigmatic signifier, offers a path into this recursive landscape. For Laplanche, the psyche is constituted by the continual return of messages from the other that cannot be fully translated—enigmatic, excessive, never entirely metabolized. The unconscious is not a reservoir of hidden content awaiting discovery, but a dynamic field in which meaning and nonmeaning circulate, echo, and transform one another. Oedipus, in this reading, is not the agent of narrative closure, but a figure caught in the recursive play of meaning and loss, translation and remainder.

This perspective finds resonance in Bersani's (2010) meditation on the "law of the father" as both a structure and an excess. For Bersani, the Oedipal drama is always already unmoored from its purported linearity: it is a myth of wandering, of detour, of desire's endless movement around the law rather than through it. Psychic life, then, is less a march toward resolution than a dance with recurrence—with the impossibility of ever "solving" the problem of desire, and the necessity of returning to it, again and again, in ever-new forms.

Benjamin (1990, 2018) similarly locates the vitality of the analytic process not in mastery or resolution, but in the mutual recognition of what cannot be known. Her model of recognition is fundamentally recursive: it is enacted in the back-and-forth, the missed encounter, the mutual openness to surprise and failure. In this frame, the Oedipal situation is not a puzzle to be solved but an invitation to live with the tension of difference, otherness, and unformulated experience.

Clinically, this curved, recursive stance changes the atmosphere of the analytic hour. Rather than striving to push the patient through a preordained sequence of developmental milestones, the analyst learns to listen for the echoes, the looping fragments, the patterns of return that mark psychic life as curved rather than linear. The past is not simply "worked through" but re-entered, inhabited, played with, and transformed in recursive acts of symbolization and encounter. The analyst, too, is drawn into this field, repeatedly unsettled in their own knowing, invited to dwell in the presence of uncertainty rather than enforce the law of sense.

Ogden's (1994) concept of the analytic third—the shared, co-created field that arises between patient and analyst—illuminates the recursive, atmospheric dimension of this work. In the recursive field, meaning is never wholly the patient's or the analyst's, never finally achieved or lost, but always in flux, hovering at the edges of articulation. Each interpretation or affective shift is a return, a re-creation, a folding back upon previous encounters. The analytic third is thus a curved space, alive with recursive possibilities, where Oedipal questions are not closed but perpetually reopened.

This recursive field is not without risk or difficulty. For both patient and analyst, it can feel disorienting, even threatening, to relinquish the security of narrative progress. The desire for closure—the fantasy of finally knowing, finally resolving—is powerful. Yet, it is precisely in resisting this fantasy that analysis opens to new forms of aliveness and creativity. The recursive approach honors the haunting, the return, the nonlinearity that marks the deepest truths of psychic life.

The myth of Oedipus, reimagined through the logic of recursion, is thus both a caution and a promise. It warns of the violence of forced resolution—of the disaster that can follow the compulsion to know at any cost. Yet it also promises the possibility of return: of circling what cannot be known, of finding new life in the very repetition that classical theory would treat as pathology. The analytic field becomes a space where the law of linearity is inverted, giving way to the ethics of return, the openness to recursive surprise, the curved temporality of ongoing psychic emergence.

What emerges from this inversion is not the collapse of structure, but a different kind of order—a living, breathing, recursive field where knowing and unknowing are in continuous relation. The Oedipal law is not abolished, but rendered permeable, flexible, responsive to the looping, affective, and symbolic textures of analytic life. The analyst's task is not to shepherd the patient to the end of the story, but to companion them in the recursive field: to witness the returns, the echoes, the moments of loss and emergence, and to trust in the curved structure of psychic growth.

In this way, the inversion of the Oedipal logic is not a negation, but an expansion—a movement from law to field, from narrative to atmosphere, from linearity to recursion. The unconscious becomes not a hidden chamber to be unlocked, but a living landscape to be inhabited: a space of endless return, looping creativity, and the radical possibility of new forms of knowing at the very heart of unknowing.

The Law, the Riddle, and the Ethics of Not-Knowing

At the heart of the Oedipal myth is an encounter with the riddle—an enigma that is neither merely an obstacle to be overcome nor a puzzle to be solved, but an event that organizes the psychic field around the limit of knowing. The Sphinx, with her inscrutable gaze and deadly question, does not simply guard the passage to Thebes; she embodies the very principle of epistemic refusal. Her riddle is not merely a test of intellect, but a summons to the limits of sense, a demand that the subject encounter what cannot be easily mastered or possessed.

In the classical telling, Oedipus's triumph lies in his capacity to answer the Sphinx, to "solve" the riddle by naming the figure of man who crawls, walks, and leans on a cane. Yet this act of knowledge is itself a kind of catastrophe: in "solving" the riddle, Oedipus sets in motion the very fate he was trying to escape. The truth revealed is not redemptive, but destructive. The Sphinx, once answered, leaps to her death; the field of ambiguity collapses, and the law—first of the city, then of the father—rushes in to fill the void. The moment of mastery is immediately haunted by loss (Freud, 1900/1953; Bersani, 2010).

This scene is not a simple allegory for the victory of knowledge over ignorance. Rather, it dramatizes the ethical ambiguity of knowing itself: what is gained and what is lost when the enigma gives way to the law. The riddle, as an event, holds open a field of uncertainty, possibility, and desire. In answering it, Oedipus closes that field—he becomes the king, but also the agent of his own destruction. The Sphinx's refusal, her demand that the subject endure the question, becomes a model for another kind of ethics: one that values the presence of the unknown, that resists the violence of forced sense, that finds vitality in the space of what cannot be said (Derrida, 1978; Glissant, 1997).

Within the clinic, this mythic drama repeats in subtle and not-so-subtle forms. Patients bring riddles—symptoms, dreams, silences—that are often less calls for solutions than gestures toward what remains unsymbolized. The analyst, positioned as the one-who-knows, is constantly tempted to "solve" the riddle, to convert enigma into law. Yet every act of interpretation carries risk: the risk of foreclosure, of narrowing the field, of annihilating the Sphinx before the question has fully formed. There is a violence in premature knowing, a danger in the analyst's desire to resolve what might be more ethically borne (Loewald, 1960; Ogden, 2005).

To reimagine the riddle as a site of epistemic refusal is to claim the value of not-knowing, not as a failure, but as a fidelity to the complexity of psychic life. The Sphinx's question is not merely a barrier, but a generative gap—a zone where language falters, where affect and symbol hover at the edge of formulation. The analytic task becomes one of dwelling with the riddle, of holding open the atmosphere in which new meanings may gather, where both analyst and patient can risk being changed by what they cannot immediately comprehend (Eigen, 1999; Benjamin, 2018).

This ethics of not-knowing runs counter to the culture of mastery that so often pervades psychoanalytic training and practice. It demands a different kind of presence: one that is willing to let the riddle persist, to allow the Sphinx her place in the analytic hour. It means listening for what is not yet sayable, noticing the tremors of affect, the unfinished sentences, the moments of confusion or contradiction that signal the field of the unknown. It is, as Bion (1962) suggested, a discipline of negative capability—the capacity to be with doubt, ambiguity, and the as-yet-unformulated.

There is, too, a particular dignity in refusing to kill the Sphinx, in honoring her riddle as an ongoing principle of psychic life. The analyst who practices this ethic is not passive but actively engaged in the work of holding, containing, and witnessing. The riddle becomes a shared space of curiosity, even play: a zone where the pressure to know gives way to the freedom to imagine, to wander, to return again and again to what is not-yet-known. In this way, the analytic field is opened rather than closed, animated by the recursive movement between question and answer, between enigma and symbol (Winnicott, 1971; D. B. Stern, 2010).

The law, in this frame, is not the endpoint of development but a mode of containment—an organization of the field that can, if rigidified, foreclose growth. The riddle resists this closure; it keeps the law permeable, provisional, subject to revision. The ethics of not-knowing thus serves as a check on the omnipotence of law, a reminder that the deepest transformations in analysis occur not through mastery, but through the recursive, affective, and symbolic play that the riddle enables.

Crucially, this ethic is not about endless deferral or avoidance. There are times when knowledge is necessary, when the field must crystallize around a new formulation, a new law. Yet even here, the recursive stance remains vital: each interpretation is provisional, each solution an opening to further questioning. The Sphinx, though momentarily silenced, will return—her riddle reappearing in new forms, demanding to be lived-with rather than solved once and for all.

In the wider cultural field, the Sphinx and her riddle symbolize not only the limits of knowledge, but the right to opacity, to secrecy, to the preservation of what cannot—or should not—be named. Glissant (1997) argues for the "right to opacity" as a principle of ethical relation: an acknowledgment that the other is irreducible, unfinalizable, always more than the law can contain. In the analytic setting, this means honoring the patient's right to ambiguity, to not-yet-knowing, to remaining, at times, a mystery even to themselves.

To refuse the fantasy of final knowledge, to dwell with the riddle and its law, is to open the analytic field to surprise, to risk, to the creative potential of what has not yet come into being. The Sphinx's gaze reminds us that every act of knowing is shadowed by what escapes, that every law is provisional, that the heart of analysis is not mastery but the willingness to return, to question, to stay with the limit.

In sum, the law and the riddle are not simply antagonists, but partners in the recursive play of knowing and unknowing. The ethics of not-knowing is a commitment to this play—to honoring the Sphinx, to living with her questions, to practicing analysis as an art of staying-with rather than solving. In this way, the analytic field remains alive, open, and attuned to the deepest mysteries of the psyche.

Clinical Vignette—The Oedipal Situation as Recursive Encounter

It is late autumn. The light is thin, slanting in through the blinds, casting long shadows across the office floor. I sit with Ethan, a man in his early forties, whose analysis has entered a period of repetition and return. Our sessions, once full of narrative, have taken on a looping quality. Ethan circles the same ground—conflict with his supervisor at work, frustration with his son's defiance, a strange sense of being "on the outside" in his marriage. As he talks, there is a rhythm to his complaint: a ritual return to scenes of rivalry, exclusion, and frustrated longing. Each telling is slightly different, yet each echoes the last.

I listen for what is new, but what emerges is something else—a sense of atmosphere, a field charged with longing and prohibition, intimacy and distance. I find myself wondering about the invisible figures populating his stories: the supervisor who seems both adversary and ideal, the son who both defies and repeats him, the wife who hovers just outside the center of his psychic drama. I am aware, too, of my own presence in the room—sometimes the rival, sometimes the judge, sometimes the absent father. The analytic third is palpable: we are both inside a story that seems to write and rewrite itself, looping back on unresolved questions, ambiguous wishes, and the ache of not-knowing (Ogden, 1994).

One morning, Ethan arrives unusually agitated. He launches into a tale of workplace conflict—a younger colleague has been promoted, and Ethan feels "bypassed." His words are sharp, defensive, almost accusatory. "It's always the same," he says, "I work hard, and someone else gets the reward. Maybe I'm just not cut out for this." He falls silent, looking at me with an intensity that feels like a challenge. I sense, in that moment, a familiar pressure: the analyst as Sphinx, holding the riddle, invited to deliver the answer.

I consider the classical frame: the temptation to interpret his experience as an Oedipal repetition, a rivalry with the father, the longing for the mother's exclusive gaze displaced onto work and marriage. I feel the urge to bring coherence, to name what is latent, to offer the resolution his suffering seems to demand. Yet as I listen more deeply, I sense the recursive field asserting itself: the story is not linear but spiral; the meaning is not fixed but shifting, always on the verge of undoing itself. My own anxiety rises—a familiar desire to "do something," to end the looping, to deliver the law. I recall Bion's (1970b) advice to be "without memory and desire," and instead, I let myself linger in the not-knowing.

"What's it like, right now, to be telling this story again?" I ask, gently. Ethan hesitates. "I don't know," he says. "I guess I want you to tell me what it means. Or maybe I want you to be angry for me. Or at me. I'm not sure." His uncertainty opens a space—an atmosphere thick with possibility.

I notice a feeling in the room: the charge of something unformulated, the gravitational pull of the unspoken.

Over the next weeks, the pattern continues. Ethan returns, again and again, to scenes of disappointment and rivalry, each time with a new detail, a new affective tone. Sometimes he rages at the injustice; sometimes he shrinks into shame; sometimes he detaches entirely. I feel the recursive tension in my own countertransference—frustration at the repetition, curiosity about what persists, a quiet awe at the subtle shifts in atmosphere. At times, the room feels dense with unknowing, a field in which both of us are suspended.

One session stands out. Ethan recounts a childhood memory: waiting for his father to come home from work, standing at the window with his mother, watching the headlights sweep across the driveway. "I always wanted to be the one he noticed first," Ethan says, his voice barely audible. "But he would go straight to my little brother, every time. I'd stand there, waiting, pretending not to care. I don't think I ever got used to it." There is a silence. I feel a wave of grief—his and, perhaps, my own.

In this moment, the Oedipal scene is not a distant myth or developmental milestone. It is alive in the room, folded into the present, returning as affect, atmosphere, and bodily memory. The recursive field is palpable: the longing for recognition, the rivalry for love, the ache of being seen and unseen. I sense that to interpret too quickly would be to foreclose something vital. Instead, I say, "It feels like that longing is still here, right now." Ethan nods, and his eyes fill with tears. The session ends in silence, both of us holding the gravity of the unsolved riddle.

Afterward, I reflect on what has transpired. The analytic process has not advanced in a straight line. Instead, we have circled the same ground, each return opening new layers of meaning, new textures of feeling. The Oedipal situation has not been resolved, but inhabited: a recursive encounter where the law, the riddle, and the ethics of not-knowing are all alive at once. My role is not to deliver an answer, but to sustain the atmosphere in which new experience can emerge—to hold the unformulated, to witness the recursive play of knowing and unknowing, to companion Ethan in his return to the scene of longing.

In subsequent sessions, Ethan begins to notice the pattern himself. "I keep bringing this up," he says one day, with a trace of wonder. "I used to think I was just stuck. But maybe… maybe it's not about moving on. Maybe it's about being here, with it." He pauses and, for the first time, does not ask for an interpretation. Instead, he sits quietly, feeling the atmosphere, the recursive rhythm of return. There is a new lightness in the room—a sense that something has shifted, even as the riddle remains.

This vignette illustrates the heart of the recursive analytic field. The Oedipal situation, rather than being a stage to outgrow or a law to submit to, becomes a site of creative possibility—a space where repetition is not mere stuckness, but a principle of return, an invitation to inhabit and be transformed by what cannot be fully known. The analyst's ethic is not to solve the riddle, but to sustain the recursive play, to hold open the possibility of surprise, movement, and emergence within the very structure of looping.

Ultimately, the analytic encounter is not about transcending Oedipal dynamics, but about learning to live with their return—their presence in the recursive atmosphere of the room, their capacity to generate new meanings, affects, and forms of relation. The law and the riddle remain, but they do so as living questions, as openings, as companions in the ongoing work of becoming. In this way, the recursive encounter with Oedipal material becomes not a sign of failure, but a wellspring of psychic transformation.

Disobedience, Detour, and the Curvature of Desire

Despite its place as the emblem of law and the teleology of knowing, the myth of Oedipus is anything but a straightforward tale. Beneath the canonical reading—child, riddle, crime, punishment—lies a deeper mythic substrate, one suffused with wandering, error, repetition, and refusal. Oedipus, before he becomes king or criminal, is above all a wanderer: a figure of exile and detour, propelled by prophecies he cannot escape, traversing the world in a spiraling search for origins and meaning. This movement is not linear but curved—an endless orbit around the unsolvable, a journey shaped less by destination than by deviation.

The classical Oedipal law prescribes a path: the child must renounce forbidden desires, submit to the authority of the father, and enter the order of symbolic law. Yet Oedipus's actual path is marked by disobedience and refusal. He flees his adoptive parents to avoid the prophecy, only to fulfill it in flight. Each effort to escape the law becomes an enactment of it; each detour is a return. The myth thus inscribes a paradox: the more Oedipus resists his fate, the more tightly he is bound to it. Disobedience is not an aberration but an engine of the drama, generating the recursive loops and curved movements that give the myth its staying power (Freud, 1900/1953; Bersani, 2010).

In this light, desire in the Oedipal field is never a simple force moving toward satisfaction or renunciation. It is shaped by detour, by missed encounters, by the impossibility of closure. The "law of the father" is not a singular prohibition but a principle of endless return: every attempt to traverse or outwit the law folds back on itself, generating new patterns of longing, fantasy, and loss. Oedipus's journey is not a model of development but an allegory of recursive desire—desire that curves around what it cannot possess, doubling back, finding new routes and new forms (Laplanche, 1999).

Anthropologically, the motif of wandering is not unique to Oedipus. In myth after myth, heroes are shaped by exile, errancy, and delay. Odysseus's return is a series of digressions; Moses leads his people not by the shortest path but through 40 years of wandering. These narratives do not celebrate the mastery of knowledge but the transformative force of not-yet-arriving, of dwelling in-between, of detour as destiny (Campbell, 1949). Desire in these stories is not defined by what is finally attained, but by the capacity to sustain the journey—to tolerate the curvature of fate, the uncertainty of what will come, the impossibility of full return.

Psychoanalytically, the logic of detour is inseparable from the logic of the unconscious. Freud's own discoveries about dreams, slips, and symptoms are founded on the principle that psychic meaning is never direct but always displaced, condensed, deferred. The unconscious "thinks" in curves and loops, in associative wanderings and enigmatic signals. Analysis is not a straight path to truth, but a recursive meandering through scenes, affects, and symbolic fields. The patient's resistance, the analyst's uncertainty, the atmosphere of unknowing—all these are signs of the curvature of psychic life (Freud, 1900/1953; Bollas, 1987).

In the clinic, the Oedipal situation rarely plays out as a drama of final transgression or resolution. More often, it appears as a mood, a set of recurring patterns, a horizon of longing and refusal. Patients may circle the same themes for years: rivalries that never resolve, desires that defy articulation, acts of disobedience that repeat without satisfaction or relief. The analyst's task, within this curved field, is not to push the patient toward law or closure, but to witness and companion the movement of desire itself—to hold open the possibility that detour is not failure, but the condition for new forms of meaning and being.

Jessica Benjamin (1990, 2018) reminds us that mutual recognition is always haunted by misrecognition—that the encounter with the other is always imperfect, asymptotic, unfinished. This, too, is a form of detour: the impossibility of full merger or perfect knowing becomes the ground for a recursive, ongoing relationship. The analytic hour is shaped by these curved movements—approach and withdrawal, contact and absence, the repetition of not-quite-meeting that generates new psychic possibilities.

The law's excess—its inability to fully contain or resolve desire—is not a flaw in the structure but its generative heart. Oedipus, in fleeing the law, enacts its recursive force; the patient, in resisting interpretation, opens the analytic field to surprise and emergence. The detour is not an evasion but a method, a way of staying in touch with what cannot be directly accessed or owned. It is, as Loewald (1960) suggests, in the movement between past and present, between the known and the unknown, that psychic life is continually renewed.

In mythic terms, the curvature of desire is reflected in the very landscape of Oedipus's story: crossroads, forks, return journeys, mistaken identities, moments of blindness and sudden insight. The myth's structure is a spiral, not a line—a choreography of errancy that refuses the finality of arrival. The analytic process, at its best, honors this structure. Rather than leading the patient out of the labyrinth, it allows for the possibility of inhabiting it: exploring its passages, dwelling in its shadows, finding sustenance in its uncertainty.

To practice analysis from this curved stance is to resist the tyranny of the straight path—the demand for mastery, resolution, or the "right" answer. It is to value the generative power of not-knowing, the creative tension of return, the ethical richness of staying-with. Disobedience and detour are not to be overcome but inhabited, made into resources for psychic transformation. The analyst becomes a fellow traveler, attuned to the recursive rhythm of desire, willing to get lost and to find meaning in the very movement of wandering.

In this way, the Oedipal myth, reread through the lens of recursion and curvature, ceases to be a story of inevitable tragedy or triumphant law. It becomes, instead, a map for living with the open field of desire—a field shaped by misrecognition, delay, and the infinite possibility of beginning again.

Closing Reflection—Refusing Linearity, Opening the Field

To traverse the Oedipal myth as it lives in psychoanalysis is to encounter a narrative that both demands resolution and eternally resists it. The enduring fantasy of the Oedipal law—the promise of knowledge, mastery, and integration—has shaped the very core of analytic theory and practice. Yet, as this chapter has unfolded, what comes most fully into view is not the authority of linear progress, but the vibrancy of its refusal. Oedipus's tragedy is less about what is known or not known than about what cannot be stilled: the force of recursive return, the pull of the riddle, the ceaseless looping of desire around its own impossibility.

Refusing linearity is not a call to abandon structure or meaning, but to reimagine the field in which they arise. When the analyst releases the pressure to shepherd the patient toward closure, the analytic space becomes more than a stage for reenacting law or transgression. It becomes a living field—a symbolic and affective atmosphere in which new forms of experience can emerge precisely because they are not prematurely foreclosed. The riddle of the Sphinx, the detour of desire, and the recursive dance with the law all become sources of psychic creativity, not problems to be solved.

In the clinical setting, this stance shifts the analyst's role from interpreter to companion, from master of knowledge to witness of unknowing. The recursive field is not a void, but a rich landscape of possibility. Patient and analyst loop together through old scenes and new feelings, returning again and again to the edge of the unsayable. Here, the unfinished and the unresolved are not failures—they are evidence of the psyche's capacity for openness, movement, and the slow work of transformation. The very resistance to final knowledge, the patience to remain in tension, is what allows the unconscious to speak in ever-new forms.

This curved temporality is both ethical and generative. By resisting the law's closure, the analyst enacts a discipline of care that values ambiguity, detour, and surprise. The field is opened to difference, to the possibility that recognition can arise in the gaps, that insight is not a conclusion but a process of ongoing becoming. As Jessica Benjamin (2018) reminds us, mutual recognition is sustained not by perfect understanding, but by the willingness to remain in relation, to encounter misrecognition, and to hold open the question of the other's alterity.

To refuse linearity is also to resist the lure of mastery—the fantasy that analysis can deliver a final answer, resolve the riddle, or legislate desire. Instead, analysis becomes a site for witnessing the irreducibility of experience, the dignity of opacity, the recursive pulse of psychic life. The Oedipal field is reimagined not as a road with a clear destination, but as a landscape of crossings, echoes, blind alleys, and sudden openings. The analyst and patient become co-travelers in this space, attuned to the emergent, the paradoxical, and the unknown.

The symbolic field, in this recursive stance, is not static but alive with the possibility of new combinations, new forms of meaning. Each return to the Oedipal scene—each looping back to rivalry, longing, and law—creates an opportunity for differentiation, elaboration, or play. The analytic process becomes less about fixing identity or resolving conflict, and more about holding space for what Loewald (1960) characterizes as a creative gap—a felt missing that keeps meaning and being in formation.

As we close this chapter, what remains is not a solved riddle or a mastered law, but a renewed commitment to the field of unknowing. Refusing linearity is a way of honoring the psyche's complexity, its capacity for surprise, and its need for symbolic and affective space. It is an invitation to live, both in analysis and beyond, with the curved, recursive, and unfinished dimensions of our experience.

In the chapters to follow, this stance will recur as method, ethic, and invitation: to revisit the classical themes of psychoanalysis not as settled truths, but as living questions—fields in which the recursive play of knowing and unknowing continues to open the possibility of transformation.

Chapter 3

Projection as Knowledge Transmission—Recursive Unknowing and the Symbolic Field

This chapter reconceives projection not merely as a defensive expulsion, but as a recursive structure of knowledge transmission that forms the very atmosphere of psychic and analytic life. Tracing the evolution from classical Freudian and Kleinian concepts of projection and projective identification, this chapter explores how these processes generate an emergent symbolic field—an affective and symbolic atmosphere in which self and other, knowing and unknowing, are in constant recursive interplay. Drawing on theorists such as Loewald, Laplanche, Ogden, Benjamin, Bollas, Eigen, and Green, this chapter shows how projection becomes not just an obstacle to be overcome, but a generative principle of creativity, surprise, and ongoing transformation. Through a detailed clinical vignette, the recursive and atmospheric dynamics of projection are brought to life, highlighting how the analyst's task shifts from interpretation and mastery to witnessing, containment, and presence within the shared field. This chapter closes by proposing an ethic of not-knowing—a discipline of analytic hospitality that values the recursive, unpredictable play of projection as the ground of new subjectivities and meanings.

The Classical Concept of Projection—Disowning, Expelling, Explaining

Projection is among the earliest and most foundational concepts in psychoanalysis. To project, in the classical frame, is to disown what is intolerable within the self and expel it onto the world or the other. Freud (1911/1958) described projection as a primary defense: a means of ridding the psyche of painful affects, impulses, or fantasies by locating them outside the boundaries of the ego. What cannot be known or tolerated within is not simply repressed but imagined as coming from without—a maneuver that

DOI: 10.4324/9781003747109-5

simultaneously relieves internal conflict and structures the subject's relationship to reality.

This movement is not merely one of fantasy, but of knowledge. In projection, the psyche engages in a paradoxical act of epistemic clarification and obfuscation. The projected content—whether anxiety, envy, hostility, or desire—is made visible, tangible, and narratively coherent, but only by being misrecognized as "other." What is most deeply one's own is now perceived as belonging to someone or something else, often with the conviction that it has always been external. As a result, projection not only organizes the subject's relationship to the world but also shapes the field of what can be known or not known about oneself.

The act of projection thus constitutes a boundary operation, policing the frontier between self and other. Freud (1915/1957—"The Unconscious"; see also 1915/1957—"Instincts and Their Vicissitudes") argued that early consciousness is marked by confusion between inside and outside (see also Freud, 1925/1961, "Negation"), with projection serving as the mechanism by which the psyche carves out an internal space by exporting unmanageable contents. This expulsion is both defensive and creative: it produces a world that appears orderly, populated by figures who embody the very qualities the subject cannot tolerate in themselves. In this way, projection is a tool for constructing reality—a technique for mapping the boundaries of the self, even as those boundaries remain porous and unstable.

Early psychoanalytic theorists expanded on Freud's formulation, emphasizing the explanatory power of projection for understanding paranoia, anxiety, and the emergence of external persecutors. In The Schreber Case, Freud (1911/1958) saw the patient's delusions as elaborate externalizations of his own forbidden desires and fears. The persecuting other, in this model, is a psychic artifact—a figure who carries the projected burden of what the subject must not acknowledge. Projection thus becomes the engine of a recursive epistemology: it produces "knowledge" of the world that is, in fact, a disguised relation to one's own internal states.

For Melanie Klein (1946/1975), projection acquires an even more central role in early development. In the paranoid-schizoid position, the infant splits experiences of good and bad, hurling intolerable feelings—envy, rage, destructiveness—into the mother or the breast. The world becomes peopled with part-objects, each saturated with affect expelled from the self. Klein's vision is not simply one of defense, but of psychic survival: the child must project to avoid being overwhelmed, even as the act of projection creates a world alive with persecutory threats and potential comfort. Here, the boundary between inner and outer is not a static line but an active, shifting zone of exchange—a zone where knowledge, fantasy, and affect are continually negotiated.

The classical psychoanalytic literature returns again and again to this fantasy of psychic clarity by offloading the intolerable. Projection promises the relief of anxiety and guilt, but it also exacts a price: the externalized affect may return in disguised form, haunting the subject as fate, enemy, or symptom. The more strenuously the self seeks to expel what is unwanted, the more it is confronted by the recurrence of that very material, now dressed in the garb of the other. Projection thus generates a recursive loop: the psyche is always in danger of encountering itself, even—perhaps especially—where it most insists on the division between self and other.

In this sense, projection is both a defense and an epistemological stance. It is an attempt to render the unknown known, to place intolerable affect "out there" in order to master or escape it. Yet it also inaugurates a new form of unknowing: by projecting, the subject ensures that what is most intimate remains inaccessible, knowable only through displacement and misrecognition. The border between self and other is stabilized at the cost of truth. The subject's world becomes, in effect, a theater of disavowed self-knowledge—a space in which what is feared, envied, or despised is always somewhere else, located safely outside.

This mechanism is not limited to pathology or early development; it persists throughout psychic life, shaping the dynamics of relationships, communities, and even cultures. In the analytic setting, projection may structure the transference, with the analyst cast as the carrier of qualities the patient cannot claim. In the wider world, projection operates as a force in prejudice, scapegoating, and the creation of collective enemies. What is remarkable is how invisible this process can become to the subject—how natural it feels to "know" the other through the lens of what has been unconsciously exported.

Classical psychoanalysis, for all its focus on interpretation and making the unconscious conscious, has often treated projection as a process to be undone: something to be analyzed, re-owned, and metabolized. The goal is to transform projected knowledge into self-knowledge, to re-integrate what has been split off, to dissolve the boundaries that have become rigid or defensive. Yet as later theorists will explore, projection is not so easily overcome. Its recursive logic resists final mastery; each attempt to "take back" the projection opens new loops, new forms of ambiguity, and new sites of unknowing.

This, then, is the paradox at the heart of the classical concept of projection: it is at once a means of knowing and unknowing, of constructing and defending the self, of mapping the border between inner and outer even as that border is constantly traversed. In the next section, we will see how the development of projective identification further complicates this picture, revealing projection as a process not of simple expulsion but of communication, entanglement, and recursive implication in the symbolic field.

Projective Identification and the Blurring of Boundaries

The concept of projective identification marks a crucial turn in psychoanalytic thinking, one that destabilizes the boundary logic of classical projection and ushers in a new understanding of psychic life as fundamentally relational and recursive. Melanie Klein (1946/1975) introduced projective identification to capture a dynamic that is more complex than mere expulsion of unwanted parts. In this process, the self not only projects intolerable feelings, fantasies, or parts of the self into another, but remains psychically invested in those ejected elements, retaining a hold on what is now "out there." The other—parent, partner, analyst—becomes not simply the passive recipient of projection, but an active participant in the drama, shaped and animated by the qualities, affects, or fantasies projected into them.

Projective identification thus blurs the boundaries between self and other, inside and outside, known and unknown. Klein's clinical vignettes are rich with examples: a child projects envy or aggression into the mother, who then comes to be experienced as envious or attacking; or, conversely, the mother may unconsciously take on the projected feelings, enacting them in her own affect or behavior. What was once clearly inside or outside is now suspended in a psychic atmosphere—shared, negotiated, and contested by both parties. The psychic field becomes a zone of entanglement, alive with currents of feeling and meaning that cannot be fully claimed by either self or other.

Wilfred Bion (1962) deepened this understanding, viewing projective identification as a primary mode of communication in infancy and analysis. For Bion, the infant projects raw, unprocessed emotional experiences—what he called "beta elements"—into the mother, who, if she is receptive and containing, transforms them through her own psychic digestion and returns them in a metabolized form. This "container–contained" relationship is not merely defensive; it is the origin of thinking, of the capacity to symbolize and know oneself. Yet when containment fails, projective identification becomes a mechanism of psychic evacuation, flooding the other with unmanageable experience and undermining both connection and knowledge.

With the advent of field theory and relational psychoanalysis, projective identification was further reimagined as a two-person, or even multi-person, phenomenon. Thomas Ogden (1994) describes projective identification as the "in-between" of analytic experience—a process by which analyst and patient co-create a third space, the "analytic third," in which feelings, ideas, and unconscious fantasies circulate, shift, and are transformed. Here, projective identification is not simply a pathology to be overcome, but a medium for mutual recognition, creativity, and growth. It is through this recursive back-and-forth that both participants may come to know, and be known by, the other.

The blurring of boundaries wrought by projective identification introduces a radical uncertainty into the analytic situation. Whose feeling is this? Who is the originator of a thought, a desire, an affect that now permeates the room? In the grip of intense projective identification, the boundaries between self and other are porous, sometimes terrifyingly so. Analyst and patient may both feel overtaken by alien affects, or may find themselves enacting roles or positions that neither consciously intended. The field becomes saturated with unformulated experience, with knowledge that is felt but not yet symbolized, owned, or understood.

This recursive movement can be seen in the clinical microprocess: the patient, unable to tolerate anxiety or despair, projects it into the analyst, who may then find herself gripped by inexplicable feelings or urges. If unrecognized, this can lead to enactment—repetition, countertransference confusion, or even rupture. Yet when held in awareness, projective identification becomes a site of analytic possibility. The analyst, by noticing what is being transmitted and metabolizing it in herself, can offer it back to the patient in a new, symbolized form. The recursive nature of the process ensures that knowing and unknowing are always entangled, always in motion.

Projective identification thus challenges the fantasy of psychic clarity and the hope of absolute knowledge. The analytic field is not a stage for uncovering hidden truths, but a living atmosphere in which affect, meaning, and identity are continually reassembled and refigured. The "truth" of the analytic encounter is not simply what can be interpreted or made conscious, but what emerges in the shifting interplay of projection, identification, and return. The recursive loop of projective identification can both trap and liberate: it may fix both parties in repetitive roles, or it may serve as the engine of transformation, generating new forms of knowing through mutual recognition and surprise.

This complexity also implicates the analyst's subjectivity. No longer the detached interpreter, the analyst becomes a participant in the recursive field, called upon to witness, contain, and sometimes bear what the patient cannot. This demands not only technical skill but affective discipline—the capacity to tolerate ambiguity, to "not know" long enough for meaning to emerge. It also requires ethical humility, as the analyst's own unconscious is drawn into the recursive loop, sometimes revealing what the analyst has herself disowned or projected.

In sum, projective identification reveals the psyche as fundamentally relational, recursive, and atmospheric. It exposes the limits of the classical boundary model, showing that self and other, knowing and unknowing, are never fully separable. The analytic field becomes a site where projection is not just a defensive expulsion, but a shared creation—a looping, generative movement in which new subjectivities can be imagined, suffered, and transformed.

Inversion—Projection as Recursive Knowledge-Transmission

To fully grasp the radical implications of projection, we must move beyond the image of psychic "expulsion" and attend to the recursive, looping movements by which the self and other become entangled in the production—and obstruction—of knowledge. The fantasy of projection as a unidirectional defense, as an act of ridding oneself of intolerable contents, begins to collapse under the weight of lived analytic experience and theoretical insight. In its place emerges a more complex, dynamic process: projection as recursive knowledge-transmission, a structure in which what is disowned does not merely vanish but returns, transformed, through the encounter with the other and the shared symbolic field.

Hans Loewald's (1960) vision of psychic life offers an early bridge from classical to recursive frames. Loewald understood the psyche not as a closed system but as a permeable field, always in relation with its objects—especially the analytic other. He described the process of symbolization as one of continual movement between inner and outer, self and other, the known and the unknown. Projection, in Loewald's framework, is not simply an act of defense but a form of communication: it is through the projected that the self reaches toward the world, tests the boundaries of reality, and invites recognition or transformation. The analyst's task, then, is not simply to "return" the projection to its source, but to witness and inhabit the recursive field in which self and other co-create meaning.

Jean Laplanche (1999) radicalizes this logic even further. For Laplanche, the unconscious is not merely a storehouse of repressed content, but a site of ongoing translation and retransmission—a dynamic "enigmatic signifier" constantly emitted by the other, especially in the asymmetrical relation of adult to child. In this model, projection is not simply an export of inner experience, but a response to the untranslatable, enigmatic messages of the other—messages that the subject cannot fully know, but must nonetheless respond to. The loop of projection and introjection becomes a recursive circuit: what is unknown in the self seeks an address in the other, but the other's own unconscious interventions and failures ensure that the process never reaches closure. For Laplanche, the unconscious is fundamentally an effect of the other within the self, and thus every act of projection is a relay, not a discharge (Laplanche, 1999).

In clinical practice, this recursive structure is palpable. A patient's anxiety or shame is felt in the analyst, who may find herself holding, amplifying, or enacting the very feeling the patient disowns. Yet, as Ogden (1994) describes in his work on the analytic third, this is not a simple matter of "catch and return." Rather, the analyst and patient are drawn into a shared symbolic field, in which meaning is continually being produced, disowned, and transformed through mutual implication. The analytic third is alive with recursive transmissions: I find myself knowing you through what you cannot bear to know; you discover yourself through what you experience in me. Each "projected" element becomes a node in a complex network, feeding back into both self and other in unpredictable ways.

Jessica Benjamin (2018) reframes this process as one of mutual recognition, but also mutual misrecognition. In her model, psychic life is not about achieving a final mastery over one's own projections, but about living with the recursive uncertainties they generate. Recognition is always shadowed by the possibility of misunderstanding, and the analyst's task is not to stabilize meaning, but to remain open to the surprise, failure, and generativity of the field. The recursive loop of projection becomes the very space in which new forms of subjectivity can be born—not through final knowing, but through the willingness to dwell with ambiguity and mutual transformation.

The recursive logic of projection disrupts the dream of psychic purity or clarity. There is no "outside" to the loop: what is expelled is never simply gone; what is taken in is never entirely other. Each attempt to clarify the boundary between self and other produces new layers of opacity, new transmissions and retransmissions that sustain the field of unknowing. In the analytic hour, this may appear as an atmosphere—an emotional weather front that passes between analyst and patient, charged with affects, images, or thoughts that cannot be fully attributed or explained. The symbolic field thus becomes a living archive of recursive transmissions, a site where knowledge and unknowing perpetually produce and unsettle one another.

Crucially, recursive projection is not only a psychic phenomenon but also an ethical one. The analyst is called to bear what the patient cannot but also to recognize their own implication in the loop. There is a humility required: the knowledge one "transmits" or "receives" is never solely one's own. As Loewald, Laplanche, Ogden, and Benjamin each remind us, analytic work is less about mastery than accompaniment—a discipline of staying with the recursive field, bearing witness to the transmission and transformation of meaning across the boundaries of self and other.

Recursive projection also destabilizes the linear temporality of classical analysis. Rather than moving from ignorance to knowledge in a straight line, the analytic process is one of circling, revisiting, and returning—loops within loops, repetitions that open new symbolic possibilities. What was projected yesterday may return in altered form tomorrow; what was "known" is always vulnerable to being unknown, unsettled by the next recursive turn. The analytic field thus becomes a space of perpetual revision, where knowledge and its limits are constantly negotiated.

This inversion of projection—from expulsion to recursive transmission—has profound clinical implications. It suggests that analytic change does not depend on the full "re-integration" of what is projected, but on the capacity to inhabit and metabolize the recursive field itself. The analyst does not "give back" what was projected in the hope of dissolving all boundaries; instead, she helps to cultivate an atmosphere in which the loops of knowing and unknowing can be tolerated, explored, and creatively transformed. The goal is not final clarity but increased capacity for complexity, ambiguity, and recursive being.

In this sense, the analytic hour becomes an experiment in symbolic ecology: the field is seeded with projections, introjections, and transmissions that generate new forms of psychic life. The recursive loop of projection becomes not a trap, but a resource—a principle of creativity and renewal, a way of living with the irreducible alterity of self and other. The field is always already in motion, animated by the energies of what cannot be fully known, contained, or mastered.

To practice analysis from this recursive stance is to surrender the fantasy of purity or omniscience, and to enter the field as a participant in ongoing symbolic transmission. The analyst and patient are both implicated in the recursive loop, both bearers and recipients of projected knowledge and unknowing. This mutual implication is not a failure, but the very condition for analytic transformation—the ground on which new subjectivities, new meanings, and new forms of psychic life can be risked and realized.

The Symbolic Field—Projective Loops, Atmosphere, and Emergence

If projection in its classical form was about managing the boundaries between self and other, the recursive and relational vision uncovers a more expansive reality: the emergence of a symbolic field, a shared atmosphere suffused with the recursive transmission of affects, images, and meanings. This symbolic field is neither strictly within the self nor simply external; it arises in the very space between subjectivities, woven from the loops and echoes of what is projected, introjected, and re-symbolized. In this space, unknowing is not an absence but a vital presence—an atmosphere that sustains creative psychic possibility.

Christopher Bollas (1987) was among the first to foreground this atmospheric dimension of analytic life, describing how the "unthought known"—those psychic elements that exist prior to conscious representation—permeate the field and shape experience long before they can be spoken. For Bollas, the analytic situation is an environment of symbolizing potential, in which unconscious transmissions, resonances, and moods pass back and forth, gradually finding form and meaning. The field is a living matrix, responsive and mutable, where subjectivities are co-created and transformed by recursive exchange.

This symbolic field is marked not only by content but also by mood, resonance, and affective weather. Michael Eigen (1999) develops this idea, emphasizing the atmospheric, even mystical, nature of analytic presence. He writes of the field of the between—a zone of psychic transmission where affect, desire, and not-knowing circulate, often beneath the threshold of articulation. The field is charged with what is not yet symbolized, animated by the recursive movements of projection, reception, reverberation, and creative return. In this view, the analytic encounter is less a dialogue between two discrete minds than a participation in an emergent, atmospheric third—a shared psychic space where new meanings become possible.

André Green (1999), in his exploration of the "dead mother" complex and the uncanny, pushes this concept further—first formulated in his essay on the "dead mother" (Green, 1983/1986) and elaborated in *The Work of the Negative* (1999)—showing how the symbolic field is sometimes saturated with the un-symbolizable—with affective residues and voids that cannot be assimilated or named. Projection here does not simply fill a gap but creates one: the field is constituted as much by absence, lack, and opacity as by shared content. This negative space is not a failure of symbolization, but its condition of possibility. Green's work reminds us that the symbolic atmosphere is always, in some sense, haunted—shaped by what is withheld, unspoken, or unformulated.

Field theory in contemporary psychoanalysis (Baranger & Baranger, 2008; Ferro & Civitarese, 2016) has systematized these intuitions, viewing the analytic setting as a dynamic, recursive matrix in which both patient and analyst contribute to the generation and transformation of the symbolic field. The field is not static; it is an emergent phenomenon, marked by constant movement, surprise, and creative turbulence. In this context, projection becomes less a unidirectional act and more a recursive, generative process—one that produces a continuously evolving psychic atmosphere.

In practice, the symbolic field is palpable. It may be sensed as a change in mood, a shared affective intensity, or a sudden shift in the "weather" of the session. Sometimes it appears as a synchronicity—an image or phrase that arises simultaneously for both analyst and patient, or a resonance that echoes across different analytic pairs in the same week. At other times, it is felt as an uncanny silence, a heaviness, or a surge of unspoken tension that both parties register without knowing its precise origin. The field is a site of emergence: new meanings, affects, and subjectivities crystallize not through conscious deliberation, but through participation in the recursive atmosphere.

The generativity of the symbolic field lies in its resistance to final mastery. The recursive transmission of projections, affects, and images ensures that the analytic encounter is always open, always subject to revision and surprise. Conversation-analytic work reinforces this view; Buchholz and Kächele (2013) show that analytic meaning emerges through turn-by-turn co-construction, each conversational move subtly reshaping the symbolic field. Even the most familiar themes—envy, longing, guilt, desire—are recast as they loop through the field, acquiring new inflections, combining in unexpected ways. The analyst's task is to remain attuned to the atmosphere, to notice the shifts in symbolic weather, and to trust that meaning may emerge where none seemed possible.

There is a discipline to this stance, a willingness to let the field "speak" in its own time. The analyst must tolerate periods of confusion, uncertainty, and unknowing—moments when nothing seems to move, when meaning is suspended in the air. These are not failures of technique, but necessary passages in the work of emergence. The recursive structure of the symbolic field means that knowledge is always provisional, always subject to interruption and renewal. The field may "clear" suddenly, offering a moment of recognition, insight, or connection; or it may deepen, becoming more opaque, saturated with affect or ambiguity.

Clinically, the field perspective transforms the analyst's approach to projection and projective identification. Rather than seeking to immediately "resolve" or "interpret" what is projected, the analyst learns to participate in the atmosphere—listening for echoes, shifts, and emergent meanings. The symbolic field becomes a resource for creativity and transformation: old patterns may be replayed and reworked, and new psychic organizations may crystallize through recursive play and symbolic improvisation. The analytic hour is thus less about following a script and more about cultivating a shared attunement to the field's potential.

This view also dissolves the fantasy of analytic omniscience. No one fully controls the field; no single subject can claim authorship of what emerges. The recursive loops of projection, reception, and transformation ensure that analytic knowledge is always partial, shared, and susceptible to disruption. The field itself may be thought of as a symbolic atmosphere—an ecology of knowing and unknowing, of explicit and implicit communication, of form and formlessness. In this sense, the work of analysis becomes less about penetrating to hidden truths and more about cohabiting the symbolic field, attending to the recursive atmospheres that shape and reshape psychic life.

Finally, the symbolic field holds ethical implications. The analyst's responsibility is not only to interpret but also to maintain the conditions for emergence: to safeguard the atmosphere in which new meanings, affects, and forms of being may appear. This requires humility, patience, and a capacity for presence that is open to surprise and interruption. The symbolic field is a space of invitation, not demand—a site where both analyst and patient can risk new ways of being and knowing, sustained by the recursive movement of the analytic field.

In sum, the symbolic field is not a background but a living atmosphere, generated and regenerated through recursive projection and participation. It is here that the recursive structure of projection reveals its most creative, enigmatic, and transformative potential—an open field in which new psychic forms, affects, and subjectivities can emerge from the ongoing dance of knowing and unknowing.

Clinical Vignette—Projection, Recursion, and Unknowing in Practice

It is a late afternoon in spring. The city outside is shedding its winter gray, and in my office, Mara arrives with a barely contained intensity. Over the course of our work, the texture of her suffering has shifted: the content of her complaints—work frustrations, fraught relationships, and a chronic sense of inadequacy—has become secondary to a persistent, almost palpable field of unease that envelops our sessions. It is as if we are both moving through a thick psychic fog, heavy with unsaid expectations, longing, suspicion, and uncertainty.

This day, Mara sits down and, with a searching look, says, "Sometimes I feel like there's something in the air—like you're waiting for me to reveal what's really wrong, but I can't quite find it. I worry I'll disappoint you." Her words hang, stirring the atmosphere between us. I notice a flutter of discomfort within myself—a tension between wanting to reassure, wanting to challenge, and the urge to retreat into professional neutrality.

As I listen, it is clear Mara is not simply describing her experience; she is transmitting it. The sense of being evaluated, of never quite measuring up, seems to seep from her into the room and, subtly, into me. I begin to question my own presence—am I somehow conveying impatience? Is my silence being read as judgment? Even as I steady myself, I feel the gravitational pull of Mara's projection drawing me into a role I did not consciously choose. The field is charged: I am at once observer and participant in the recursive loop that Mara and I are co-creating.

Over the weeks, this loop intensifies. Mara alternates between anxious confession ("I know I go over the same ground… You must be tired of hearing it") and moments of prickly accusation ("Are you even listening? Sometimes it feels like you're far away"). My countertransference oscillates in response—at times defensive, at times subtly drawn to enact the very distance she fears. Rather than immediately interpreting, I find myself practicing a kind of atmospheric listening, letting the recursive structure of the field register in my own affect, body, and reverie.

One session, Mara brings a dream that crystallizes our recursive dynamic. She recounts:

> I'm in a forest at dusk. I'm trying to find my way home, but the path keeps splitting and turning back on itself. Every time I think I recognize a tree or a landmark, it shifts—the way forward becomes the way back. I can hear someone calling my name, but I can't see who it is. The sound echoes. I keep walking, feeling lost, but also strangely comforted by the trees around me, as if they're watching over me. I never find my way out, but I'm not panicked. It's more… suspended. Like waiting for something to emerge.

The dream's motifs—the looping paths, the ambiguous presence calling her, the eerie blend of lostness and subtle containment—mirror our analytic field. Instead of rushing to interpret, I share my sense that the dream evokes both her anxiety and the possibility of being held, even in confusion. Mara nods, sitting with the reverberations. "I think that's what it's like here sometimes," she says quietly. "I keep circling, hoping to arrive somewhere, but maybe I'm meant to linger in the not-knowing."

This acknowledgment marks a subtle shift. Our sessions retain their recursive atmosphere, but the affect begins to change. Mara becomes more able to name the tension in the room, and I feel less compelled to fill silences with explanations or solutions. Together, we begin to treat the analytic field less as a problem to be solved and more as a space to inhabit. The looping, affect-laden exchanges are no longer evidence of analytic failure, but signs of a living, emergent process.

There are regressions and moments of difficulty—days when Mara arrives angry or withdrawn, convinced I am judging her, or when I notice myself growing impatient or discouraged. But gradually, a new relational texture emerges: silences become less threatening; Mara occasionally wonders aloud what I am feeling, rather than assuming she knows. At times, I share my own experience of the atmosphere: "It feels like we're both waiting for something to reveal itself, and that can be unsettling, but it also feels alive."

Through this mutual attention to the symbolic field, the recursive loop becomes less claustrophobic and more creative. Mara begins to risk curiosity about my inner world and her own, noticing how her assumptions about my judgments echo old relational patterns. I become more attuned to how my countertransference is not just a private reaction but an atmospheric signal—evidence of our shared participation in the recursive field.

Looking back, what feels most striking is not a linear movement toward insight or resolution, but the emergence of a new way of being-with: a cohabitation of the analytic atmosphere. The "problem" of projection is not solved or eliminated but lived-with, explored, and transformed into a resource for deepening contact and symbolic play. The field itself becomes a kind of holding environment—capacious enough for both of us to bear uncertainty, echo, return, and unknowing.

In the final months of this phase of our work, Mara brings another dream:

> I'm by a river, watching leaves swirl in the current. I want to pick out a single leaf, but every time I reach for one, it spins away. But I also notice the pattern the leaves make together—a kind of dance I never saw before.

She laughs, a bit self-consciously, and says, "Maybe it's okay not to catch every leaf. Maybe just watching them is enough." I feel a corresponding lightness and say, "There's a beauty in letting things move together, even if we don't pin them down." In the field between us, a new possibility is present: the capacity to linger, to notice, and to find meaning in recursive, emergent forms rather than in closure.

This vignette enacts the recursive, atmospheric logic of projection. What is projected is never simply expelled or returned but shapes the field, generating new affective and symbolic possibilities. The analytic task is not mastery, but accompaniment—witnessing, containing, and participating in the creative emergence of meaning from the recursive loops that constitute psychic and relational life.

Closing Reflection—Projection, Recursion, and the Symbolic Atmosphere

As this chapter draws to a close, what stands out is not a theory to be settled or a mechanism to be finally mastered, but an atmosphere: the subtle, living field generated by projection's recursive movements—its loops, transmissions, and creative gaps. Throughout analytic history, projection has been cast as a defense, a problem to be overcome, or a process to be exposed and reversed. Yet, when viewed through a recursive lens, projection emerges not only as an obstacle but as the very condition of psychic life: a principle of creativity, a generator of symbolic atmosphere, and a key to inhabiting the analytic field as a space of surprise, renewal, and transformation.

The classical wish for mastery—whether in the form of insight, re-integration, or boundary clarification—gives way, here, to something both more humble and more profound: a practice of living with loops, returns, and irreducible uncertainties. The analytic encounter becomes less a journey toward final knowledge and more a practice of accompaniment and attunement. The recursive field, shaped by the atmospheric transmission of affect, image, and desire, is the ground on which new subjectivities may emerge. The task is not to "take back" every projection or to finally distinguish the self from the other, but to remain present with what passes between, through, and beyond both.

The symbolic atmosphere—so easily missed by a technique overly focused on interpretation—becomes, in this recursive stance, a central analytic reality. It is a space of weather, mood, and resonance: sometimes charged with longing, grief, envy, or hope; sometimes marked by silence, opacity, or waiting. The field's atmosphere is alive with transmissions that cannot be directly attributed, explanations that remain partial, and patterns that return with new inflection. The analyst's challenge is not only to interpret but also to dwell in and with this atmosphere: to allow meaning to emerge in its own time, to notice how surprises and shifts in the field open space for psychic movement, and to honor the symbolic as a site of continual transformation.

In this way, projection ceases to be a static defense or pathology and becomes a dynamic, generative movement—a form of psychic weather, animating the analytic situation and opening it to the possibility of real encounter. Recursion, far from indicating mere repetition or stasis, becomes the logic of emergence: through each return, the field is subtly altered;

through each loop, a new form of knowing or being becomes available. The symbolic field is not an object to be grasped but a space to be inhabited—one whose richness depends on the ongoing interplay of knowing and unknowing, presence and absence, form and atmosphere.

This closing reflection is, itself, a recursive gesture: a return to the themes that have animated this chapter, but with an altered perspective. The limits of mastery are not the limits of creativity; the opacity of the field is not a void, but the condition for surprise. The analyst's fidelity to not-knowing, to remaining present in the recursive field, is an ethical stance that honors the irreducibility of the other, the provisional nature of meaning, and the ongoing possibility of psychic renewal.

As the recursive structure of projection unfolds, new ethical and clinical possibilities arise. The analytic encounter becomes a site for dwelling-with: with mystery, with affect, with the symbolic weather of the field. The analyst and patient together inhabit a space where projections may be suffered, played with, relinquished, or transformed—not through the force of interpretation alone, but through the atmospheric discipline of shared presence. The task is not to expel or conquer the unknown, but to invite it, to linger with it, to welcome its creative returns.

Looking forward, this recursive and atmospheric approach to projection sets the stage for future chapters—on fantasy, introjection, destruction, or other forms of epistemic inversion. Each will carry forward the same discipline: an attunement to loops, to atmospheres, and to the surprising ways in which the symbolic field sustains psychic life. The ethic of unknowing, here, becomes the ground for analytic hospitality—a willingness to receive what comes, to accompany what cannot be resolved, and to participate in the generative play of the analytic field.

In the end, projection is neither a failure nor a final truth, but a movement—an ongoing invitation to enter the atmosphere of the analytic field, to risk surprise, and to discover, in the very act of not-knowing, the possibility of new forms of subjectivity and relation.

Part II

The Recursive Field

Return as deepening, circuit by circuit.
Each pass alters the space between us and what we're seeing.
Form breathes; meaning ripens in the re-encounter.
Listening becomes the method by which the field thinks.

DOI: 10.4324/9781003747109-6

Chapter 4

Recursive Interiors—Self-Structure, Temporality, and the Symbolic Logic of Linking

This chapter advances **recursive interiority** as a missing axis of self-structure. It proposes that inner continuity is not simply narrated or defended—it is generated through recursive linking among partially dissociated self-states. Where recursive linkage fails (as in trauma, psychosis, or structural dissociation), inner time collapses.

Synthesizing Donnel Stern's concept of unformulated experience, Philip Bromberg's dissociated self-states, Hans Loewald's symbolization, Thomas Ogden's analytic third, and Wilfred Bion's attacks on linking with Gödel's incompleteness theorem, Russell's paradox, Hofstadter's strange loops, Derrida's différance, and Levinas's ethics of infinite responsibility, I argue that recursive temporality constitutes the gravitational topology of the psyche.

Clinically, this requires a shift toward **recursive listening**: sustaining loops, tolerating remainder, and *holding the loop open* rather than foreclosing experience through premature coherence. This chapter explicitly differentiates recursion from rumination, memory retrieval, and simple integration; specifies operational hallmarks of recursion (state–state mapping, iterability, time-generation, non-closure, symbolic elevation, resonant containment); and offers clinical vignettes illustrating how recursive collapse and repair manifest in analytic work.

This chapter also addresses the **training and supervisory implications** of recursive listening. Analysts-in-training often seek closure too quickly—whether in case write-ups, supervision narratives, or clinical interventions. A recursive orientation reframes training as learning to tolerate suspended loops and supervisors as sustaining recursive potential rather than demanding premature synthesis.

Finally, I point to **future research directions**: how recursion might be studied phenomenologically (through first-person reports of recursive depth),

DOI: 10.4324/9781003747109-7

clinically (tracking temporal anomalies as diagnostic markers), and theoretically (mapping recursion's intersections with topology, physics, and aesthetics).

By formalizing recursion as an orthogonal dimension of structure, this chapter reframes classical models (psychotic, borderline, neurotic) as distinct recursive disturbances and proposes a psychoanalysis oriented less toward resolution than toward recursive survival—continuity through loops that never fully close.

Core Contributions

1. **Axis**: Introduces recursion as an orthogonal dimension of self-structure (distinct from content/organization).
2. **Temporality**: Defines inner time as the sum of links, not a property of states.
3. **Failure modes**: Reinterprets trauma, dissociation, and psychosis as attacks on recursive temporality.
4. **Clinical ethic**: Specifies recursive listening ("hold the loop open") as a technique and stance.
5. **Training and supervision**: Frames analytic education as learning to sustain recursion rather than forcing coherence.
6. **Formalism**: Offers a symbolic condensation of temporality as link-summation.
7. **Topology**: Replaces static structure with gravitational orbit across self-states.
8. **Future research**: Suggests empirical, phenomenological, and theoretical pathways for extending recursion into psychoanalysis and beyond.

Fractured Mirrors and the Descent into Self

> When I take ketamine, I experience myself like a mirror endlessly reflecting itself. I fall deeper into myself as I let each image pass over me and I deepen into myself until there is the sensation of free fall but no image left.

This phenomenological report is not a pharmacological curiosity; it is a condensed articulation of psychic structure. What it reveals is **recursive interiority**: the self encountering itself through layered reflection—loops within loops, each iteration both shaping and being shaped by its remainder.

Freud, Ferenczi, and beyond the Archaeological Model

Freud's (1937/1964) archaeological metaphor pictured psychic depth as stratification—layer upon layer beneath the surface. But recursion is not mere vertical excavation. It is curvilinear folding: images folding into images, spirals rather than strata.

Ferenczi's (1932/1988) "confusion of tongues" adds a necessary resonance. Trauma is not simply an event but a collapse of recursive linkage: the child's language of tenderness invaded by the adult's passion interrupts the very loop by which the child's self might safely fold back into itself. Instead of recursive layering, recursive rupture.

Clinical Interlude: A Dissociative Loop

A patient once said: "When panic hits, I watch myself scream from the corner of the ceiling." This is more than defense. It is a recursive fracture: two layers of self, co-present yet temporally estranged. Later she added: "I know it's me, but it doesn't feel like my time." The analytic task was not to enforce unity but to sustain the bridge long enough for temporality to resume.

Here supervision played a crucial role. A candidate initially interpreted this dissociation as "avoidance of affect." In supervisory dialogue, we reframed it as a recursive fracture—two states unlinked in time. The supervisory task became recursive itself: holding open the candidate's oscillation between competing frames until a new temporality of understanding emerged.

Recursive Selfhood as Ontological Form

Multiplicity (Bromberg, 1998), fragmentation (Ferenczi, 1932/1988), and the unformulated (Stern, 1997) are well theorized. Recursion isolates a different axis: not how many selves exist, but how self-states link across time.

Heidegger (1927/1962) argued that time is not a neutral container but the horizon of self-relation. Recursion carries this into psychoanalysis: inner time arises only through self-folding. The self does not precede time; time is generated in the act of recursive relation.

Attacks on Linking as Attacks on Time

Bion's (1959) "attacks on linking" can now be specified: what is destroyed is the recursive bridge that metabolizes continuity. Without recursion, memory and symbol disintegrate; the psyche becomes stranded in simultaneity or void.

Eigen (1993) reminds us that recursion is never neutral: every loop is charged with resonance, tremor, and risk. Linking shakes both patient and analyst. When resonance becomes unbearable, loops sever, leaving fragments unlinked in time.

Recursive Depth and Mathematical Paradox

Gödel (1931/1962) showed that every formal system contains truths unprovable within itself. Likewise, every self-state contains remainder irreducible from within.

Russell (1903) demonstrated the paradox of the set that cannot contain itself: self-states cannot hold their contradictions alone.

Hofstadter (1979) extended this into aesthetics: strange loops generate coherence that is never complete. Escher's staircases ascend while returning to origin. So too the self—paradoxical, recursive, inexhaustible.

Recursive Descent as Ontology

The ketamine free fall is a limit case: recursion iterated until the image dissolves—continuity distilled as pure looping. Continuity is not given; it is generated. Collapse means loss of time itself.

For the analyst, the task is not coherence at all costs but recursive listening: attending to loops attempted, severed, or sustained, and **holding the loop open** long enough for time to gather.

Recursive Temporality, Inner Time, and the Linking of Self-States

If, by analogy with modern physics, time is grasped relationally—measured through relations among moving bodies—then inner time—psychic temporality—must likewise be relational. It is not linear but recursive. Not a single thread but a spiraling motion between self-states, observers, dissociated fragments, and symbolic echoes that bind them. Time arises not as a passive flow but as an active linking of recursive layers—each reflecting and temporally situating the other. The self is not only fragmented; it is interfragmented by recursive temporality.

Stern and the Unformulated: Time as Latency

Building on Donnel Stern's[1] (1997) account of unformulated experience, we can understand such states as *un-timeable*—they belong to no sequence until looped back into symbolic form. What is "unformulated" is not outside meaning—it is suspended in recursive latency. In the analytic hour, a sudden image or bodily sensation often feels as if it has "always been there," even though never articulated. This emergence is recursive: the psyche loops back, linking present self-state with prior unformulated depth, thereby generating continuity.

A patient once whispered: "It feels like I'm remembering something I never lived." Such paradox captures recursion's temporality. It is not recovered memory, nor fantasy, but the shimmer of recursive linking—the self folding back to make time where none had existed.

Bromberg and Dissociation: The Collapse of Recursive Time

Bromberg (1998) reframed dissociation as multiplicity: we live our lives in different self-states and feel unitary only when we can move fluidly among them. From a recursive view, this fluidity is precisely the capacity for linking. Dissociation is not only the presence of multiple states but also the *collapse of their bridges.*

A traumatized patient may recount an event as though it "just happened yesterday," despite decades having passed. What is missing is not memory but recursive temporality—the looping motion that situates one state in relation to another across time. Trauma is not simply the past in the present; it is the failure of recursive time to hold.

In clinical training, candidates often interpret this kind of "time collapse" as resistance or repression. Supervision reframes it: the event is not simply repressed but unlinked. The supervisory dialogue becomes a recursive act—looping the candidate's present understanding back into the patient's dissociative temporality, thereby opening new continuity.

Gödel, Russell, and Recursive Residues

Recursive temporality resonates with mathematics. Gödel's (1931/1962) incompleteness theorem shows that every system contains truths unprovable within itself. Likewise, every self-state harbors residues irreducible from within. Continuity requires looping to another self-state capable of retroactive witnessing.

Russell's (1903) paradox—that a set cannot contain itself—illuminates recursion further. Each self-state is a temporal set: it cannot hold its own contradiction. Continuity arises only in the loop between states.

Derrida and Slippage: The Asymptotic Loop

Derrida's (1967/1997) slippage—the impossibility of signifiers coinciding fully with what they represent—becomes temporal here. Recursive temporality is never complete. Each loop leaves a remainder. We never fully retrieve a prior self; we approach it asymptotically.

When patients revisit traumatic memories, the present articulation is both continuous with and different from earlier ones. There is no recovery, only recursive approximation. Continuity is sustained not by closure but by loops that tolerate slippage.

Ringstrom and Analytic Play: Reactivating Recursive Time

Philip Ringstrom's[2] (2014, 2025, in press) work on analytic play situates recursion in the clinical field.[1] Play suspends linear time, allowing dissociated states to circulate in provisional orbit. Past and present interlace, fantasy mingles with memory, and recursive temporality reactivates.

A patient dreams her childhood home is simultaneously her current apartment. The analyst responds, "What does it feel like to live in both at once?" This sustains recursive temporality: it allows states across time to loop into symbolic space without collapse into narrative clarity.

Play, then, is recursion enacted. It keeps loops open long enough for continuity to form.

Recursive Temporality and Physics

By analogy with modern physics, time can be treated as relational: in relativity, duration depends on relative motion; in some quantum-gravity proposals, time is emergent at fundamental scales. By analogy, inner time may likewise emerge from relations among self-states. On this metaphor, recursive temporality is orbital rather than linear: self-states exert a kind of "gravitational" pull on one another. When that binding weakens, experience can scatter into dissociation; when it over-concentrates, experience can collapse toward psychotic simultaneity. The analyst's presence supplies stabilizing mass—"recursive gravity"—that helps keep loops in orbit long enough for continuity to form.

Clinical Interlude: A Shattered Clock

A patient once described his inner world as "a room full of clocks, each set to a different time." At first, he experienced this as madness. When the analyst suggested: "Perhaps the clocks are not broken—they just don't yet tick together," the metaphor shifted. Over months, the patient began to weave these clocks into stories, linking them. Continuity emerged not by resetting the clocks but by allowing them to loop.

Definition: Recursive Temporality

- Not linear progression but spiraling loops of self-states.
- Time arises through recursive linking, not pre-given flow.
- Clinical markers of collapse: timeless trauma, dissociation as parallel worlds, psychosis as simultaneity.
- Restoration through play and witnessing: sustaining loops without premature closure.

Operational Hallmarks of Recursion

- **State–state mapping**: explicit bridges formed between self-states.
- **Iterability**: capacity to return and repeat without erasure.
- **Time-generation**: continuity emerges as recursive product, not a precondition.
- **Non-closure**: loops leave residue; incompleteness is preserved.
- **Symbolic elevation**: loops metabolize raw affect into symbol while retaining resonance.
- **Resonant containment**: analyst functions as a recursive node, holding loops open.

Note: "Symbolic elevation" *refers to the process by which raw affect or fragmented experience is lifted into symbolic form while retaining its vitality.* "Resonant containment" *refers to the analyst's capacity to absorb and reverberate affective intensity, holding it within recursive circulation without prematurely foreclosing it.*

Recursion vs. Rumination

- **Recursion**: dynamic linking of self-states across time; generative, symbolic, and temporality-producing.
- **Rumination**: repetitive cycling within a closed loop; static, self-sealing, temporality-collapsing.
- Distinguishing the two is crucial: recursion opens continuity; rumination forecloses it.

When Recursion Pauses: Flow, Meditation, and Annihilation

Not all suspensions of recursive temporality are pathological. In certain states, the psyche becomes so fully identified with a single self-state that recursion momentarily halts. Csikszentmihalyi's (1990) description of *flow* exemplifies this: time seems to vanish, awareness is absorbed, and the recursive motion of linking is unnecessary because the self-state is experienced as complete. Crucially, when the flow state is later recalled or narrated, recursion resumes—folding the "timeless" immersion into broader continuity. Unlike dissociative rupture, flow does not foreclose recursive potential; it suspends it provisionally.

Meditative absorption offers another mode of recursive pause. Here, recursive latency is cultivated deliberately, as the practitioner sustains identification with breath, mantra, or awareness itself. Time suspends, not through collapse but through intentional containment. Psychoanalytically, this resembles Stern's (1997) unformulated: experience hovers, awaiting recursive re-entry into symbolization.

By contrast, ketamine's "hole" can feel like recursion run to its limit case. The descent through recursive reflections culminates in imagelessness, where no self-state remains available to fold back into relation. This is annihilation of recursive temporality—an experience of pure suspension where continuity is not generated but dissolved. Yet even here, recursive narration afterward reintroduces temporality: the hole becomes an event folded back into the orbit of self.

The Missing Dimension of Self—Recursive Linking and Symbolic Continuity

Psychoanalysis has long theorized the self in terms of structures, organizations, and relational matrices. Freud's metapsychology introduced psychic topographies and economic balances of energy; later developments emphasized object relations, defenses, and levels of structural integration. Kernberg (1975) formalized distinctions between borderline, neurotic, and psychotic organizations, while McWilliams[3] (2011) extended these clinical portraits into richly textured accounts of personality. These frameworks remain indispensable, yet they leave something unformulated: not another level or category of structure, but a dimension that makes all structures viable. This missing axis is recursive linking—the motion by which self-states fold back upon one another, generating symbolic continuity across time.

Without this recursive axis, structural models are incomplete. They describe positions, not movements; defenses, but not the temporal bridges that allow a fragmented self to persist. They map psychic terrain but omit the gravitational field that binds terrains together. Recursive interiority names that binding field: the self's capacity to return to itself across layers, to relink dissociated states, to survive temporal rupture by looping through it.

We might even attempt a symbolic condensation:

$$\mathbf{T}_{\text{self}} = \sum \mathbf{L}\left(s_i, s_{i+1}\right)$$

where

- $\mathbf{T}_{\text{self}}$ = psychic temporality
- $\mathbf{L}(s_i, s_{i+1})$ = recursive linking between self-states s_i and s_{i+1}

This formulation suggests that psychic temporality does not inhere in any isolated self-state but arises only from the summation of recursive linkages across them. Continuity is the emergent property of linkage, not of content.

Because each recursive link not only connects but transforms, the self is never a stable entity. The moment a self-state is observed, it shifts from n to $n + 1$—a new state that folds back upon the prior one but is never identical to it. What is examined is already altered by the act of examination. **Subjectivity is therefore an *unstable object*:** the self can only appear in recursive relation, never as a fixed essence. This instability is not pathology but condition—it is what allows continuity to be generated through loops that both preserve and transform.

Loewald and the Transformative Loop

Hans Loewald (1978) gestured toward this recursive dimension when he described symbolization as the transformation of undifferentiated experience into a new psychic reality. For Loewald, symbolization is never simply a one-way translation from raw affect into thought; it is a looping process in which the psyche revisits and reconstitutes its own depths.

Consider how this appears in analytic supervision: a candidate presents a session in which a child's cry was "translated" into an interpretation about separation anxiety. The supervisor intervenes, noting that the cry must first be *returned* to the child—held and reverberated before it is named. This is

Loewald's recursive loop: the cry folded back into psychic life at a higher order, not simply replaced by interpretation.

Loewald (1978) suggests symbolization transforms undifferentiated experience into a new psychic reality; I extend this to argue that symbolization is best understood as two-directional—downward into the unformulated and upward into articulation. The recursive link is what ensures that the symbol remains alive rather than ossified. When symbolization fails, it is not because representation is absent but because recursion is broken—the loop back to unformulated depth is severed. Loewald's vision thus anticipates the recursive dimension: symbolization as ongoing re-linking, continuity as recursive resonance.

Eigen and the Affective Charge of Recursion

Michael Eigen[4] (1993) brings intensity into view. His work reminds us that recursive linking is never neutral. Each fold across self-states carries affective charge, resonance, and risk. To relink dissociated states is to risk re-encountering psychic fire—unbearable grief, terror, or ecstasy. Recursive continuity is less about calm integration and more about the capacity to survive recursive reverberation without collapse.

In candidate training, this is often the hardest lesson: that analysis is not a gentle smoothing of ruptures but a survival of recursive shakenness. Supervision encourages tolerance for trembling links: the iterability of returning to what was unendurable, the non-closure of loops that preserve residue, and the demand for resonant containment, where analyst and supervisor together hold intensity without extinguishing it.

Eigen's insistence on psychic shakenness reframes recursion not as abstract topology but as lived survival. The recursive bridge is not a smooth passage but a trembling threshold. Each loop is a return to what could not be borne, now borne differently.

Ogden and the Recursive Third

Thomas Ogden's[5] (1994) concept of the analytic third crystallizes recursion in the relational field. The third is not simply the sum of analyst and patient but a new psychic structure generated between them—a recursive co-construction that neither party controls. Within the analytic third, temporalities overlap: past and present, fantasy and reality, dissociated self-states and newly symbolized ones.

The third is a recursive site par excellence. It allows the patient to encounter aspects of self otherwise inaccessible, precisely because the analyst co-inhabits the loop. When recursive linking within the self has collapsed, the analytic third sustains an external recursive structure in which re-linking becomes possible.

Here, the hallmarks are evident: state–state mapping between analyst and patient, the time-generation of shared experience, and the symbolic elevation of fragments into the relational field. In this sense, recursion is not only intrapsychic but also intersubjective.

Bion and Attacks on Recursive Temporality

Bion's (1959) idea of "attacks on linking" acquires new depth in recursive perspective. In trauma, it is not only thought that is attacked but also the recursive scaffolding that sustains psychic time. When linking collapses, the self becomes stranded in a perpetual present, unable to loop back into its own history. The recursive bridge is destroyed, and with it, temporal continuity.

From this angle, psychotic fragmentation and dissociative ruptures can be seen as recursive failures: not merely splits or defenses, but breakdowns in the looping motion that binds states across time. The patient may appear coherent in one self-state but unable to feel the temporal gravity of another. What is lost is not content but recursion: the possibility of re-linking across temporal folds.

Recursive Reverberation as Depth of Self

Taken together, Loewald, Eigen, Ogden, and Bion point to a dimension of self that psychoanalysis has intuited but never formalized. Symbolization, intensity, the analytic third, and attacks on linking all presuppose recursive motion. What appears as linear continuity is in fact recursive re-linking—a dialogue between the unformulated and the symbolized, the dissociated and the integrated, the unbearable and the borne.

The depth of self, then, is not a matter of content or category but of recursion. Without recursive reverberation, symbols are flat, intensity is uncontainable, the third collapses, and linking is severed. With recursion, the self lives—not as a unitary whole, but as a gravitational orbit of states folded within one another, sustained by looping motion.

This "missing dimension" is therefore not another structural category but an axis of recursive temporality and symbolic linkage. To theorize the self without recursion is to miss the very motion that makes selfhood possible. Recursive interiority is not an accessory to existing models but their unseen foundation—the gravitational topology that binds psychic life together across time.

Recursive Failures, Dissociation, and Attacks on Linking

If recursion is the missing dimension of selfhood, then its collapse reveals the most devastating disruptions of psychic continuity. Trauma, dissociation, and psychosis can all be read as recursive failures: the breakdown of the self's capacity to loop back into its own depths and sustain inner temporality. When recursive bridges collapse, the subject loses the ability to metabolize experience across self-states, and with that loss, time itself fragments.

In the symbolic condensation introduced earlier,

$$\mathbf{T}_{\text{self}} = \sum \mathbf{L}\left(s_i, s_{i+1}\right)$$

recursive failure is precisely the diminishment or destruction of the linking function $\mathbf{L}(\mathbf{s}_i, \mathbf{s}_{i+1})$. Without links, there is no sum. Without the sum, temporality collapses into simultaneity or void. The hallmarks of recursion vanish: state–state mapping breaks down, iterability collapses into frozen repetition, time-generation halts, symbolic elevation flattens, and resonant containment becomes impossible.

Bromberg and Worlds Apart

Philip Bromberg's (1998) clinical portraits of dissociated self-states remain among the most vivid accounts of recursive failure. His patients do not merely shift between moods or roles; they inhabit distinct "worlds" that cannot coexist in temporal relation. One self-state does not know, or cannot tolerate knowing, the existence of another. What results is not only fragmentation of subjectivity but also a foreclosure of recursive time.

For Bromberg, dissociation is not just defensive avoidance but a structural reality: each state functions as if the others did not exist. In recursive terms, the bridge between states has collapsed. The patient is unable to loop back, unable to feel the temporal gravity of the self that exists elsewhere.

What is lost is not simply memory or continuity of narrative but the recursive motion that would link one state to another.

When analysts encounter these "worlds apart," the temptation is to seek integration by insisting upon coherence. Yet Bromberg teaches us that the task is not to collapse multiplicity into unity but to cultivate recursive possibility: to allow states to circulate in relation, however fragile, rather than remain sealed off. Recursion reframes dissociation not simply as fragmentation, but as the collapse of looping motion itself.

Stern and the Temporality of the Unformulated

Donnel Stern's (1997) concept of unformulated experience offers another lens on recursive breakdown. These are experiences not yet symbolized, not yet held in temporal relation. They hover in latency, awaiting recursive re-linking. When a recursive function is intact, unformulated experiences can be revisited and symbolized—folded back into psychic continuity. When recursion fails, these states remain suspended, neither integrated nor erased.

Stern's model implies that unformulated states are inherently temporal: they carry the potential to become symbolized in the future, but only if recursive motion loops back to retrieve them. Trauma interferes with this process by freezing recursive time. The unformulated becomes unformulatable, suspended in an endless present. In such cases, recursive failure manifests as temporal foreclosure—the psyche is unable to fold back upon itself to metabolize the experience.

From this angle, the analyst's role is not to impose form prematurely, but to sustain recursive potential—to hold open the possibility that the unformulated may one day be re-linked. This patience with temporal suspension is itself an ethical stance, one that recognizes the recursive dimension as foundational to continuity.

Bion and Attacks on Recursive Temporality

Bion's (1959) notion of "attacks on linking" takes on new resonance when reframed through recursion. In trauma, what is attacked is not only thought, but the recursive scaffolding that sustains psychic time. Attacks on linking destroy the bridges between self-states, leaving the subject stranded in isolated moments. The recursive loop collapses, and with it, the continuity of temporal experience.

Consider the traumatized patient who cannot link a present trigger with a past event. The recursive bridge that would allow temporal integration has been obliterated. Instead, the traumatic fragment erupts as if it were happening now. Time collapses into simultaneity; recursive depth gives way to temporal flatness. The attack is not on content but on structure: the recursive dimension itself is destroyed.

Bion's emphasis on the analyst's function as a container resonates here. To contain is to hold recursive possibility when the patient cannot. It is to provide the scaffolding for recursive time to be reactivated. Without this holding, attacks on linking persist, and the self remains stranded in fractured temporality.

Derrida and Slippage without Continuity

Where recursion collapses, Derrida's (1967/1997) notion of slippage becomes pathological. Normally, the slippage of signifiers is constitutive: it ensures that meaning is never closed, that recursive loops always contain remainder. But in recursive failure, slippage ceases to generate symbolic resonance and instead produces psychic free fall.

In trauma and psychosis, signifiers slip without anchoring to recursive loops. The patient cannot revisit a prior self-state to retroactively symbolize the residue; instead, meaning disintegrates into endless drift. The recursive structure that would metabolize slippage into symbolic continuity is absent. What remains is not *différance* but collapse: slippage without orbit, fragmentation without recursive return.

Eigen and the Collapse of Resonance

Michael Eigen (1993) reminds us that recursive folds are never neutral. They are charged with intensity—grief, terror, ecstasy—that must be metabolized through recursive motion. When recursion fails, this intensity cannot be borne. It erupts as dissociative rupture, somatic implosion, or psychotic overwhelm.

Eigen's language of resonance captures the affective dimension of recursion. When recursive linking collapses, resonance collapses with it. The psyche becomes mute, unable to reverberate with its own depths. In analytic work, this often appears as deadness, numbness, or affective flatness. What is missing is not feeling per se, but recursive reverberation—the capacity of affect to circulate across self-states, to be borne and transformed in recursive loops.

The analyst's role, in Eigen's vision, is to serve as a resonant node: to reintroduce recursive possibility by reverberating with the patient's un-metabolized intensity. This is not simply empathy but recursive survival: the analyst absorbs and amplifies intensity without extinguishing it, allowing recursive continuity to slowly reemerge.

Clinical Implications of Recursive Failure

Clinically, recursive failure reveals itself in temporal anomalies. Patients may describe time as collapsed, looping, or frozen. They may feel stranded in the traumatic present, unable to revisit dissociated states without retraumatization. What is striking is not only their fragmentation but also their inability to recursively revisit their own history.

In such moments, the analyst's task is not to restore coherence directly but to sustain recursive potential. This may mean tolerating suspended temporality, bearing the gap between self-states, or listening for recursive echoes that remain inaudible to the patient. The ethic here is one of restraint: to hold loops open without forcing closure.

Recursive Breakdown as Revelation

Ultimately, recursive failures reveal that the self's integrity depends less on singularity and more on recursive temporality. Trauma, dissociation, and psychosis are not merely disruptions of content or narrative; they are collapses of recursive dimension. They show us that continuity itself is recursive: it arises from the looping motion that binds self-states across time.

When recursion collapses, the self fragments into isolated moments. When recursion is sustained, even in fragile form, the self survives its own folds. Dissociation, trauma, and psychosis therefore expose the recursive axis not as a theoretical abstraction but as the lived condition of continuity. They remind us that selfhood is not given but looped into existence, sustained by recursive linking that can collapse—and be rebuilt—at any moment.

Recursive Play, Symbolization, and the Ethics of Witnessing

If recursive failure manifests as temporal foreclosure, recursive repair takes shape through play, symbolization, and witnessing. These are not ancillary activities of the psyche but the very conditions through which recursive temporality can be reopened after collapse. To engage in play, to symbolize, or to witness is to restore the looping motion of the self—the recursive circulation that binds dissociated states into temporal relation.

Play as Recursive Suspension

Philip Ringstrom (2014, 2025, in press) places play at the center of analytic process, describing it as the locus where past, present, and fantasy converge without requiring premature resolution. In play, time bends. Memories do not remain locked in linear sequence but slip into present associations; fantasies do not displace reality but interweave with it. Play enacts recursive temporality: it creates the conditions under which one self-state can loop into another without collapse.

Analytic play is not simply a technique; it is a temporal structure. It suspends the demand for linear time and allows self-states to circulate in relation. In terms of the hallmarks, play restores state–state mapping by allowing estranged parts of self to recognize one another provisionally. It reactivates iterability by creating fresh contexts in which states can return differently. It re-generates inner time itself, sustaining time-generation through orbit.

Ringstrom's emphasis underscores the ethical stance embedded in recursion: the analyst must tolerate paradox, contradiction, and incompleteness rather than impose premature coherence. Play is recursive precisely because it sustains open loops.

Symbolization as Recursive Re-Linking

Hans Loewald's (1978) vision of symbolization is particularly resonant when read recursively. For Loewald, symbols do not merely represent experiences; they transform them, ushering undifferentiated psychic material into a higher order of organization. Symbolization is not a one-way process but a looping motion: raw experience is folded back into the psyche in symbolic form, reshaping both the experience and the subject who receives it.

From a recursive perspective, every act of symbolization is a re-linking. An unformulated or dissociated state loops into a symbolic register, establishing continuity across temporal gaps. This restores symbolic elevation, lifting fragments into forms that can reverberate across states. The symbol thus carries a dual temporality: born of a prior state and yet belonging to the present moment of articulation.

Loewald's notion that symbols enliven psychic reality helps us see why recursion is necessary for continuity. Without recursive re-linking, symbols remain inert. They may exist as linguistic markers, but they do not reverberate across self-states. With recursion, however, symbols come alive—circulating across layers and transforming dissociated fragments into living continuity.

Derrida, Slippage, and the Remainder

Derrida's (1976) account of slippage complicates this process by reminding us that symbols never fully coincide with the experiences they represent. Every loop leaves a remainder. Recursive linkage is always asymptotic, never complete. From the perspective of hallmarks, this is non-closure: the loop sustains itself precisely by not exhausting its origin.

To symbolize recursively is to accept that there will always be residue, excess, or unformulated remainder. The recursive loop does not close seamlessly; it sustains openness. Derrida's *différance* becomes temporal: every recursive return differs from its origin, every loop produces slippage. Continuity is thus not seamless integration but recursive resilience—the capacity to survive, and even be constituted by, remainder.

Clinically, Derrida's insight cautions against the fantasy of full recovery or total integration. The analyst's task is not to close loops but to sustain their circulation. Recursive temporality thrives on slippage; it lives in the space where remainder persists.

Levinas and the Ethics of Recursive Witnessing

Emmanuel Levinas (1969) offers a crucial ethical lens. For Levinas, responsibility is infinite, an obligation to the other that cannot be exhausted or finalized. Applied recursively, this translates into a temporal ethic: the analyst must sustain loops of witnessing without collapsing them into mutuality or recognition prematurely.

In *Post-Mutuality Ethic* (Anderson, 2025), I argued that psychoanalysis must at times resist the demand for recognition. To witness recursively is not to provide immediate symbolic closure but to bear rupture without forcing it into coherence. Levinasian ethics reframed in recursive temporality suggests that the analyst's task is to "hold the loop open."

This means listening across self-states, tolerating suspended time, and accompanying recursive circulation even when it remains incomplete. In terms of hallmarks, recursive witnessing restores resonant containment: the analyst absorbs and reverberates the patient's intensity without collapsing it, sustaining a loop that can eventually bear symbolic form.

Eigen and the Intensity of Recursive Survival

Michael Eigen (1993) emphasizes that psychic life is marked by intensity—tremors of ecstasy, terror, or annihilation that the psyche must bear. Recursive linking is charged with this intensity. Each recursive fold is not a neutral bridge but a trembling connection across discontinuity.

When the analyst bears witness to recursive folds, they do not simply provide continuity; they absorb and amplify intensity. To sustain recursive temporality is to survive its affective force. Eigen's emphasis on shakenness highlights that recursive repair is not about smoothing over ruptures but about resonant containment—the trembling survival of affect in recursive orbit.

Clinical Illustrations

Consider a patient who alternates between states of despair and manic activity. Each state disavows the other, creating recursive collapse. In analytic play, fragments of humor or metaphor may allow these states to circulate provisionally. A dream about a collapsing building might be interpreted not as a singular symbol but as a recursive bridge: despair and mania both loop into it, each refracted in altered form. Here, state–state mapping and iterability begin to revive.

Or consider the patient whose traumatic memories remain unformulated. Recursive witnessing requires that the analyst sit with latency, sustaining the possibility of future symbolization without forcing articulation. Continuity is maintained not through closure but through recursive patience—holding the loop open until it can be re-linked. This demonstrates time-generation: temporality begins to return when loops are tolerated.

Recursive Continuity as Ethical Practice

Recursive repair is thus not a matter of achieving synthesis but of sustaining circulation. Continuity is not seamlessness but recursive resilience: the ability of the self to loop through rupture and return altered but intact.

This reframing has ethical consequences. It resists the fantasy of mastery, insisting instead on accompaniment. It honors remainder, slippage, and the unformulated as constitutive of psychic life. To practice psychoanalysis recursively is to engage in a form of ethical patience: to accompany loops that never close, to sustain temporality where it collapses, to dwell in recursive circulation as a mode of life.

Recursive Topologies of the Self—Toward a New Structural Model

Classical psychoanalytic theory has long organized psychic life into categorical structures. Following Freud's structural turn (1923/1961) and his distinctions between neurosis and psychosis (1924/1961), later theorists—most notably Kernberg (1975) and McWilliams (2011)—elaborated the now-familiar spectrum of personality organization (neurotic, borderline, psychotic). These models remain invaluable, offering ways to differentiate forms of conflict, defense, and psychic organization. Yet they share a blind spot: they describe positions of structure but not the recursive motion that animates continuity across them. They provide static portraits of self-organization but omit the recursive temporality that sustains and disrupts them.

Recursion as an Orthogonal Dimension

The recursive dimension is not another structural level, but an axis that cuts across all levels. It describes how the self sustains continuity through recursive linking—how self-states fold back into one another across time. Without recursion, psychotic, borderline, and neurotic structures appear as discrete strata, each with its defenses and relational patterns. With recursion, these structures reveal themselves as temporally dynamic: each is defined not only by its content and form but also by its recursive capacity.

We might return to the symbolic condensation introduced earlier:

$$\mathbf{T}_{\text{self}} = \sum \mathbf{L}\left(s_i, s_{i+1}\right)$$

where

- $\mathbf{T}_{\textbf{self}}$ = psychic temporality
- $L\left(s_i, s_{i+1}\right)$ = recursive linking between self-states s_i and s_{i+1}

Continuity arises not from the self-states themselves, but from the summation of recursive linkages across them.

Recursive Hallmarks across Structures

- **Psychotic organization:** recursion collapses into uncontained simultaneity. State–state mapping is absent; iterability is broken (returns as raw intrusion rather than altered revisitation); time-generation fails, producing simultaneity or void; symbolic elevation cannot lift fragments; resonant containment is unavailable without an external holder.
- **Borderline organization:** recursion is unstable. Loops form but rupture, leaving continuity fragile. State–state mapping flickers; iterability emerges but collapses before resonance can accumulate; non-closure becomes chaotic rather than creative; resonant containment is precarious and often borrowed from the analyst.
- **Neurotic organization:** recursion is over-constrained. Loops are closed too tightly; non-closure (normally vital) is foreclosed; symbolic elevation persists but risks ossification; iterability returns as rigid repetition rather than transformed re-encounter.

Thus, recursion reconfigures structural models. It does not replace them but provides a dimension that reveals their temporal underpinnings. Psychic survival is less about static structure and more about recursive motion.

Dissociation, Trauma, and Recursive Rupture

Bromberg's (1998) dissociated self-states become failures of $L(s_i, s_{i+1})$: bridges between states are down. Trauma is Bion's (1959) attack on linking reframed as an attack on recursive temporality itself. The self loses the ability to loop back into dissociated layers, becoming temporally stranded. From this perspective, structural breakdowns are failures of recursion: psychotic disorganization reflects collapsed recursion; borderline fragmentation reflects unstable recursion; neurotic rigidity reflects over-constrained recursion.

Symbolization and Recursive Reverberation

Loewald (1978) shows that symbolization transforms undifferentiated experience into living psychic reality. Read recursively, symbolization is a reverberation: unformulated states loop into symbolic form, altering both the material and the subject who receives it—*symbolic elevation in action.* Eigen (1993) adds the affective register: each fold carries intensity; resonant containment metabolizes it when recursion holds and collapses when it fails. Recursive survival therefore depends not on integration alone but on the trembling reverberation of affect across loops.

Recursive Paradoxes: Gödel, Russell, Hofstadter

Gödel's incompleteness theorem (1931/1962) implies that every self-state harbors residues it cannot prove or symbolize alone; linkage to another state is needed for retroactive witnessing. Russell's (1903) paradox—that no set contains itself—illuminates why no state can hold its own contradiction without a loop to another state. Hofstadter's (1979) "strange loops" show continuity generated by self-referential yet incomplete patterns—coherence that never fully closes. Together, they underscore recursion as a logic of necessary incompletion.

Ringstrom, Ogden, and the Recursive Third

Ringstrom's play (2014, 2025, in press) enacts recursive temporality by suspending linear time and inviting multiple self-states into circulation—reviving iterability and time-generation. Ogden's (1994) analytic third is a recursive structure co-created by analyst and patient where loops are sustained, slippages acknowledged, and remainders held—restoring state–state mapping, symbolic elevation, and resonant containment. Both highlight recursion as not only intrapsychic but also intersubjective: a looping field sustained across two subjectivities.

Toward a Recursive Topology of the Psyche

Traditional models chart vertical levels (psychotic, borderline, neurotic). Recursion adds a horizontal, temporal axis: the motion of the self folding back upon itself—linking, unlinking, re-linking. In this topology:

- **State–state mapping** sustains distinctiveness across folds,
- **Iterability** ensures returns are altered, not frozen,
- **Time-generation** prevents collapse into simultaneity or void,
- **Non-closure** preserves openness to remainder,

- **Symbolic elevation** animates symbols across states, and
- **Resonant containment** enables affective survival.

The self is not a fixed structure but a recursive gravitational field, where depth arises from repeated folding.

Clinical and Ethical Consequences

Clinically, the task shifts from premature integration to sustaining recursive motion—holding loops open until they can be symbolized. Dissociation, trauma, and psychosis are read as recursive ruptures; play, symbolization, and witnessing as recursive restorations. Ethically, recursion resists mastery, honoring slippage and remainder as constitutive of psychic life.

Recursion as Foundational Axis

In sum, recursion is not an accessory to psychoanalytic theory but its missing axis. It reframes structure as dynamic topology and offers guidance for practice: listen for loops, sustain circulation, and honor remainder.

Conclusion—Recursive Listening, Recursive Life

The argument advanced here is that psychoanalytic theory has overlooked a fundamental dimension of psychic life: the recursive axis. Structural models—whether Freud's tripartite organizations (1923/1961), Kernberg's (1975) levels of personality organization, or McWilliams's (2011) elaborations of character structure—have provided invaluable maps. But these maps are incomplete. They chart defenses, affects, and object relations, yet they do not account for the recursive motion that makes temporality, continuity, and symbolic depth possible.

The Recursive Axis across Structures

By proposing recursion as an axis orthogonal to existing models, we gain a way to understand phenomena that otherwise evade theory. Psychosis, borderline instability, and neurotic rigidity each manifest not only as structural configurations but also as recursive disturbances. Psychosis collapses recursion into simultaneity without differentiation; borderline states fracture loops, leaving temporal continuity unstable; neurosis constrains loops too tightly, denying remainder and slippage. Recursion thus reframes structure as dynamic topology rather than static category.

In this light, dissociation can be understood as a rupture in recursive linking (Bromberg, 1998). Trauma, as Bion (1959) recognized, attacks not only thought but also the recursive scaffolding that sustains inner temporality. Loewald's (1978) symbolization becomes the recursive re-linking of unformulated states, and Eigen's (1993) trembling intensity becomes the affective force carried across recursive folds. Ringstrom's (2014, 2025, in press) play appears as recursive suspension, where loops can be reopened and temporality restored. Ogden's (1994) analytic third becomes a recursive structure that patients and analysts co-inhabit, sustaining linkage across dissociation. Each of these theorists, in their way, circled recursion without naming it.

Continuity as Recursive Resilience

Philosophically, recursion reframes continuity. Continuity is not seamless coherence but recursive resilience—the self's ability to loop through rupture and return altered but intact. Continuity is survival by means of recursive depth, not erasure of difference.

This recursive resilience is enacted through six hallmarks:

- **State–state mapping:** the capacity to link distinct self-states without collapse.
- **Iterability:** the ability to return to prior states in altered form, rather than static repetition.
- **Time-generation:** the production of inner temporality through recursive looping, preventing collapse into void or simultaneity.
- **Non-closure:** the openness to remainder and slippage, ensuring continuity remains alive rather than ossified.
- **Symbolic elevation:** the transformation of raw states into symbolic forms that reverberate across time.
- **Resonant containment:** the capacity to bear affective intensity across folds, allowing survival of recursive reverberation.

Gödel's incompleteness theorem (1931/1962) teaches that no system can contain all of its truths within itself; so too, no self-state can resolve its own remainder without recursive linkage. Russell's (1903) paradox—of the set that cannot contain itself—illuminates the impossibility of any self-state fully enclosing its temporal contradiction. Derrida's différance and slippage (1976) extend the point: every recursive link leaves excess. Continuity is recursive not because it resolves contradiction, but because it sustains it without collapse.

Recursive continuity is thus paradoxical. It survives by folding difference into orbit. It is not the straight line of linear time but the spiral of recursive temporality—forever looping, never closing.

Recursive Listening as Clinical Ethic

For the analyst, this perspective demands a different listening. To listen recursively is not merely to follow content, but to attend to loops, reverberations, and missed linkages. It is to hear when one self-state speaks without resonance from another; to notice when temporal continuity collapses; to hold open recursive potential without demanding premature integration.

Recursive listening requires patience and restraint. The temptation to unify or narrativize too quickly risks collapsing recursive motion. The ethic of recursive listening is to sustain loops provisionally—to witness one self-state while allowing another to hover in latency, to honor the slippage that prevents seamless closure. This is what I have elsewhere described as a *post-mutuality ethic* (Anderson, 2025): recognition that does not demand reciprocity, witnessing that sustains recursive depth even when coherence cannot yet be restored.

Here Levinas's (1969) notion of infinite responsibility acquires a temporal inflection. Responsibility is not only to the other's presence but also to their recursive temporality—their unfinished loops, their dissociated folds, their unformulated residues. The analyst becomes the guardian of recursive possibility, bearing the ethical weight of time that is not yet linkable.

Atmosphere, Topology, and the Recursive Psyche

Recursion is more than model or method. It is an atmosphere, a topology of psychic life. To fall into recursive interiority is to experience the self as descent through mirrored images, as in the ketamine free fall: each loop reflecting the last, each fold deepening into imageless recursion. To witness another recursively is to enter this atmosphere with them—to sustain their looping motion when it threatens to collapse.

This atmosphere is not reducible to cognitive process or symbolic structure. It is the lived texture of recursive temporality—the mood of slippage, remainder, and intensity. It is the gravitational pull of self upon itself, the orbit of psychic life.

Implications for Training and Supervision

If recursion is a missing dimension of structural theory, then training and supervision must adapt. Supervisors can model recursive listening by slowing the impulse to provide explanations, instead attending to loops in the trainee's clinical material. Rather than rushing to integration, supervisors can ask: *What states are speaking here? What loops are attempted or broken?* Training curricula might explicitly differentiate recursive linking from integration, teaching analysts to hear looping temporality as a distinct phenomenon. Supervision becomes a recursive space itself—a place where the loops of analytic work are revisited, sustained, and borne with resonant containment.

Directions for Future Research

Future research might examine how recursive temporality manifests across different cultural, developmental, and neurodiverse contexts. Autism, for example, may provide a privileged site for understanding bottom-up recursive assembly, while psychedelic states highlight recursive depth in its imageless form. Empirical work could study how recursive listening shapes outcomes in trauma treatment, and theoretical work might integrate recursion with models of affect regulation, attachment, or neural network dynamics. These expansions could further situate recursion as a cross-disciplinary axis linking psychoanalysis, philosophy, and physics.

Closing

Psychoanalysis, at its most vital, is recursive listening. It is the willingness to hear the self as it folds back upon itself, to accompany its loops through rupture and return, to sustain its remainders without forcing closure. Recursive analysis is not about coherence alone but about recursive survival—the capacity of the psyche to live by folding, looping, and surviving itself again and again.

The recursive axis is the missing dimension of structural theory. To name it is to reveal the gravitational depth of the psyche, to propose that selfhood is less a straight line than an orbit, less a structure than a recursive topology. By recognizing this, psychoanalysis can more fully honor the complexity of psychic life—not as seamless continuity but as recursive resilience, not as resolution but as survival through loops.

Notes

1 I am indebted to Donnel Stern, whose act of seeing me in my earlier work has itself become part of the recursive field that allows me to descend more deeply into these notes. Like Orpheus returning from the underworld, I bring them back only partially intact, carrying their shimmer and their remainder.

2 I acknowledge here the influence of Philip Ringstrom's evolving work on recursive play and altered temporality (2025, in press). His articulation of play as recursive suspension helped clarify the clinical bridge between recursive collapse and recursive repair.

3 I am grateful to Nancy McWilliams, whose recognition of the clarity and depth of my work has offered a stabilizing counterpoint. Her attunement affirmed that recursive writing can remain accessible without losing its complexity, and her confidence in me has been a crucial support in continuing this work.

4 I am deeply appreciative of Michael Eigen, whose excitement about the importance of my work extended a resonance that fueled my recursive descent. His willingness to tremble with psychic intensity encouraged me to stay with the shakenness of recursion, to treat it not as a threat but as generative survival.

5 I extend thanks to Thomas Ogden, whose perception of value in my writing inspired how this work might be written. His attunement to the atmospheric qualities of analytic experience granted me permission to write in recursive form, to risk style as a mode of transmission.

Chapter 5

Introjection as Hospitality—Containment, Curvature, and the Limits of Psychic Welcome

This chapter reconceives introjection not merely as a process of psychic acquisition or internalization, but as an ongoing, recursive discipline of hospitality: a radical openness to being changed by the other. Moving beyond the classical model in which the analyst contains and returns the patient's projected experience, this chapter reframes introjection as a field phenomenon—a shared atmospheric process shaped by curvature, surprise, and the unpredictability of psychic life. Drawing on Derrida's philosophy of hospitality, Laplanche's enigmatic signifier, Green's "dead mother," and the contemporary psychoanalytic literature on field theory, this chapter explores how the limits of containment—moments of deadness, opacity, and unassimilable otherness—are not analytic failures, but sites of ethical encounter and psychic creativity. Through detailed clinical vignettes, recursive reflection, and attention to the atmosphere of analytic work, this chapter advances an ethic of not-knowing: the analyst and patient dwell together in a field where hospitality is always provisional, containment is recursive, and the deepest transformations emerge not from mastery or integration, but from the willingness to stay with what cannot be fully known, received, or metabolized. In this curved, generative field, the limits of psychic hospitality become a wellspring for new forms of relation, meaning, and analytic presence.

The Classical Concept of Introjection—Taking in, Making One's Own

Introjection, in its earliest psychoanalytic usage, was conceived as the psychic process of taking in aspects of the other—objects, persons, qualities, affects—and making them one's own. If projection is the psychic motion of exporting what is intolerable, introjection is its apparent opposite: the

DOI: 10.4324/9781003747109-8

absorption, internalization, and sometimes idealization of what comes from outside. Yet from the beginning, introjection has been more than a simple reversal; it is a mysterious, often ambiguous movement that destabilizes the boundaries between self and other, inside and outside, known and unknown.

The term "introjection" was first introduced by Ferenczi (1909/1994), who sought to distinguish it from identification. For Ferenczi, introjection was an active psychic process—an "extension of the boundaries of the ego" to encompass the loved or needed object. It was a form of psychic hospitality: the self becomes porous, open to the presence and influence of the other. Freud, meanwhile, spoke of introjection as a necessary mechanism for the formation of the superego and the structuring of the ego itself. In *Mourning and Melancholia* (1917/1957), Freud described how the lost object is "set up again inside the ego," its qualities and affects internalized and worked over as part of the subject's own psychic life.

In the early Freudian tradition, introjection is inseparable from the work of mourning, loss, and love. When the external object is lost—whether by death, absence, or emotional rupture—the psyche seeks to preserve it by internalizing its features, thereby transforming absence into psychic presence. Following Abraham and Torok, I distinguish **incorporation**—a crypt-like, undigested installation of the lost object that bypasses symbolization—from **introjection**, the ego's symbolizing expansion that metabolizes loss. Thus the melancholic "incorporates" while the healthy mourner "introjects," allowing new identifications and symbolic capacities to form (Freud, 1917/1957; Abraham & Torok, 1978/1994).

Melanie Klein expanded the reach of introjection, situating it at the heart of early psychic life. For Klein (1946/1975), the infant's world is organized around the primal movements of projection and introjection—expelling what is unbearable, taking in what is nourishing or idealized. The breast, as the first object, is both introjected as a good internal object and projected onto as a source of envy or aggression. The psychic world is populated by these internal objects—part-mother, part-breast, part-fantasy—each coloring the child's experience of self and world. Klein's vision is thus fundamentally recursive: the self is never fully separate from the objects it takes in; psychic life is a looping, atmospheric dance of identification, envy, idealization, and loss.

Wilfred Bion's concept of "container-contained" further complicates the classical account. For Bion (1962), introjection is not simply the passive absorption of the other, but a dynamic process in which raw, unprocessed emotional experiences ("beta elements") are projected into another for digestion, then reintrojected in a transformed, symbolizable form. The mother's function as "container" is crucial: she receives, metabolizes, and returns what the infant cannot yet bear, thereby enabling introjection to serve psychic growth rather than confusion or fragmentation. The analytic situation, in Bion's model, recapitulates this early process. The patient projects unformulated affect into the analyst, who must hold and transform it before it can be safely introjected.

In this frame, introjection is at once a movement of psychic nourishment and of psychic risk. To take in the other is to risk confusion, contamination, or even psychic "deadness" if what is taken in cannot be metabolized. The boundary between self and other is made permeable, porous, and ambiguous—a site of recursive return, not simple mastery. André Green's "dead mother" complex (1983/1986) illustrates the danger: when the object is unresponsive or unavailable, what is introjected is not life but deadness, absence, or the uncanny echo of loss. Introjection is never only creative; it is haunted by the possibility of emptiness, foreclosure, or melancholic stasis.

The classical concept of introjection is thus already marked by paradox and reversal. It is the movement by which the self is constituted, but also the route through which the other's absence, trauma, or psychic opacity is carried into the heart of the subject. In its most generative forms, introjection enables the psyche to grow, to elaborate new identifications, and to sustain the symbolic capacity for differentiation and play. In its more defensive or pathological forms, introjection can become a means of psychic foreclosure, swallowing the other whole or installing deadness where life might have been.

Throughout, introjection operates as a recursive process: what is taken in is never identical to what is outside; it is transformed, symbolized, or sometimes rendered enigmatic in the passage through the psychic membrane. Loewald (1960, 1978) emphasized this dynamic, arguing that introjection is the foundation of symbolization itself. For Loewald, the child's capacity to take in the other—first in fantasy, then in symbol—makes possible the growth of the ego, the emergence of psychic space, and the creation of new forms of meaning. The analytic encounter, in this frame, becomes a recursive laboratory: the analyst is introjected, digested, and remade by the patient, just as the patient is taken in and transformed by the analyst's presence and reverie.

The limits of introjection are also the limits of psychic hospitality. To take in the other requires both openness and boundary, both creative receptivity and the capacity to metabolize difference. Where the field is too rigid, introjection becomes impossible—new experience bounces off the closed psychic surface. Where the field is too porous, the self is overwhelmed, invaded, or lost. The work of analysis becomes a negotiation of these boundaries, a recursive attunement to the field's oscillations between openness and closure, creativity and defense.

In sum, the classical concept of introjection is anything but simple. It is a movement of psychic hospitality and risk, a recursive process through which the self is formed, deformed, and transformed by the taking-in of the other. The analytic field is constituted by these looping movements of projection and introjection—giving, receiving, metabolizing, and sometimes failing to contain. Even at its most "classical," introjection is an invitation to rethink the boundaries of self and other, the meaning of containment, and the recursive dance of knowing and unknowing that animates analytic life.

Containment, Metabolization, and the Limits of Classical Containment

If the classical concept of introjection centers on taking in and making one's own, then the idea of psychic containment represents its dynamic infrastructure—the means by which the psyche, and later the analytic field, metabolizes what has been received. In the second half of the 20th century, psychoanalytic theory became increasingly preoccupied with the question of how the self can bear, transform, and survive what is taken in from the other. The work of Bion, Loewald, and their interlocutors recasts introjection not as a given but as a capacity: something enabled or thwarted by the atmosphere of the field, the qualities of the container, and the recursive oscillations of affect and symbol.

Wilfred Bion's (1962) paradigm of "container-contained" is foundational here. For Bion, the mother (and, by extension, the analyst) is tasked not merely with receiving the projections of the infant, but with transforming them—holding the raw "beta elements" of unprocessed affect and returning them, through reverie, in a form that can be introjected and symbolized. The function of the container is not passive: it is an active psychic labor, a metabolization of experience that allows what is foreign, overwhelming, or terrifying to become thinkable. When containment succeeds, the infant (or patient) can reintroject what was projected, now rendered less toxic and more capable of psychic elaboration.

Yet Bion is explicit about the limits of this process. Containment can fail. The mother who cannot receive or metabolize the infant's projections may become an object of terror, emptiness, or persecution; the analyst who cannot contain the patient's unformulated experience may return it untransformed, or even unconsciously "project it back." In these failures, introjection becomes impossible, or worse, pathogenic: the psyche is left with untransformed fragments, psychic toxins, or alien elements that cannot be digested (Bion, 1962; Ogden, 1994). The recursive movement—projection, containment, introjection—collapses, and the field becomes saturated with dread, deadness, or repetition compulsion.

Hans Loewald's (1960) theory of symbolization also centers on the metabolization of what is taken in. For Loewald, the psychic field is alive when it can metabolize difference, when what is introjected is not simply absorbed, but transformed—given new symbolic texture and integrated into the self's ongoing story. The analytic setting is, in this sense, a crucible for transformation: the patient brings unprocessed, sometimes unformulated psychic matter; the analyst holds, bears, and dreams it; and, through the recursive oscillation of presence, absence, and reverie, the field gradually generates new symbolic form.

Yet Loewald, too, is attentive to failure. When the analytic field becomes too rigid, too defended, or too saturated with trauma, the capacity to metabolize is blocked. What is introjected may remain inert, undigested, or even toxic. The risk of deadness is ever-present: what cannot be symbolized may be buried, acting as a psychic tomb that exerts gravitational pull on the analytic hour (Green, 1997). In such moments, containment is not a comfort, but a prison; introjection is not nourishment, but foreclosure.

The classical model of containment and metabolization presupposes a certain linearity: projection occurs, containment is provided, introjection follows, and the self grows. But clinical experience repeatedly exposes the limits of this sequence. In the lived field of analysis, these moments rarely unfold in neat succession. Instead, they loop and repeat, dissolve and reappear. Containment is not an achievement to be secured once and for all, but an ongoing, recursive labor—a discipline of presence, attunement, and revision.

In the analytic hour, containment is experienced less as a function and more as an atmosphere: the mood of the room, the density or spaciousness of affect, the rhythm of movement between openness and closure. Sometimes, containment is palpable—an enveloping sense of safety or being held, in which the patient dares to risk new forms of psychic life. At other times, the atmosphere is brittle, tense, or dead, and the analytic pair struggles to metabolize what is present. The recursive field of containment is marked by these oscillations: moments of resonance and rupture, cycles of openness and withdrawal, affective weather that shapes the very possibility of introjection.

The limits of classical containment also show themselves in moments of analytic failure. The analyst may miss, misread, or be unable to bear what the patient brings; the field may become saturated with uncontained affect, flooding both participants with anxiety, despair, or numbness. At times, the very attempt to contain becomes defensive—a way to keep the other at bay, to wall off what is most intolerable or unassimilable. The analyst's effort to metabolize can itself become a form of resistance, a flight from the not-knowing that is the condition for genuine transformation.

Yet it is precisely in these recursive failures that the potential for new forms of containment—and new psychic life—arises. The analytic field is not static; it is animated by repetition, return, and the creative play of surprise. Containment, then, is best understood not as a fixed capacity but as a dynamic field phenomenon: an ongoing negotiation of boundaries, openness, and the recursive play between what can and cannot be metabolized. The very limits of containment—the points where the analytic pair cannot yet bear, symbolize, or integrate what is present—are often the sites of greatest creative potential.

Clinical examples abound. A patient, Callum, enters the room in a mood of dense anxiety, his speech fragmented and urgent. He projects overwhelming affect onto me; I feel the pull to reassure, explain, or interpret, but notice a kind of "psychic indigestion" in myself—a feeling that I cannot quite metabolize what is being projected. In this moment, containment fails. The room feels crowded, breathless; the atmosphere is saturated with untransformed fear. We loop through this pattern for weeks: Callum's anxiety, my struggle to contain, the repeated collapse of symbolic space. Yet gradually, as I become more able to bear the failure—naming it, staying with it, risking my own uncertainty—the atmosphere shifts. Containment is not "achieved" once and for all but emerges in the recursive process of trying, failing, and trying again.

The limits of classical containment are also the limits of introjection. What cannot be metabolized cannot be truly taken in; what remains uncontained becomes an excess, a symptom, or a dead spot in the field. The analyst's stance thus becomes one of recursive hospitality—an openness to return, to repetition, to the possibility that what is intolerable now may become symbolizable in another loop, another field configuration. Containment is revealed as a discipline of waiting, of presence, of risking surprise.

Bollas (1987) reframes this as the analyst's capacity for "receptive unconsciousness"—the willingness to let the field do its work, to wait for the unthought known to emerge in its own time. Ferro and Civitarese (2016) describe the analytic field as a space of "narrative co-construction," animated by the recursive interplay of containment and emergence. What is metabolized is not only the patient's affect, but the field's atmosphere itself—a living weather that shapes what can be taken in and what must remain, for now, outside.

In sum, the limits of classical containment invite a turn toward recursion, atmosphere, and creative failure. Containment is not a linear function but a recursive process, shaped by the ongoing, affectively charged interplay of projection, metabolization, and introjection. The analytic field thrives not on perfect containment, but on the shared discipline of staying-with: risking failure, returning again, and holding open the possibility of transformation where the boundary between self and other, known and unknown, is at its most permeable.

Inversion—Introjection as Psychic Hospitality and Epistemic Reversal

To invert the classical model of introjection is to move from a story of psychic acquisition—taking in, assimilating, and owning the other—toward a radically different ethical and epistemic stance: one of hospitality, porousness, and a willingness to be changed by what remains irreducibly other. In this frame, introjection is not simply the internalization of qualities, values, or objects, but an opening to difference, ambiguity, and even the destabilization of the self's own boundaries. The analytic field becomes not a site for the secure integration of experience, but a space where self and other, knowing and not-knowing, are continually unsettled by recursive invitation and reversal.

Jacques Derrida's (2000) meditation on "hospitality" serves as a conceptual bridge here, extending psychoanalytic concerns into the philosophical domain of ethics and otherness. For Derrida, true hospitality is not the mastery of the guest by the host, but a radical openness to the stranger—an invitation that risks the boundaries of home, comfort, and self-certainty. In the analytic situation, this ethos of hospitality is enacted whenever the analyst makes psychic space for the unformulated, the unpredictable, or the unassimilable in the patient. The analyst's own self-experience is exposed to alteration; introjection becomes less a defensive maneuver and more an encounter with otherness that cannot be fully tamed or possessed.

Laplanche (1999) offers a psychoanalytic parallel in his theory of the enigmatic signifier. For Laplanche, the unconscious is not simply a product of repression, but the effect of "messages from the other"—inscriptions, affects, and desires that originate outside the self and remain partially untranslated. Introjection, in this light, is not the domestication of the other, but a creative encounter with the surplus, the enigmatic, and the as-yet-unformulated. The child, and later the patient, is continually addressed by the other's unconscious and must take in what cannot be fully metabolized. This process is recursive: what is introjected is always already marked by ambiguity, difference, and the ongoing demand for symbolic work.

Jessica Benjamin (1988/2018) frames this process as one of mutual recognition—not mastery or perfect understanding, but a willingness to welcome what is not oneself, to remain in contact with alterity even when it cannot be resolved. Psychic hospitality, in this sense, is not a gesture of generosity from a secure self, but an ethical discipline of staying open to the stranger within and without. The analytic field becomes a laboratory for this ongoing negotiation: a site where introjection means risking surprise, uncertainty, and transformation, rather than the secure accumulation of internal objects.

This reversal is not without anxiety. The porous self—the self open to introjective hospitality—faces the risk of confusion, loss, and even psychic disorganization. André Green's (1997) work on the "dead mother" complex and the "unrepresentable" points to the dangers inherent in radical openness: what is taken in may overwhelm, deaden, or annihilate the self's organizing capacities. Yet it is only by risking this openness that the field remains alive; only by welcoming the unassimilable that psychic transformation becomes possible.

The recursive structure of introjection as hospitality is evident in the microdynamics of analytic process. A patient brings a mood, a fantasy, or a fragment of dream; the analyst is moved, unsettled, altered—sometimes in ways that defy conscious understanding. The analyst's reverie, affect, or countertransference becomes a site where the patient's experience is received, but not merely assimilated. Instead, something is held, played with, and sometimes returned in a new form—an interpretation, a silence, a gesture of empathy or shared confusion. This loop—of taking in, being altered, and re-encountering—creates an atmosphere of mutual becoming, where both analyst and patient are changed by the encounter.

Thomas Ogden (1994, 2004) describes this as the work of the "analytic third"—a co-created psychic field in which both participants introject aspects of the other, not as static objects but as living, recursive invitations to symbolic work. The analytic third is neither the analyst nor the patient alone, but an emergent field that shapes, and is shaped by, the ongoing loops of hospitality, reversal, and mutual transformation. Ogden's clinical vignettes are full of moments when the analyst finds herself speaking, dreaming, or feeling in ways that reflect the patient's unformulated experience—yet these are not mere reflections, but co-created, atmospheric phenomena that re-enter the field as new opportunities for introjection and symbolization. In a similar vein, Buchholz reconceives the working alliance as a "Doing We"—a recursively built accomplishment of the pair—linking our ethical stance of hospitality to observable interactional practices across the hour (Buchholz, 2022).

The recursive logic of hospitality means that the field is never finished. Every act of taking in—the patient's experience of the analyst, the analyst's reception of the patient's projection, the shared reverie of the analytic third—creates new psychic configurations, new opportunities for surprise, disruption, and growth. The process is not linear or cumulative, but looping, spiraling, and unpredictable. Sometimes, what is taken in at one point cannot be metabolized until much later; sometimes, the hospitality of the field is overwhelmed and must be rebuilt through mutual recognition and repair.

This model also complicates the analyst's role. No longer the secure container or expert interpreter, the analyst is called to participate in the field's openness—to risk her own boundaries, to acknowledge the ways in which she is changed, challenged, or even wounded by the encounter. The analyst's vulnerability is not a failure, but a resource: it allows for the emergence of new symbolic forms, for the shared elaboration of experience that neither participant could create alone. The ethic of hospitality is recursive: it invites both self and other into a dance of reversal, where knowing gives way to not-knowing, and certainty is exchanged for the possibility of surprise.

At the same time, this model clarifies the limits of hospitality. There are experiences, affects, or forms of otherness that cannot be taken in—at least not yet, or not by the analytic pair as currently constituted. Trauma, deadness, or radical difference may resist introjection, remaining as residues or symptoms that haunt the field. The analyst's task is not to force hospitality, but to bear witness to its limits, to honor the zones of opacity and unassimilability as part of the field's recursive life.

A clinical example: Sasha, a patient with a history of profound relational trauma, finds it nearly impossible to "take in" the analyst's presence. Weeks pass in silence or with minimal contact. When moments of connection arise—a shared laugh, a brief glance, a sudden surge of affect—they are quickly foreclosed, leaving an atmosphere of loss and longing. As an analyst, I notice my own impulse to "fill" the space, to offer interpretations or reassurance. But over time, I learn to risk a different stance: to let the field remain open, to welcome what can be taken in without forcing what cannot. Slowly, the atmosphere changes. Sasha begins to ask, tentatively, about my experience of the sessions; I share my own sense of uncertainty, of not-knowing. The field becomes more hospitable, not through mastery but through mutual risk and the recursive return to what is possible in the present.

The ethic of hospitality, then, is inseparable from the ethic of unknowing. To invite the other in is also to invite the unknown, the unpredictable, the as-yet-unformulated. Introjection as reversal is not the end of psychic work, but its beginning: an ongoing commitment to welcome, to risk, and to be changed by what comes. The analytic field thrives on this recursive openness, finding its richest creativity not in the secure ownership of meaning, but in the ongoing dance of invitation and surprise.

In summary, to invert the classical account of introjection is to recognize that psychic life is sustained by the recursive play of hospitality and reversal. The self is constituted not by the secure possession of internalized objects, but by an ongoing, looping engagement with otherness—an openness to being altered, surprised, and even undone by the encounter with what is not-yet-known. In this sense, the analytic field is not only a site of containment, but a site of hospitality: a space where the limits of self and other are tested, stretched, and renewed in the recursive ethic of analytic life.

The Uncontainable Other—Opacity, Deadness, and the Limits of Hospitality

If introjection as psychic hospitality gestures toward a radical openness to otherness and surprise, it also exposes the analytic field to its own intrinsic limits: zones of opacity, deadness, and unassimilable alterity. No matter how capacious the self or how recursive the analytic field, there exist forms of experience, trauma, and psychic deadness that cannot be taken in, metabolized, or symbolized—at least, not on demand or according to analytic intention. The work of hospitality is thus always shadowed by a remainder: a kernel of the other that resists introjection, that remains irreducibly outside, haunting the psychic field with absence, silence, or uncanny repetition.

André Green (1983/1986) named this remainder the "dead mother" complex—a figure for the object that, once vital and sustaining, has become psychically absent, impenetrable, or cold. The dead mother is not simply a lost object, but an uncontainable otherness that settles in the field as an atmosphere of lifelessness, silence, or dread. Green's clinical descriptions are vivid: the patient finds herself unable to take in comfort, vitality, or recognition from the analyst; the analytic hour is pervaded by a sense of deadness, a failure of hospitality at the most fundamental level. What is introjected is not nourishment but psychic emptiness—a "blank," as Green puts it, that cannot be symbolized or metabolized.

This figure of uncontainability is not confined to catastrophic maternal loss or trauma but recurs in every analytic field as a limit phenomenon. There are always aspects of the other—patient or analyst—that resist being taken in, that remain opaque, enigmatic, or even menacing. Laplanche's (1999) "enigmatic signifier" describes precisely this: the residue of the other's desire or unconscious communication that can never be fully translated or appropriated. No matter how recursive, how symbolically attuned, the analytic field cannot absorb the entire force of alterity. The presence of the unassimilable is not a failure, but a structural feature of psychic life.

Opacity, then, is not simply a defensive posture, but an ethical and structural fact. Édouard Glissant's (1997) "right to opacity" insists that the other's irreducibility is both dignified and necessary: a demand that the subject not be reduced to what can be known, introjected, or symbolized. In the analytic field, this right to opacity is mirrored in the moments when the analyst cannot enter the patient's world, when the patient's experience remains sealed off, untranslatable, or enigmatic. There is dignity in this unknowability—a resistance to being swallowed, digested, or rendered transparent for the sake of analytic understanding.

The uncontainable also emerges as deadness in the field—a felt absence or inertness that can become as much an atmosphere as any explicit content. Michael Eigen (1999) writes movingly about analytic deadness: those sessions, hours, or even entire analytic relationships where the field seems frozen, thick with silence, affectively flat, or stuck in endless repetition. Here, the effort to take in or metabolize fails; what is introjected is not aliveness but a kind of psychic death. Yet even here, the recursive stance offers a resource: deadness is not the end of analytic work, but a condition to be inhabited, witnessed, and, at times, even shared.

For some patients, the experience of deadness or opacity is a defensive construction—a way to protect the self from the risks of hospitality, openness, or new experience. For others, it is an inherited psychic legacy—a trauma that cannot be borne, a loss that cannot be grieved, an absence that cannot be symbolized. The analytic pair may circle these zones for months or years, oscillating between efforts to enliven the field and moments of surrender to what cannot be changed. The recursive, atmospheric approach to containment means learning to wait, to bear the deadness, to risk not-knowing, and to trust that something may eventually move—even if that movement is slow, uncertain, or only partially formulated.

The limits of hospitality also have cultural and intersubjective dimensions. There are forms of otherness—rooted in history, language, race, sexuality, or collective trauma—that cannot be fully taken in by the analyst or the field. The attempt to "contain" these differences may become, unintentionally, an act of appropriation, erasure, or even violence. The analytic ethic here is not to press for assimilation, but to honor the inassimilable: to grant opacity, to hold space for what cannot be symbolized or known within the available frame.

In analytic practice, the encounter with the uncontainable other often produces intense countertransference. The analyst may feel useless, blank, deadened, or even persecuted by the field's refusal to move. These experiences are challenging and humbling—testing the analyst's capacity for hospitality, presence, and patience. At times, the analyst's own deadness is called into the field, as a response to the patient's trauma or as a reactivation of the analyst's own unformulated experiences. The recursive ethic does not ask for perfect containment or infinite hospitality; it asks only for a willingness to stay with, to accompany, and to bear witness to the zones where hospitality fails or is refused.

A clinical example illustrates these dynamics. Julia, a patient with a history of profound emotional neglect, finds it almost impossible to feel received or "taken in" by me. Our sessions are often silent; when she does speak, her words feel hollow, as if rehearsed or borrowed from someone else. I notice my own affect flattening, a sense of fatigue or boredom creeping into the room. Attempts to enliven the field—interpretation, humor, shared reverie—fall flat. For months, we dwell in this deadness together. Only gradually, and sometimes only in retrospect, do I notice subtle shifts: Julia asks about my experience of the silence; I acknowledge my own difficulty finding words. The field does not come alive all at once, but the shared willingness to bear deadness opens the possibility for something new. Our mutual recognition of opacity, of what cannot be contained or introjected, becomes a fragile ground for future hospitality.

The limits of hospitality thus become a resource, not a sign of analytic failure. In honoring the opacity, deadness, or uncontainable otherness in the field, analyst and patient resist the drive for premature understanding or assimilation. They learn to wait, to witness, to bear what cannot be metabolized—trusting that the recursive atmosphere of the analytic hour will, in its own time and fashion, generate new possibilities for movement, contact, and transformation.

The ethical implications are profound. To respect the limits of hospitality is to respect the dignity of the other's opacity, trauma, and irreducibility. It is to resist the temptation to "fix" deadness, to rush past silence, or to claim understanding where there is none. The recursive stance—staying-with, returning, inhabiting the atmosphere—creates space for the unknown to persist, for the inassimilable to be held, for surprise to emerge without demand.

In the recursive analytic field, hospitality is always partial, always provisional. There will always be aspects of the other that cannot be taken in, that resist containment, that remain enigmatic, uncontained, or dead. But it is in the very willingness to stay with these limits that the most radical forms of hospitality are enacted. To welcome what cannot be metabolized; to bear witness to deadness; to grant the other their right to opacity—these are the hallmarks of an analytic ethic that honors not only the possibility but also the impossibility of introjection.

In summary, the uncontainable other marks the boundary of the analytic field—an edge that cannot be crossed but must be respected, inhabited, and even cherished. The recursive ethic of hospitality finds its deepest meaning not in endless openness or infinite receptivity, but in the courage to stay with what cannot be known, contained, or taken in. The analytic field thus becomes not a site of perfect integration, but a living, breathing space in which the limits of hospitality are witnessed, honored, and gently, recursively transformed.

Clinical Vignette—Introjection and the Atmosphere of Psychic Welcome

It is late winter, the city gripped by a persistent grayness that seems to seep into the consulting room. I have been working with Alan for nearly two years. His early sessions were characterized by a wary distance—a constant scanning for judgment or disappointment, a reluctance to trust that anything could be truly "taken in" without distortion or harm. He is reserved, intelligent, quick to anticipate interpretations, and often apologizes for "taking up too much space." In the beginning, the analytic field was taut, thin, as if stretched over the surface of an emptiness neither of us could yet acknowledge.

Alan grew up in a household dominated by volatility and inconsistency—a mother whose love arrived unpredictably, a father whose moods governed the atmosphere without warning. As a child, Alan became an expert at reading the room, attuning himself to subtle shifts in tone or affect, always strategizing about how to minimize disruption. Safety, for him, meant invisibility. The very idea of being "received" or "taken in" was freighted with anxiety: to be seen was to risk annihilation or engulfment; to make contact was to court the unpredictable.

In the early phase of our work, Alan often spoke in the language of defense. He described himself as "armored," his affect shielded by wit, intellect, or, at times, icy detachment. He listened for hidden meanings, dissected my words, and often preempted my questions. Our exchanges, though lively, circled the same patterns—a recursive repetition of approach and retreat, anticipation and withdrawal. When I invited him to reflect on our process, he would say, "I can hear what you're trying to do, but it feels like you're just doing your job. I don't know if I really believe any of this can matter."

I felt the weight of Alan's skepticism—a mood that would settle in the room, dampening my curiosity, rendering my interventions limp or formulaic. There were hours when I felt the analytic atmosphere thicken into a kind of psychic fog. I worried that I was failing him, or worse, replicating the deadness he feared. At times, my reverie was haunted by a sense of futility—a repetitive echo of "nothing gets in, nothing comes out." I noticed myself growing self-conscious, hyper-aware of my own desire to be helpful, to be the "good container," to offer some evidence of welcome.

A turning point arrived, as such moments often do, in the most ordinary of ways. Alan entered one day in an uncharacteristically agitated state. He described a difficult encounter with a colleague, the sudden memory of a childhood humiliation, and the acute sense of being "contaminated" by the other's opinion. "I know I shouldn't care," he said, "but it's like I let them get inside me, and I can't get it out. I feel invaded, like I swallowed something poisonous."

For the first time, I felt Alan speaking from within his own body, rather than about it. The words "let them get inside me" lingered in the air, vibrating with anxiety and longing. I reflected back: "It sounds unbearable to feel so affected by someone else—almost as if being open means risking being poisoned." Alan nodded but then added, "It's not just them. I think I feel that way with you too. Sometimes I worry that if I let anything in, I'll lose myself. But if I don't, then I feel nothing at all."

This admission marked a subtle shift in the analytic field—a thinning of the defenses that had kept both of us safe but isolated. I could feel my own affect come alive, a mix of tenderness and sorrow. I found myself saying, "It sounds like it's very hard to trust that anything could be received without harm, but also that the alternative—total self-protection—can feel lifeless, empty." Alan looked at me for a long moment, as if weighing the risk of continuing. He said quietly, "I wish it was different. I want to feel something get through."

Over the next several weeks, our sessions became increasingly saturated with this longing and ambivalence. Alan oscillated between moments of openness—sharing memories, reflecting on dreams, risking curiosity about my experience—and sudden withdrawals, shutting down, or retreating into sarcasm. At times, he would challenge me: "Are you just going to sit there and nod? Doesn't this get boring for you?" I recognized these challenges as tests—efforts to discern whether the analytic field could survive disappointment, anger, or even contempt.

I responded as honestly as I could, acknowledging when I felt confused, discouraged, or moved by his vulnerability. Rather than striving to offer perfect containment, I allowed myself to be present in the uncertainty, to welcome what could be received, and to name what felt blocked. “There are times I feel far away,” I said once, “like we’re both watching this from a distance. And there are times, like now, when I feel closer, even if that’s risky for both of us.” Alan responded with a faint smile: “Yeah. I can feel that. It’s weird, but not bad.”

A striking dream emerged in this phase. Alan described being in an old library, its shelves endless and shadowy. He searched for a particular book, but every time he reached for it, the shelves rearranged themselves. The librarian—a faceless figure—offered him a cup of tea. Alan hesitated but accepted, noticing the warmth in his hands. “I never found the book,” he said, “but the tea was good. I woke up feeling… calm, which is not normal for me.”

We lingered over the image of the librarian and the cup of tea. I wondered aloud whether the dream might represent the analytic process itself—not a quest for the “right” answer or interpretation, but an invitation to find nourishment, warmth, and welcome in the midst of uncertainty. Alan nodded, “Maybe it’s not about finding the book. Maybe just having someone offer me something, and me taking it in, is enough.” The field felt lighter, the air less charged.

From this point, the rhythm of our work became less about mastery and more about shared presence. There were setbacks: weeks when Alan would return to defensive vigilance, or when my own countertransference would tip toward irritability or disengagement. Sometimes, he would accuse me of being “too nice” or of hiding my real feelings. At other times, he asked about my experience of silence or my own strategies for coping with uncertainty. Our roles began to blur, each of us bearing witness to the field’s oscillations between welcome and refusal, contact and withdrawal.

Gradually, Alan began to describe moments outside analysis when he noticed a new capacity to receive—to allow himself to feel affected by others without immediate retreat or collapse. He described listening to music and “letting it get inside me,” or allowing a friend’s compliment to linger, rather than brushing it away. He even described moments with me—pauses in the session, subtle shifts in mood—when he felt “almost like it’s safe to just be here, even if I don’t know what happens next.”

One session stands out. After a particularly charged silence, Alan said, “I used to think you had to earn being welcomed, or that it was always conditional. But lately, I wonder if it's something that just… happens, when the atmosphere is right." I replied, "That feels important—the idea that hospitality isn't something you force, but something that arises between us, sometimes unpredictably." We sat quietly, both aware of the novelty and fragility of this insight.

Throughout this process, the analytic field became less a site of achievement and more an atmosphere—an emergent quality that neither of us could produce alone, but that we could recognize, honor, and cohabit. At times, the old patterns would return: Alan would recoil, I would feel deadened, and the field would contract. But with each recursive return, our capacity to dwell in the ambiguity, to risk not-knowing, and to tolerate the limits of hospitality grew.

Looking back, what feels most striking is not a linear progression toward integration, but the recursive looping through approach, refusal, contact, and withdrawal. The moments of hospitality—when Alan could "take in" something from me or from the field—were not always predictable or sustained. They arrived as surprises, often after periods of deadness or silence, and receded again as the field shifted. What mattered was not the permanence of welcome, but the shared willingness to return, to try again, to risk surprise and disappointment.

In the final phase of this clinical moment, Alan reflected on the paradox of hospitality. "I used to think being affected was dangerous, that you had to protect yourself at all costs. But now I see there's something alive in letting yourself be changed, even if it's just for a moment." I echoed his reflection, noting that the field itself seemed to pulse with this movement—opening, closing, returning, looping through new forms of contact and refusal. "Maybe," I offered, "what we're doing is learning to be affected together, even when it's uncertain."

This vignette enacts the recursive atmosphere of introjection and hospitality. It is not a story of triumph or mastery, but a living demonstration of how the analytic field sustains and is sustained by the unpredictable emergence of welcome, the discipline of staying-with, and the courage to risk being changed by what can and cannot be taken in.

Recursive Containment—Atmosphere, Curvature, and the Ethics of Not-Knowing

As the analytic process unfolds, the limits and possibilities of introjection, containment, and psychic hospitality come to hinge less on technique or interpretation and more on the recursive atmosphere generated by the analytic field itself. Containment is no longer simply a function, an act performed by an analyst for a patient, but a shared atmospheric phenomenon—a living, breathing field shaped by the ongoing oscillations of contact, withdrawal, openness, and refusal. In this atmosphere, introjection becomes not a final achievement, but a recursive discipline: the work of welcoming and re-welcoming, metabolizing and re-metabolizing, what the field brings forth, what it cannot yet bear, and what it must leave opaque.

The concept of **recursive containment** invites us to see the analytic situation as inherently non-linear, curved, and affectively charged. Rather than tracing a straight line from projection to containment to introjection, recursive containment attends to the way psychic life doubles back on itself—looping, revisiting, repeating, and transforming. Each moment of contact or rupture is not an endpoint, but a node in an ongoing network of returns. The atmosphere of the analytic field is charged with these loops: silences that return with new meaning, resistances that open into possibility, deadness that is gently endured until life reemerges.

This curved temporality transforms our understanding of both containment and introjection. Where classical models envision the analyst as a static container—receiving, holding, and returning the patient's affect—recursive containment sees the analyst as a participant in an evolving field, shaped as much by her own openness and not-knowing as by any technical intervention. Bion's (1962, 1970a) discipline of negative capability—the willingness to bear confusion, uncertainty, and the absence of meaning—becomes the hallmark of this stance. The analytic atmosphere is not controlled or managed; it is inhabited, sensed, and held open, even when the contents are ambiguous or disturbing.

The ethic that emerges from this recursive stance is one of humility and hospitality toward not-knowing. The analyst does not seek to dominate the field or to impose coherence; instead, she welcomes the indeterminate, the opaque, the as-yet-unformulated. In this sense, containment is not only a psychic act but an ethical one—a discipline of refraining from forced interpretation, premature knowing, or the foreclosure of surprise. The analyst learns to risk the discomfort of her own ignorance, to allow space for the field's unpredictable generativity, and to trust that meaning, if it is to emerge, will do so in its own time.

Crucially, recursive containment is also a relational achievement. Both patient and analyst contribute to the atmosphere, bringing their histories, resistances, vulnerabilities, and openness to being affected. The recursive field is alive with the traces of past analytic hours, the moods and affects that linger across sessions, the echoes of what has not yet found symbolic form. Ogden's (1994) concept of the analytic third comes most fully into view here: the field is a "between" that neither participant owns, yet both co-create and sustain. In recursive containment, the field is allowed to do its work—generating moments of contact, withdrawal, and unexpected movement.

The curvature of psychic space is felt most acutely at these boundaries: the places where the field bends back on itself, where the past repeats as atmosphere, and where the limits of containment are recognized and honored. The analytic field is never a blank slate, nor a linear progression; it is a looping, recursive environment marked by surprise, repetition, and affective weather. The willingness to return—again and again—to what cannot be known, to what resists assimilation, is the very essence of analytic hospitality.

The **ethics of not-knowing** arises in this curved, recursive field. Rather than a posture of resignation or defeat, not-knowing is an active, courageous stance: the analyst and patient together create a space where mystery, opacity, and the unformulated are not rushed or erased but welcomed as part of the field's vitality. Derrida's (2000) hospitality becomes, in the analytic setting, a discipline of staying open to what cannot be predicted or managed—a generosity toward the other's irreducibility, and toward one's own capacity for surprise. The field thus becomes a living demonstration of ethical presence: staying-with, enduring uncertainty, and refraining from colonizing the unknown with explanation or interpretation.

Clinical moments bring this ethic into focus. After months of looping through deadness and silence, a patient, Rosa, brings a sudden, vivid memory: her grandmother's perfume, the warmth of a kitchen in winter, a moment of unspoken comfort. The field shifts; the atmosphere is suddenly fragrant, alive with the possibility of welcome. Yet rather than grasping for meaning or rushing to interpret, I find myself pausing—letting the atmosphere do its work, trusting that what is needed is presence, not mastery. We sit quietly, both sensing the change, both unsure what it will mean. In the days that follow, the field loops back to deadness, then opens again to new images and affects. The recursive discipline is one of patience, humility, and attention to the field's own timing.

This ethic of recursive containment is not without its perils. The analyst may be tempted to "solve" the problem of opacity, to fill silence with words, or to force an opening where the field remains closed. Yet the recursive stance teaches a different discipline: to let surprise, disruption, or even boredom be lived-with, to wait for the field's own curvature to create openings. In this way, recursive containment preserves the dignity of the patient's experience, the other's right to opacity, and the field's capacity for generative movement.

In addition, recursive containment extends beyond the dyad, carrying implications for the wider culture of analytic practice. Supervision, consultation, and analytic training can all become sites of recursive hospitality—places where not-knowing is honored, where the "container" is the field itself, and where the unpredictability of emergence is valued over rigid adherence to theory or protocol. The ethic of recursive containment thus infuses the broader analytic community, modeling a form of symbolic and affective welcome that is generative, flexible, and attuned to difference.

A final note on surprise: the recursive analytic field is perhaps most alive in those moments when something truly unexpected emerges—a new association, a shift in mood, a sudden sense of recognition or contact. These surprises are not engineered; they are invitations, generated by the recursive discipline of staying-with, waiting, and welcoming what the field brings forth. In this way, the analytic hour becomes not just a site of containment, but a laboratory for creativity, emergence, and the birth of new forms of meaning.

In summary, recursive containment is less an act than an atmosphere, less a technique than an ethic. It is the discipline of staying-with: looping through openness and closure, honoring the limits of hospitality, and welcoming the unknown as the condition for psychic transformation. The curved, recursive field of analysis becomes a space where self and other, knowing and unknowing, are held together—not in static containment, but in the dynamic atmosphere of surprise, hospitality, and the ongoing play of emergence.

Closing Reflection—Hospitality, Limits, and the Generativity of the Field

As this chapter draws to a close, the recursive logic of introjection and containment reconfigures what it means to practice psychoanalysis—not as a linear technique for integrating the other, but as a field-based, ethically attuned discipline of hospitality, humility, and surprise. Throughout the preceding sections, we have traced a movement from classical models of taking-in and metabolizing, through the recursive reversals of psychic hospitality, to the existential and ethical boundaries where opacity, deadness, and the uncontainable other shape the analytic hour.

The heart of this reimagining is not a repudiation of the classical frame, but its recursive transformation. What begins as a question—How do we take in the other?—becomes, in the atmosphere of analytic hospitality, a living inquiry: how do we dwell together in the unfinalizable field of psychic difference, surprise, and refusal? The answer is not a technique, but a stance: a recursive discipline of staying-with, of returning again and again to the field's limits, openings, failures, and emergent surprises.

Hospitality in the analytic field is never absolute; it is always provisional, shaped by the capacity and willingness of both analyst and patient to risk being changed, surprised, and even wounded by what cannot be assimilated. To welcome the other—whether as projection, affect, or enigmatic signifier—is to grant a space for difference that may not be resolved, digested, or made fully one's own. The analytic field's true vitality is found in these recursive movements: the opening and closing of contact, the looping through deadness and renewal, the repeated invitation to surprise.

The **limits of hospitality** are not obstacles to be overcome, but necessary conditions for the work of analysis. The patient's resistance, the analyst's failures, the zones of opacity or uncontainability—all these are not marks of analytic deficiency, but the atmosphere in which real transformation can occur. It is only in risking the acknowledgment of what cannot be known, taken in, or symbolized that the analytic pair finds their way to new forms of relation. In this sense, the right to opacity, to psychic deadness, and to unassimilable difference is an ethical cornerstone—not only protecting the dignity of the other, but also sustaining the generativity of the analytic field.

This generativity is, above all, **atmospheric and recursive**. The most profound changes in analysis often occur not through acts of will or insight, but through the unpredictable emergence of new psychic weather—a shift in mood, a return of feeling, a sudden image or dream. These surprises arise from the recursive discipline of hospitality: the shared willingness to stay with what is, to bear what cannot be contained, and to allow the field to generate new forms on its own terms. The analyst and patient do not create these moments by force; they participate in a field where surprise, affect, and meaning can appear, be welcomed, and sometimes slip away.

The recursive field, then, is not a site of mastery but of humility. It is a space where analyst and patient alike must relinquish fantasies of omnipotence, control, or perfect understanding. Each act of introjection, containment, or hospitality is always incomplete, always subject to revision, return, or refusal. The analyst's ethic is not to solve the problem of the other, but to remain open, porous, and willing to be affected, even—especially—by what cannot be assimilated. This discipline of humility is itself generative: it makes room for surprise, for new forms of being-together, and for the unpredictable creativity of the analytic field.

The closing reflection is itself a recursive gesture—a looping return to the central motifs of this chapter, each time with a slightly different inflection, shaped by what has transpired in the atmosphere of writing and reading. This recursive movement enacts the very ethic it describes: a willingness to risk repetition, to stay with what remains unresolved, and to allow the field's limits to become sites of new possibility. In analytic work, as in life, the most fertile ground is often found not in final knowing, but in the ongoing practice of welcoming what comes, bearing what cannot be borne, and remaining present to the unpredictable play of difference and return.

Looking ahead, the recursive logic of hospitality, limits, and field generativity reframes all the subsequent concepts of psychoanalysis—fantasy, destruction, reparation, aggression—not as stable structures, but as dynamic processes, always looping back, always transforming in the presence of the other. The analytic field is never closed, never completed; it is a living, recursive space where new meanings, affects, and forms of relation can be risked, welcomed, and sometimes lost.

In closing, the analytic ethic is not to strive for a final integration of the other, nor to banish opacity or deadness from the field. Rather, it is to accompany the other, to honor the unpredictable movements of the analytic atmosphere, and to trust that what cannot be contained may, in its own time, become a site of welcome, surprise, and renewal. The recursive field, with all its risks and refusals, is not a detour from analytic work, but its very heart—the atmosphere in which both analyst and patient can find themselves changed by what arrives, and by what can never be fully taken in.

Chapter 6

Fantasy as Recursive Field—Atmosphere, Emergence, and the Ethics of Not-Knowing

This chapter reimagines fantasy not as a solitary wish or defensive fiction, but as a recursive field: an atmosphere of symbolic transmission, affective play, and creative emergence that animates the analytic situation. Moving beyond the classical dichotomy of fantasy versus reality, this chapter explores how fantasy loops through the analytic field—structuring and destabilizing knowing, mediating the unformulated, and inviting both analyst and patient into ongoing symbolic co-creation. Drawing on Freud, Winnicott, Lacan, Bollas, Bromberg, Eigen, Green, Ferro, Civitarese, and Benjamin, this chapter shows how fantasy's recursive structure both sustains and unsettles the analytic process. Through clinical vignettes and theoretical reflection, it articulates an ethic of not-knowing—a discipline of analytic presence that holds open the possibility for reversal, surprise, and psychic transformation. In this recursive, field-based approach, fantasy becomes not a barrier to reality but the very medium through which the analytic field remains alive, generative, and open to new forms of psychic life.

The Classical Frame—Fantasy as Wish and Defense

Fantasy, in the classical psychoanalytic canon, is both the engine of psychic life and the guardian of its mysteries. Freud's earliest clinical writings are saturated with the presence of fantasy—phantasy, in the British spelling that would later distinguish Melanie Klein's contribution. From the primal scene to the daydream, fantasy stands at the threshold of desire and defense, endlessly reworking what can be wished, known, or suffered.

For Freud, fantasy was first and foremost a matter of wish-fulfillment. The 1900 publication of *The Interpretation of Dreams* marks the scene: dreams, like daydreams and neurotic symptoms, are the disguised fulfillment of unconscious wishes (Freud, 1900/1953). The logic of fantasy is

DOI: 10.4324/9781003747109-9

both compensatory and creative. What reality cannot provide, fantasy supplies—first in the veiled form of the dream, then in more elaborate, conscious reverie. The neurotic, said Freud, "builds castles in the air"—the daydream as compromise between forbidden desire and psychic censorship.

Yet fantasy was never merely an escape from reality; it was also a site of compromise, negotiation, and defense. In *Formulations on the Two Principles of Mental Functioning* (Freud, 1911/1958), Freud describes the emergence of fantasy as a psychic adaptation: when reality fails to satisfy, the mind generates fantasies to sustain desire and regulate disappointment. The child's early, omnipotent wishes—fantasies of mastery, reunion, or revenge—are gradually modulated by reality-testing, yet fantasy life persists, reshaped by the demands of the external world and the internal dictates of the superego.

As psychoanalytic theory developed, fantasy's role became both more central and more ambiguous. In *A Child is Being Beaten* (Freud, 1919/1955), Freud observed that the structure of fantasy is itself layered: the same scene may be repeated, revised, and reenacted across the span of development, accruing new meanings and defenses at each iteration. Fantasy is not simply a repository of forbidden wishes, but a theater in which the drama of self and other, love and aggression, is continually played out. The "primal fantasies"—of the primal scene, seduction, and castration—are, Freud argued, universal psychic structures: myths that organize subjectivity, regardless of the individual's actual experience (Freud, 1918/1955, 1919/1955).

The epistemic status of fantasy, even for Freud, remained uncertain. Fantasies are both true and not-true, anchored in desire but often divorced from external reality. They bear a relation to the unconscious that is at once expressive and defensive: they reveal what cannot otherwise be known, but always in disguise. In the *Wolf Man* case, Freud famously oscillated between interpreting the patient's primal scene as a historical event and as an expression of universal fantasy (Freud, 1918/1955). The analyst's task, in the classical frame, is to interpret fantasy—to render its meaning conscious, to trace its origins in lived experience or infantile desire, and to help the patient distinguish between internal and external reality.

British analysts would take up the ambiguity of fantasy and radicalize it. Susan Isaacs (1948) famously insisted that unconscious *phantasy* is the continuous mental representation of instinct. Building on this, Hanna Segal (1957) clarified how symbol formation depends on the transformation of unconscious phantasy into representational thought, while reserving "fantasy" for conscious daydreams and stories. This distinction, while subtle, has profound implications: fantasy is not only a defense against reality, but the very medium through which reality is experienced, interpreted, and symbolically reworked.

For Melanie Klein (1946/1975), unconscious phantasy is the foundation of psychic structure itself. The infant's relation to the breast, the mother, the world, is always already mediated by phantasy—by imagined scenes of attack, fusion, loss, and reparation. Phantasy is at once bodily and symbolic: the sucking of the breast is inseparable from the fantasy of taking in goodness, or from the terror of being invaded by envy or destruction. Klein's world is peopled by part-objects, animated and organized by unconscious phantasy. Psychic reality, in this frame, is constituted as much by phantasy as by perception.

Klein's emphasis on the reality of phantasy led to a new appreciation of its epistemic ambiguity. Phantasy is not "false" in the ordinary sense; it is the "reality" of the psyche, structuring experience, meaning, and even identity. The child's fantasy of the bad breast is not simply an error, but a living, affectively charged reality—one that organizes anxiety, defense, and the patterns of relating that persist throughout life. For Klein, as for Isaacs and Segal, the analyst's task is not merely to "correct" fantasy but to enter its world, to bear witness to its force, and to help the patient symbolize and transform its power.

The classical literature thus locates fantasy at the heart of both knowing and not-knowing. Fantasy allows the psyche to process and manage experiences that are overwhelming, forbidden, or unsymbolizable. It is a defense, but also a generative principle—a way of creating psychic space for desire, mourning, aggression, and play. At the same time, fantasy can serve to obscure, disguise, or fixate: it can become a closed loop, a defense against the very realities it was designed to process.

In clinical practice, fantasy is everywhere. Patients bring dreams, stories, images, and private reveries—fantasies of triumph, seduction, punishment, rescue, or annihilation. The analyst listens for the wishes, fears, and unconscious meanings embedded in these productions, interpreting their symbolic logic and tracing their links to childhood or transference. Yet even the most sensitive interpretation cannot fully resolve the paradox of fantasy: it is at once a truth and a fiction, a vehicle for knowing and for refusing to know.

This tension is especially acute in the analytic situation itself. The transference-countertransference field is saturated with fantasy: the patient's expectations of the analyst, the analyst's reverie, the shared creation of meaning and atmosphere. Fantasy is the medium of analytic play, but also the ground of misunderstanding, misrecognition, and resistance. The analytic hour thus becomes a site where fantasy is lived, enacted, and sometimes transformed—but never wholly mastered.

In sum, the classical frame establishes fantasy as the psychic space of wish and defense, of knowing and not-knowing. It is the scene where desire is staged, disguised, and negotiated; where the self is both revealed and concealed. The recursive, looping quality of fantasy—its capacity to return, shift, and transform—remains latent but untheorized. In the sections that follow, we will trace how this classical inheritance is inverted and expanded, as fantasy becomes a recursive field, an atmosphere, and a principle of epistemic and symbolic reversal.

The Inversion—Fantasy as Field and Recursive Loop

The classical model established fantasy as a largely intrapsychic theater—a stage for wish and defense, populated by private dramas and symbolic actors. Yet, as psychoanalytic thought evolved, so too did the understanding of fantasy's topography and structure. The notion that fantasy unfolds solely within the boundaries of the self has been repeatedly challenged by developments in field theory, relational psychoanalysis, and the study of analytic process itself (Baranger & Baranger, 2008). In these contemporary currents, fantasy emerges not as a private script but as a recursive, co-constructed field—an atmosphere of shared and shifting meanings that permeates the analytic encounter.

Thomas Ogden (1994) stands as a pivotal figure in this shift. In his work on the "analytic third," Ogden described how patient and analyst do not simply exchange fantasies but together generate a third, emergent psychic space—a symbolic field in which new forms of experience, meaning, and play can arise. This "analytic third" is not owned by either party; it is the field itself, animated by the recursive movement of fantasy, affect, and reverie. The field becomes the locus of transformation, surprise, and recursive return: what was private fantasy becomes a shared atmosphere, a space in which self and other, knowing and unknowing, are continually negotiated.

Wilfred Bion (1962) anticipated aspects of this shift with his concept of "reverie." For Bion, the analyst's receptive, dream-like state is a medium for the patient's unconscious phantasy life to be contained, metabolized, and returned in new symbolic forms. The analytic setting is thus an atmospheric field, charged with unconscious transmissions and recursive loops. The analyst does not merely interpret fantasy from a distance; she enters the field and becomes part of the recursive circulation of affect, image, and meaning.

The Italian field theorists, notably Antonino Ferro and Giuseppe Civitarese (2016), have made the recursive, field-based nature of fantasy central to their approach. They describe the analytic session as a "field of dreaming," a zone in which patient and analyst co-create a narrative, a mood, and an affective atmosphere that is at once shared and ungraspable. The field is suffused with unconscious fantasy—not just as content, but as process, as weather, as the very texture of analytic presence. Here, fantasy is no longer only the property of the patient's mind but an emergent property of the analytic dyad—a recursive play of meanings that takes shape in the between.

What emerges from these developments is an inversion of the classical fantasy paradigm. Rather than treating fantasy as an inner theater to be deciphered, the analytic stance shifts toward participating in, and witnessing, the recursive field. Meaning arises in the play of resonance, echo, and return. The analyst's reverie, the patient's free association, the shared dream-like mood of the session—all are elements of a field in which fantasy loops between subjects, generating both surprise and repetition, rupture and renewal.

Crucially, this recursive field is not static. It is animated by affective and symbolic currents that double back, shift, and reformulate. A fantasy first articulated by the patient may be metabolized in the analyst's reverie, returned as an image or mood, and then reworked by the patient in a new story or dream. These loops are not mere repetitions; they are creative recursions—movements that can generate new meaning, insight, or forms of experience that would be impossible for either party alone.

This shift to a recursive field also destabilizes the traditional distinction between conscious and unconscious fantasy. In the analytic field, fantasies are not always spoken; they are felt, enacted, atmospherically transmitted. Michael Eigen (1999) describes the analytic encounter as a field of the between—a psychic climate in which both analyst and patient are continually surprised by what emerges. This atmospheric looping aligns with Buchholz's (2019) account of how therapeutic dialogue generates new symbolic possibilities through recursive sequences of speaking and hearing. Fantasy becomes an event, an atmosphere, a force that shapes the session even in silence or confusion. The recursive play of fantasy is thus experienced as mood, tension, symbolic image, or even as a kind of collective dream.

This perspective finds resonance in the writing of Ogden (2005), who highlights the analytic session as a space of "undreamt dreams"—phantasies that have not yet been articulated, but that circulate in the atmosphere between analyst and patient. These "undreamt dreams" are recursive: they appear and reappear in shifting forms, awaiting symbolization. The analyst's task, in this field, is less to interpret and more to attune—to participate in the recursive flow, to sense the symbolic weather, to hold open the space in which new forms of fantasy may be dreamed into being.

The recursive structure of fantasy is also evident in the phenomenon of "shared fantasy." In some analytic dyads, a particular theme or image will recur, shifting in form or affective valence as it is played with by both participants. A patient's fantasy of abandonment, for example, may be echoed in the analyst's reverie as a dream of exile and then return in the session as a shared feeling of absence or longing. These recursions are not accidents; they are the field's way of metabolizing unformulated experience, generating symbolic life out of what was previously unthinkable.

This recursive, field-based view does not eliminate the defensive function of fantasy, but it complicates it. Fantasies can serve as defenses—loops that protect against contact, that stabilize anxiety or shame—but they can also serve as bridges, invitations to new experience, or as means of creative surprise. The field is never neutral; it is charged with risk, aliveness, and the unpredictable emergence of meaning. What is most vital is the analyst's capacity to stay with the recursive loops, to resist the pressure for premature closure, and to accompany the patient as new symbolic possibilities take shape.

In practice, the recursive field can be sensed in the changing weather of the analytic hour: moments of clarity and confusion, sudden shifts in mood, images that reverberate for both patient and analyst. Sometimes the field feels saturated—thick with unsymbolized feeling; other times, it feels porous, alive with the potential for play. The recursive movement of fantasy animates the field, generating new forms of contact, difference, and symbolic hospitality.

The ethics of this stance are profound. The analyst does not claim to know the meaning of every fantasy, nor does she seek to master the field. Instead, she inhabits the recursive atmosphere, bearing witness to what emerges, allowing for surprise, rupture, and transformation. This discipline of attunement—of recursive presence—replaces the fantasy of interpretation with the hospitality of the field. Meaning, in this register, is always provisional, always open to further looping and return.

In sum, the inversion of the classical fantasy paradigm reveals fantasy not as a private escape but as the very substance of analytic atmosphere—a recursive, co-constructed field in which self and other, knowing and unknowing, are continually produced and undone. The analytic hour becomes an experiment in living with recursivity: an invitation to dwell in the loops, to bear the surprises and anxieties of unknowing, and to trust in the generativity of the symbolic field.

Fantasy, Reality, and the Ethics of Unknowing

Fantasy has always troubled the boundaries between reality and imagination, presence and absence, knowing and not-knowing. In the classical frame, as we have seen, fantasy occupies an ambiguous position: it is both a psychic compromise and a creative act, a defense against suffering and a mode of symbolization. But as psychoanalytic thinking has become more attuned to the recursive, field-based structure of fantasy, the distinction between fantasy and reality grows increasingly porous. Rather than serving as a mere screen for unfulfilled wishes or unintegrated traumas, fantasy emerges as an ongoing, co-constructed event—one that both sustains and unsettles psychic life and demands an ethics of analytic presence rooted in not-knowing.

The analytic encounter is suffused with the force of fantasy—not only the patient's, but the analyst's as well. Each session is a living experiment in negotiating reality and fantasy: stories are told, images emerge, affects surge and recede, often in ways neither party can fully anticipate or control. The analytic field becomes a liminal space, suspended between the "real" and the "fantastic," in which old dramas are revived, new scenes are imagined, and the boundaries between what "actually happened" and what is psychically real blur. The recursive atmosphere of fantasy is thickest precisely at those moments when what is "known" feels unstable, when the analyst's own certainties falter and something new begins to take shape in the gap between experience and interpretation.

Freud's early awareness of this ambiguity is striking. In his analysis of the Wolf Man, Freud (1918/1955) admits to a persistent uncertainty: was the patient's primal scene a real memory, or a fantasy constructed to organize his suffering? Freud's answer is, ultimately, both evasive and profound. He concludes that the truth of fantasy is not reducible to historical fact; its psychic reality is formative, shaping not only symptom and suffering but the very contours of identity. This recognition, sometimes lost in the drive for clinical "truth," anticipates the later analytic focus on the recursive play between fantasy and reality as a site of transformation.

As analytic theory evolved, this paradox deepened. Donald Winnicott (1971) famously explored the "transitional space"—the zone between inner and outer reality, where play, creativity, and symbolization arise. Fantasy, in Winnicott's view, is not an escape from reality but a vital, intermediate area of experience, a space in which the self can safely experiment, imagine, and risk surprise. This transitional space is inherently recursive: the child's play loops between the real and the imagined, the found and the created, generating a symbolic world in which both self and other can come alive in new ways. For Winnicott, the analyst's role is to protect and inhabit this space of potentiality, not to foreclose it by demanding final truths or definitive interpretations.

Jacques Lacan, in *Seminar VII: The Ethics of Psychoanalysis* (1992/2008), also insists on the recursive, looping nature of fantasy. For Lacan, fantasy is the screen that structures desire; it organizes the subject's sense of what is possible or forbidden, known or unknowable, and his "ethic of desire"—to not give ground on one's desire—asks the analyst to sustain the loop rather than foreclose it. The analyst's interpretation, in this frame, is always at risk of becoming another fantasy, another screen. Lacan's "ethic of desire" is thus paradoxically an ethic of limit: the analyst is called to sustain the loop, to "not give ground" on the radical openness of the field, and to allow the fantasy to circulate, to transform, and sometimes to reveal its own emptiness.

In the contemporary clinical situation, these themes come alive in the moment-to-moment work of analysis. Consider the patient who brings a dream, vivid and disorienting, in which the analyst appears as a menacing figure—authoritative, withholding, or perhaps secretly benevolent. The temptation for the analyst is to interpret: to anchor the dream in the patient's history, to explain its origins, to offer clarity. Yet often what is most powerful is to allow the dream to resonate in the field, to let its fantasy life unfold recursively, shifting meaning and affect over time. The analyst's willingness to "not know"—to refrain from closure, to resist the fantasy of omniscience—is itself a form of ethical containment, a discipline that holds open the space for surprise, ambiguity, and psychic growth.

Jessica Benjamin (2018) deepens this ethic in her work on mutual recognition. Fantasy, for Benjamin, is always at risk of collapse into domination or misunderstanding: the analyst's unconscious fantasy life can become entangled with the patient's, generating loops of enactment, resistance, or even impasse. Yet it is precisely in the willingness to dwell with these recursive patterns, to notice and reflect on the misrecognitions and misunderstandings, that new forms of relational knowing can emerge. The analyst's task is not to master the field, but to accompany the patient in the recursive movement of fantasy—bearing witness to the uncertainty, the emergent meanings, and the potential for transformation that arise in the space between knowing and not-knowing.

Michael Eigen (1999) offers a kindred perspective. He describes the analytic encounter as a space of "shared madness," in which patient and analyst risk entering each other's fantasies—not as delusions to be corrected, but as creative spaces to be explored. For Eigen, the field of analytic presence is animated by recursive transmissions: moods, images, and fantasies that move between participants, sometimes without words. The analyst's containment is less about explanation and more about presence—a willingness to bear, to "hold," and to dwell in the uncertainty that fantasy generates. The discipline of not-knowing, for Eigen, is not a passive withdrawal but an active receptivity to surprise, rupture, and emergence.

The ethics of not-knowing becomes most vital at those moments when fantasy and reality threaten to collapse into each other, when the difference between the two seems momentarily unsustainable. A patient who insists, with conviction, that the analyst is angry, bored, or secretly critical, may be voicing both an unconscious fantasy and an attuned perception. The analyst's task is not to hastily clarify or deny, but to inquire: "What is it like to feel that I am angry?"; "How does that belief come alive in the room between us?"; "What possibilities open when we dwell with this fantasy together?" This approach honors both the psychic reality of fantasy and the unpredictable generativity of the analytic field.

The recursive structure of fantasy also complicates the work of interpretation. The analyst's own fantasies—about the patient, the process, the possibility of healing—are always in play, shaping and being shaped by the field. This mutual, recursive entanglement can be a source of difficulty or confusion, but it is also a site of creative potential. When the analyst is able to reflect on her own fantasies, to bring them into the light of the analytic hour, the field becomes more hospitable to ambiguity, difference, and transformation.

At the same time, there are ethical dangers. The analyst who interprets too quickly, who demands resolution or mastery, risks foreclosing the space of fantasy, imposing their own meanings where ambiguity is most needed. This is a form of analytic violence: the refusal of surprise, the closing of the recursive loop. The ethics of unknowing, by contrast, is an ethic of patience, humility, and symbolic hospitality—a willingness to accompany the patient in the looping, recursive journey of fantasy, without insisting on arrival.

This ethic is not without risk or pain. There are times when the recursive play of fantasy is experienced as confusion, stuckness, or even despair. Analyst and patient may feel lost together, unsure how to proceed, gripped by the sense that meaning has stalled or that nothing new can emerge. Yet even here, the discipline of not-knowing can be sustaining: the willingness to linger in the discomfort, to trust in the generativity of the field, to bear witness to the possibility of surprise. The analytic hour becomes a space of ongoing experiment, a field in which fantasy loops and unloops, generating new forms of experience, relation, and symbolic life.

Ultimately, the porous boundary between fantasy and reality is not a flaw but a resource—a site of creative potential, ethical engagement, and recursive emergence. The analyst who learns to dwell in the loop, to inhabit the space of not-knowing, becomes a companion in the ongoing, unpredictable work of psychic transformation. Fantasy is no longer only a defense or escape, but the field in which the self and the other, the real and the imagined, are continually remade.

Fantasy and the Limits of Interpretation

If the analytic field is thick with fantasy—shifting, looping, resisting closure—then the practice of interpretation must also confront its own limits. Classical psychoanalysis often casts interpretation as the royal road to psychic truth: the analyst, with disciplined attention, deciphers the code of fantasy and reveals its latent meaning. To interpret is to illuminate the unconscious, dissolve the veils of phantasy, and move the patient toward greater reality-testing and self-knowledge. Yet, as our recursive frame has already suggested, the fantasy of interpretation itself can become another loop—one that risks foreclosing the very generativity, play, and surprise that fantasy enables.

Freud's ambivalence about the power of interpretation is present from the beginning. While his early model placed great weight on making the unconscious conscious through interpretation, Freud (1937/1964) later described the analyst's work as an "endless approximation"—an activity that can never fully grasp or exhaust the complexity of psychic life. Dreams, symptoms, and fantasies yield to interpretation, only to generate new forms, new symptoms, new riddles. The analyst is always at risk of being seduced by the illusion of mastery, of "solving" the riddle once and for all, even as the unconscious invents new disguises. The recursive return of fantasy is thus both the object of analytic work and the limit of interpretation's reach.

Contemporary theorists have elaborated these limits, emphasizing the ways in which interpretation itself can become a fantasy—a defense against uncertainty, ambiguity, or the analyst's own anxieties. Thomas Ogden (2005) writes that every interpretation contains within it the analyst's unconscious fantasy life: what the analyst sees, what is named or not named, is shaped by her own histories, countertransference, and symbolic investments. Interpretation is thus a double-edged sword: it can clarify, but it can also impose, limit, or even obscure. The patient's fantasy life is never merely an object to be interpreted; it is a living, shifting presence, animated by the recursive interplay of both participants' desires, fears, and creative energies.

Sometimes, the analytic process becomes stuck precisely because of interpretation's limits. A patient's fantasy is named—"You wish to destroy me because I am experienced as a rival for your mother's love"—but the affect does not shift. The loop persists. The field feels heavy, inert, as if the interpretation itself has become a defense: a way of pinning down what needs to remain in play. The urge to interpret, to *get it right*, can foreclose the more vital work of staying-with, of letting fantasy loop and return until it is metabolized in a new way.

This phenomenon is evident in moments of "wild psycho-analysis"—a term Freud (1910/1957) used to describe analysts who interpret too eagerly, too omnisciently, without sufficient attunement to the timing, affect, or relational context. The fantasy here is not only the patient's but also the analyst's: a fantasy of rescue, mastery, or authority, enacted through premature or overly elaborate interpretations. Such interventions often miss the field's recursive reality, where what is most transformative is not the analyst's brilliance, but the shared capacity to dwell in unknowing, to tolerate tension, and to bear the uncertainties that fantasy generates.

The field perspective, in contrast, invites a different discipline. The analyst learns to sense the symbolic weather: when the field is ripe for interpretation, when silence or reverie is more generative, when to risk naming, and when to let the loop return. Interpretation is reimagined as a creative, participatory act—one that emerges from the recursive play of affect, image, and shared reverie, rather than from the analyst's authority alone. The patient's fantasy is not a puzzle to be solved but an atmosphere to be inhabited, a movement to be accompanied.

A clinical illustration may clarify this process. Consider a patient, Eli, who recurrently dreams of losing his way in a vast library—corridors of unread books, dimly lit passageways, voices echoing from unseen rooms. Each dream session, Eli brings new details, yet the core feeling remains: confusion, curiosity, longing for an answer that is never quite revealed. The analytic hour takes on a similar texture; Eli circles the question of "what it means," but each interpretation seems to lead only to further recursion. "Maybe the library is your mind," I offer once, "and the unread books are parts of yourself you haven't discovered." Eli nods, but the field remains thick with uncertainty.

Over weeks, I notice my own urge to solve the riddle, to supply a master interpretation that will break the loop. But each effort to do so only intensifies the recursion; the dream returns, with new variations, and the analytic process feels suspended. I shift my stance: rather than seeking resolution, I begin to wonder with Eli about the experience itself. "What's it like to wander through the library, not knowing what you'll find?" I ask. Eli hesitates, then begins to describe the sensation of searching, the pleasure of possibility, the anxiety of endlessness. The field shifts; the atmosphere becomes lighter, more playful, as if the dream's power lies not in its answer, but in its invitation to explore.

This shift illustrates the limits of interpretation and the generativity of recursive engagement. The analyst's willingness to remain in the loop—to join the patient in the wandering, the not-knowing—opens the field to new meanings, affects, and forms of play. The fantasy becomes less a symptom to be decoded and more a landscape to be inhabited together. Sometimes, a wordless understanding or a moment of shared laughter does more than any brilliant interpretation: it marks a change in the field, an emergent recognition that cannot be fully articulated or pinned down.

Other clinical moments illustrate the dangers of interpretive foreclosure. In a case presented by Ferro and Civitarese (2016), the analyst's repeated attempts to link the patient's fantasy life to early trauma are met with increasing resistance and withdrawal. The patient begins to experience the analytic space as stifling, his fantasies flattened or pathologized rather than explored. Only when the analyst shifts from an interpretive to a "dreaming together" stance does the field open again: the analytic process regains its aliveness, and the patient's fantasy life can be played with, not simply explained.

The recursive, field-based view also acknowledges that interpretation is itself a fantasy—one that organizes the analyst's experience, sustains her hope for change, and sometimes protects against the discomfort of uncertainty. The analyst's interpretations are products of her own mind, shaped by her history, training, and unconscious investments. To recognize this is not to abandon interpretation, but to practice it more reflexively, with humility and openness to surprise. The analyst's willingness to reflect on her own interpretive fantasies—the need to know, to fix, to heal—becomes a vital resource in sustaining the analytic field as a site of unknowing and emergence.

In some sessions, the limits of interpretation are felt as a loss—a mourning for the fantasy of mastery, of analytic omnipotence. Yet in relinquishing the drive to interpret, a new freedom may be found. The analytic field becomes a site of encounter, not only with the patient's suffering but also with the unpredictable, creative, and symbolic life of the psyche itself. The loop of fantasy is not something to be conquered but a movement to be trusted, an invitation to dwell together in the unfinished, the recursive, and the not-yet-known.

This approach does not mean abandoning all interpretation or analytic activity. Rather, it calls for a discipline of timing, attunement, and hospitality—a willingness to let fantasy circulate, to sense when the field is ready for intervention, and to allow for periods of silence, return, or surprise. The most powerful interpretations are often those that arise naturally from the recursive field: an image that resonates for both, a shared reverie, a question that opens rather than closes. These moments do not deliver the patient to reality; they invite both participants into deeper contact with the symbolic, the affective, and the creative.

The ethics of this stance are demanding. The analyst must tolerate the anxiety of not knowing, the discomfort of waiting, and the risk of being wrong or misunderstood. Yet it is precisely this discipline that opens the analytic field to true transformation. Fantasy is not a riddle to be solved but a companion on the analytic journey—its loops, returns, and surprises marking the path of psychic growth.

In the recursive, field-based model, the limits of interpretation become resources, not failures. The analyst's humility, patience, and symbolic attunement make space for the fantasy life of both patient and analyst to be lived, explored, and played with. The analytic hour is no longer a march toward resolution, but a dance with the unknown—a recursive, generative movement in which fantasy finds its form, loses it, and finds it again.

Clinical Vignette—Fantasy as Recursive Field

It is midwinter, and the city outside is enveloped in a dense, metallic quiet. The windows of my office collect condensation as dusk falls early, thickening the boundary between the analytic space and the world beyond. Mara arrives with a shiver—her coat held tightly, as if bracing herself against more than just the cold. Her sessions have for months been marked by a recurring texture: looping stories of disappointment and longing, flashes of magical hope, and an undercurrent of restless ambivalence toward me and the analytic process itself.

Mara's opening words are both plaintive and slightly performative: "Sometimes I wonder if you're really here with me, or just watching, waiting for me to tell the right story." The question is both direct and, I sense, rehearsed—a familiar overture in the symphony of our work. Yet the affect in the room feels newly charged, a kind of low-grade static electricity that hints at something emergent.

We settle into silence, which grows heavy and then curiously light, as if the gravity of the analytic hour is shifting, seeking a new center. I notice in myself a subtle longing—for Mara to break the pattern, to bring something startlingly new. I realize, with a twinge, that I am caught in the same recursive hope as she is: waiting for transformation, for a new chapter in our analytic narrative.

After several minutes, Mara begins to speak about a recurring daydream.

> It's always the same: I'm walking through a house that's both familiar and strange. There are endless corridors and closed doors. I hear music coming from somewhere, sometimes a piano, sometimes a distant radio. I keep opening doors, hoping to find the source, but each room is empty. The only thing that changes is the light—sometimes golden, sometimes cold, sometimes everything is cast in shadow.

As she speaks, the atmosphere in the room thickens, as if the analytic field is absorbing the imagery, lending the fantasy its own gravity. I find myself drawn into her daydream, images of labyrinthine passageways flickering behind my eyelids. I notice a subtle resonance between Mara's experience and my own—my wish for analytic progress echoing her search for the source of the music.

I ask, "What's it like to keep searching, to open each door and find only light or shadow?" Mara looks thoughtful.

> It's frustrating, but it's also…strangely comforting. The house feels alive. Even though I never find what I'm looking for, I keep going. Sometimes I think the music is moving away from me on purpose. Sometimes it feels like you're the music—just out of reach, but always present.

This admission brings a new warmth to the room. The boundary between her fantasy and our analytic relationship grows porous. I sense that Mara is offering not just a narrative, but an atmosphere—a recursive field in which her longing, my presence, and our shared not-knowing swirl together. My own reverie is now animated by echoes of childhood memories: wandering my own childhood home at dusk, searching for the sound of a parent, the comfort of a familiar voice. The recursive structure is palpable; Mara's fantasy becomes our shared mood, looping through both our psychic fields.

As the sessions unfold in subsequent weeks, Mara's daydream recurs, morphs, and returns. Sometimes the music is louder, sometimes there are shadows that frighten her, sometimes a door opens onto a sunlit garden, but she is unable to step outside. My countertransference is equally fluid. At times I feel bored or impatient, as if we are circling the same unresolved theme. At other times, I am suffused with a kind of analytic awe—a sense that something new is gathering, that the field is quietly reorganizing itself in the very act of repetition.

One afternoon, Mara arrives in a mood of bright irritation.

> I had a dream last night. I was playing hide and seek with a group of children in a vast building. Every time I found a hiding place, someone else would take it over, and I'd have to keep moving. Eventually I hid behind a velvet curtain and felt safe, but then I realized everyone else had left. I was alone, but I could hear you in another room, playing the piano. I wanted to come out and join you, but I was afraid I'd be invisible.

I listen, struck by the dream's recursive architecture: the looping movement through rooms and roles, the search for contact, the oscillation between presence and absence. The motif of the piano returns, now explicitly linked to me. Mara's fantasy, far from being static, is alive, looping, and improvisational, its meaning continually reworked by the field.

I refrain from immediate interpretation. Instead, I wonder aloud, "What's it like to hear the piano, to know I'm there but to feel invisible?" Mara's face softens. "It's lonely, but it's also… familiar. I think I want you to find me, but I'm hiding too well. Or maybe I want to stay hidden, so I can keep listening."

The recursive play between visibility and concealment, searching and waiting, becomes the atmosphere of our sessions. There is no master narrative, no final interpretation. Instead, the field becomes a site of symbolic play—fantasy as a principle of relation and emergence rather than defense alone.

My own analytic presence is transformed in this recursive process. At times, I notice myself wanting to "rescue" Mara from her loop, to deliver an interpretation that would break the cycle. But each time I resist, something shifts: Mara risks more, brings new images, voices her frustrations and her pleasures in the analytic field. We begin to comment on the very texture of the analytic hour—how our mutual longings, disappointments, and fantasies move between us, sometimes clearly spoken, sometimes barely perceptible.

Midway through this period, Mara brings another dream:

> I'm in a room filled with mirrors. Every mirror shows me at a different age—sometimes a child, sometimes an old woman. You're there too, but your reflection changes every time I look. Sometimes you're smiling, sometimes you look worried, sometimes you disappear completely. I keep moving between mirrors, trying to find the 'real' me, but the images keep shifting.

We spend several sessions exploring this dream, not as a code to be cracked, but as a recursive field of possibilities. I notice the temptation to interpret—"perhaps the shifting images reflect your uncertainty about self and other, about your sense of being seen"—but instead, I ask, "Is there a mirror you like best? Or one you avoid?" Mara laughs. "The ones where you're smiling. They make me feel safe, but also suspicious—like I'm missing something." We dwell in this ambiguity, honoring the recursive movement of comfort and mistrust, the field's play of recognition and doubt.

The analytic atmosphere thickens and thins, moves and pauses, as we return again and again to these images. Mara begins to bring fragments of other fantasies—brief, flickering reveries in which she is both audience and performer, witness and secret-keeper. She notices patterns in our work: "Sometimes I think I'm telling you the same story over and over, but each time it feels a little different." I echo her, "Yes, it seems like the story is always returning, but always changing, too." Our analytic space becomes a site of looping, recursive emergence—fantasy not as a closed circuit, but as a field of continual transformation.

In one particularly charged session, Mara says,

> It's strange, but I don't want to know the answer anymore. I used to hope you'd tell me what it all means, but now I just want to keep exploring. It's like the house in my daydream—the music is always moving, and maybe that's the point.

I feel a rush of gratitude for her trust in the process, and I realize that the recursive play of fantasy has opened a new dimension in our work. The field is more hospitable, more alive; the anxiety of not-knowing has been transmuted into curiosity and creative engagement.

Looking back, what stands out is not a linear progression or a single, clarifying interpretation, but a series of recursive loops—fantasies that return and shift, moods that animate the analytic hour, images that gain and lose meaning as the field evolves. The analyst's discipline is to stay with the loop, to resist premature closure, to witness the field's capacity for surprise and symbolic play.

This vignette enacts the central thesis of this chapter: fantasy, far from being merely defensive or regressive, is the recursive field in which new subjectivities, meanings, and forms of relation come into being. The analyst's role is less to decode than to accompany, to dwell with the recursive, looping movements of the field, and to trust that transformation may arise in the very heart of not-knowing.

As Mara's analysis continues, the recursive structure endures. Fantasies return in new forms, the music of her daydreams remains elusive but generative, and our analytic field becomes ever more capable of holding difference, surprise, and symbolic emergence. The recursive atmosphere is now less a site of anxiety than a medium of creativity—a space where knowing and unknowing, longing and presence, can be played with, suffered, and transformed together.

Fantasy, Symbolic Transmission, and Unformulated Experience

If the analytic field is, as we have traced, a recursive space where fantasy loops and transforms, it is also a medium for something even more elusive: the transmission of what has not yet taken form. Psychoanalytic thinking has always circled the edges of the "unformulated"—that liminal zone where affect, image, and symbol are not yet, or perhaps never fully, articulated. Fantasy, in its recursive movement, is not just a stage for wish or defense, but a conduit for these inchoate experiences: a symbolic atmosphere through which the unformulated moves, seeks shape, and is sometimes, though never fully, brought to life.

Philip Bromberg (1998) described the analytic encounter as a site where "multiple self-states" coexist—shifting, intersecting, at times colliding or harmonizing. These self-states are not always available to conscious reflection; they appear first in fantasy, dream, mood, or sudden shifts of atmosphere in the analytic field. The recursive structure of fantasy means that these emergent self-states may be "played with" in the loop of analytic presence: a patient brings an image or a phrase, the analyst responds with reverie or bodily sensation, and together they trace the contours of something previously unformulated, hovering at the edge of symbolization.

Christopher Bollas (1987) gives this process a language of "atmosphere" and "unthought known." For Bollas, the analytic field is not just populated by explicit interpretations or conscious narratives but animated by the presence of what has not yet been thought: moods, gestures, and the silent transmission of affect. Fantasy, in this sense, is not only the mind's creation but also its medium for receiving and transmitting the not-yet-known. The looping movement of fantasy between patient and analyst becomes the space in which the "unthought known" may slowly gather shape—sometimes as an image, sometimes as a felt sense, sometimes as a moment of mutual reverie.

Michael Eigen (1999) radicalizes this insight by treating the analytic field as a kind of "psychic weather system," animated by the recursive transmission of fantasy, affect, and presence. For Eigen, the analyst's "participatory imagination" is not a mere tool, but a primary mode of being-with the patient. Fantasy is not just interpreted; it is suffered, witnessed, played with, and sometimes endured as a storm of feeling. The unformulated experience finds provisional shape in fantasy, but just as often slips away, leaving a residue—an atmospheric trace—that animates further analytic loops.

In these accounts, the symbolic function of fantasy is not to bring the unformulated fully into form, but to keep the field open for emergence. The "dreaming together" of analyst and patient is a recursive practice: each fantasy, dream, or reverie invites a new response, a shift in affect or imagination, a risk that something inchoate may find shape. Antonino Ferro and Giuseppe Civitarese (2016) describe this as a process of "narrative co-construction"—an ongoing, recursive interplay in which symbolic fragments are offered, responded to, and reassembled, not as final meanings but as provisional forms.

The analyst's discipline here is twofold: first, to attune to the atmosphere of the field, noticing when a fantasy is charged with the energy of the unformulated; and second, to resist the pressure to interpret too soon, to allow the recursive play to continue until something more differentiated can emerge. This often means tolerating periods of confusion, uncertainty, and affective ambiguity—moments when both participants feel "in the dark," yet remain together in the not-knowing. These are not failures of technique but conditions for creativity and symbolic birth.

Clinical practice is rich with examples of this process. A patient, Jamie, brings a series of fragmented images—waves crashing against a seawall, a child's hand reaching for a balloon, the sudden hush of snowfall outside the window. Each week, these images recur, sometimes in dreams, sometimes in the flow of conversation. Jamie is frustrated by the lack of narrative coherence: "I don't know what any of this means. I feel like I'm just talking in circles." As an analyst, I notice my own impatience, my desire to interpret or impose meaning. But when I resist, and simply echo or amplify the images—"What's it like to watch the waves?" "Can you feel the cold of the snow?"—the atmosphere in the room shifts. The images begin to acquire affective resonance: the waves evoke a sense of threat and beauty; the snow brings peace and isolation; the hand reaching for the balloon calls up longing, hope, and loss. The field is thick with unformulated experience, gradually, recursively, finding provisional symbolic life in our mutual play.

Jessica Benjamin (2018) describes this capacity as "symbolic hospitality"—an ethic of welcome for the unformulated, the not-yet-said, the affect that cannot yet find words. Fantasy is not merely a matter of the patient's private wish; it is an invitation for the analytic field to hold what cannot be contained elsewhere. The recursive loops of fantasy, dream, and reverie create a symbolic home for the unformulated—allowing it to be played with, suffered, and sometimes transformed.

The risks and gifts of this stance are substantial. When the analyst is too quick to interpret, the unformulated may be foreclosed—shut down before it can find shape, its creative energy lost to anxiety or defense. Conversely, when the field is too loose, the unformulated may become overwhelming, flooding the analytic hour with undifferentiated affect. The recursive structure of fantasy offers a way through: by looping, repeating, and returning, the field creates a rhythmic container, a holding environment where the unformulated can circulate, gradually gathering symbolic and affective texture.

André Green's (1983/1986) work on "the dead mother" and the uncanny underscores the complexity of this process. Sometimes, the unformulated is experienced as absence, void, or a kind of psychic deadness. Fantasy here is both a defense against this emptiness and the very medium through which new symbolic life may be kindled. The analytic task is to accompany the patient through the recursive cycles of presence and absence, to dwell together in the symbolic field until the unformulated begins to pulse with new possibility.

In the analyst's own process, this stance demands ongoing self-reflection—a willingness to attend to one's reveries, affects, and bodily sensations as data about the field's symbolic weather. The "participatory imagination" of the analyst is not an act of fantasy in the ordinary sense; it is a mode of symbolic transmission, a way of feeling-with the patient as the field's atmosphere shifts and new forms beckon. Sometimes, this means noticing the sudden emergence of an image or phrase in the analyst's mind, or the subtle movement of mood or energy in the room. These moments can be shared—tentatively, symbolically—with the patient, offering further loops, further opportunities for emergence. The discipline of "not-knowing" is thus not a passive state, but an active, recursive participation in the symbolic field. The analytic hour becomes an experiment in form and formlessness: fantasy as a medium for the unformulated, a stage for symbolic emergence, a field for the creative play of knowing and not-knowing. What is most transformative is not the final arrival of meaning, but the ongoing willingness to let the unformulated find its way into the symbolic atmosphere, however partially, however provisionally.

In sum, fantasy in the analytic field is never simply a private wish or defensive script. It is the recursive medium through which the unformulated—affect, self-state, symbol—may circulate, gather texture, and find provisional form. The analyst's task is to maintain the atmosphere of symbolic hospitality, to tolerate the uncertainties and surprises of the field, and to accompany the patient as fantasy becomes a site for the creative birth of new psychic life.

Closing Reflection—Unknowing, Reversal, and the Analytic Field

As we draw this chapter to a close, the recursive logic of fantasy reveals itself not as a niche curiosity or a theoretical embellishment, but as the pulse of the analytic field itself. What began as an exploration of fantasy's classical status—private, defensive, a wishful antidote to reality—has become a meditation on the field's irreducible complexity: a living, looping, and creative atmosphere in which fantasy, affect, and symbolic life continually unmake and remake the boundaries of knowing.

If fantasy, in its classical psychoanalytic guise, aimed to restore order in the face of conflict and absence, its recursive structure in the analytic field reverses this movement. Fantasy becomes less the solution and more the means of keeping the question open—an engine of return, surprise, and productive uncertainty. The field is never stilled; its atmosphere is shaped by the movement of fantasy across boundaries, by the unformulated that finds provisional form, and by the shared discipline of not-knowing that both analyst and patient must learn to inhabit.

Throughout, the ethic of unknowing emerges as the analytic stance most capable of honoring the recursive and generative potential of fantasy. To "know" in the classical sense—to pin down, to decode, to translate fantasy into a single, masterful interpretation—always risks foreclosing the very psychic movement that analysis seeks to animate. Instead, the discipline is one of staying-with: to remain in the loop, to witness the return of themes, affects, and images, and to trust in the creativity of the symbolic field.

What does this look like, in lived analytic practice? It means approaching each fantasy as a potential site of reversal, transformation, or emergent meaning. When the field thickens with repetition—when a dream recurs, a mood lingers, a story seems endlessly retold—the recursive perspective invites curiosity rather than impatience. The question becomes not "How do we end this loop?" but "What is being created, protected, or suffered here, in the very act of repetition?" It means noticing how fantasy both reveals and conceals: how it carries the trace of what cannot be formulated directly, how it shelters vulnerability, how it invites the analyst and patient to linger together at the edge of new symbolic possibility.

This ethic also calls for a radical humility. The analyst's interpretations, reveries, and even her theories are always caught in the same recursive logic. To interpret is itself an act of fantasy; to theorize is to loop meaning through the field, risking both contact and distortion. The analyst must be willing to have her knowing reversed: to discover that what seemed like an answer is, in fact, the beginning of a new question; to learn that the field's surprises and failures are not detours but the very route of analytic growth.

The recursive atmosphere of the field is never neutral—it is charged with the energies of desire, loss, hope, and ambivalence. At times, the field feels generative, alive with symbolic emergence; at others, it may stagnate, thickening into repetition compulsion or deadness. The analyst's discipline is to remain present even when the field feels opaque or hopeless, to bear witness to the possibility that the loop itself is a site of psychic work. What appears as "stuckness" may be the slow, recursive fermentation of the unformulated, the necessary waiting for something new to arise.

A central lesson of this chapter is that fantasy is not only a representation of the patient's inner world, but also a structure for analytic relation. It organizes how both participants imagine, feel, and symbolize what is possible in the encounter. The recursive structure of the field means that fantasy cannot be attributed solely to one party; it is a product of the between, shaped by mutual transmission, symbolic play, and the shared discipline of unknowing. Analyst and patient become co-dreamers, co-witnesses, co-creators of the psychic field's weather.

This recursive, field-based stance is more than a technical refinement—it is a revision of the very aims of psychoanalytic work. The goal is no longer to shepherd the patient from fantasy to reality, or from ignorance to knowledge, but to sustain a living field in which new forms of knowing, being, and relating can emerge. The reversal is crucial: instead of treating fantasy as the problem to be overcome, the analytic field honors fantasy as the space of possibility, the generator of surprise, and the means by which the psyche remains unfinished, alive, and open to transformation.

Practically, this means the analyst must learn the timing of the field: when to interpret, when to dream, when to remain silent, when to risk presence even in confusion or mutual opacity. The recursive ethic is one of patience, curiosity, and symbolic hospitality—a willingness to let the atmosphere shift, to let the loop return, to trust that meaning and transformation may arise from the ongoing interplay of knowing and unknowing.

Finally, the recursive approach to fantasy invites a new kind of analytic hope. In a culture obsessed with answers and closure, the field becomes a sanctuary for return, for creative reversal, for living with the unfinished. The analyst's presence, marked by humility and the discipline of unknowing, offers the patient not a pathway out of fantasy but an invitation deeper into its field—where what is most vital is not the answer, but the possibility that the next loop will bring something new.

As the book continues, the recursive, field-based approach elaborated here will serve as a foundation for the exploration of further inversions—of introjection, destruction, and other psychoanalytic concepts—each opened to the creative potential of reversal and the ethics of not-knowing. The analytic field, shaped by the recursive play of fantasy and its atmospheres, is thus revealed as a living laboratory for the ongoing creation of psychic life.

Chapter 7

Destruction as Inversion—Aggression, Ruin, and the Ethics of Refusal

This chapter reimagines destruction and aggression as inverted forms of psychic knowing, refusing their traditional psychoanalytic status as failures of integration or mere forces of unbinding. Instead, destruction is approached as a recursive ethic—a refusal of premature synthesis, false repair, or closure that sustains the possibility of unknowing and symbolic surprise. Drawing on clinical and cultural material, this chapter explores how aggression and ruin generate zones of psychic intensity where the familiar collapses and new forms of meaning threaten, or promise, to emerge. Destruction is neither pathology nor pure negation, but an agent of generativity and ethical stance: it interrupts the fantasy of mastery, exposes the limits of containment, and marks a refusal to be reconciled to inherited narratives of healing. The analytic task, then, is not to subdue or "repair" destruction, but to bear witness to its recursive presence—to trace the contours of breakdown, withdrawal, and refusal and to recognize in these sites the raw conditions for future psychic life. This chapter closes by considering the analyst's own relationship to destruction: as both a threat and a resource for hospitality, surprise, and the ongoing discipline of unknowing.

Introduction—Destruction and the Refusal of Repair

Destruction occupies an ambiguous, even forbidden, place in psychoanalytic thought. From Freud's earliest meditations on the death drive to Klein's evocations of envy and reparation, destruction has appeared as both an unmanageable threat and a mysterious wellspring within psychic life. It is often cast in the role of pathology—an unbinding force that undoes integration, the force behind breakdowns, regressions, and ruptures that analytic technique is called upon to contain, repair, or redeem. Yet beneath these habitual framings, destruction harbors another potential: it is not

DOI: 10.4324/9781003747109-10

simply the antithesis of psychic growth, but sometimes its very ground, an agent of surprise and the precondition for the emergence of something new.

The psychoanalytic tradition, for all its investment in transformation and healing, has always circled around destruction as a kind of negative gravity. We are drawn to the fantasy of repair—the idea that wounds can be healed, that the psychic fabric can be sutured, and that violence or loss can be metabolized into meaning. Analysts and patients alike long for the restoration of coherence, for integration after fragmentation. But this longing, necessary as it is, can become its own defense: a refusal to acknowledge the generativity of breakdown, the creative necessity of ruin, and the value of what cannot be resolved. In privileging repair, psychoanalysis sometimes risks obscuring the deeper ethical and symbolic work that only destruction can perform.

This chapter is an invitation to invert the usual perspective: to see destruction not as a failure to be overcome, but as a recursive ethic, a site where unknowing and symbolic surprises are sustained. What would it mean to bear witness to destruction, not as a mistake or deficiency, but as a refusal of premature synthesis—a force that resists the false comfort of closure? In analytic work, there are moments when the urge to repair becomes not only impossible but also ethically suspect. To rush toward integration is sometimes to betray the atmosphere of psychic intensity that emerges in collapse, to foreclose the possibility of new forms of meaning, or to silence what refuses to be tamed by narrative or interpretation.

Aggression, ruin, and the acts of psychic undoing that populate analytic life are thus repositioned here as zones of possibility rather than mere problems to be solved. Destruction interrupts the fantasy of mastery that can inhabit both the analytic frame and the wider cultural imagination. It exposes the limits of containment, reveals the porousness of the boundaries we so carefully construct, and marks a refusal to be reconciled to inherited narratives of healing. In the recursive logic of the psyche, destruction can be the very site from which future life will be drawn—not through the comfort of restoration, but through the opening of new psychic space.

To approach destruction as a recursive ethic is to invite a shift in clinical presence: to relinquish the analyst's role as healer-in-chief and to occupy, instead, the position of witness and companion at the threshold of breakdown. This means resisting the pressure to integrate too quickly, to hold what cannot yet be held, and to recognize the value of withdrawal, non-repair, and refusal as forms of ethical fidelity. It means tracing the contours of psychic ruin with curiosity rather than dread and remaining open to the possibility that what seems like negation or absence may, in time, become the raw condition for new psychic life.

In what follows, I aim to unravel the recursive textures of destruction in psychoanalysis: tracing its genealogy, articulating its ethical stance, and illuminating the clinical atmospheres where aggression, ruin, and refusal signal not the end of meaning but its radical beginning. If destruction is to be reimagined as a generative force, then the analytic task is not to subdue or "fix" it, but to learn how to bear its presence—welcoming surprise, sustaining unknowing, and inhabiting the creative risk at the heart of psychic undoing.

The Genealogy of Destruction in Psychoanalysis

Destruction has haunted psychoanalytic theory from its earliest articulations, evolving through multiple conceptual idioms and historical moments. Freud's late turn to the death drive marked a decisive reframing of psychic life: in *Beyond the Pleasure Principle* (1920), destruction emerges not only as aggression turned outward but also as a drive toward unbinding, repetition, and psychic dissolution. This "daemonic" force, distinct from Eros, seeks a return to an inanimate state—a proposition that would fracture the optimism of classical psychoanalysis and mark the beginning of its engagement with the negative (Freud, 1920/1961).

Building on this, Melanie Klein positioned destruction as the linchpin of her theory of object relations. For Klein, primitive aggression is bound to the infant's earliest fantasies, suffusing both love and hate and requiring continual processes of reparation and symbolization. In her classic papers, the destructiveness of envy, rage, and persecutory anxiety is never fully outgrown but must be "worked through" repeatedly in the psyche's internal world (Klein, 1946). Reparation, in her schema, is the subject's attempt to mend what aggression has shattered—a moral, affective, and symbolic labor that underwrite psychic development (Klein, 1937).

Winnicott, too, brought destruction to the foreground, but with a distinctive inflection. For Winnicott, aggression is not simply pathology nor always in need of repair. In *The Maturational Processes and the Facilitating Environment* (1965), he describes the child's "destruction" of the object as a developmental necessity: only in surviving the child's aggression does the object become real and reliable in the psychic field. Winnicott's "use of an object" framework reimagines destruction as creative—a risk and a test, not just an act of violence (Winnicott, 1969/1971). Where Klein's focus is on the reparative drive, Winnicott privileges the space of destruction as a zone of encounter and authenticity.

Throughout these lineages, destruction has often been viewed as pathology—an indicator of failure to integrate, of drives run amok, or of a breakdown in the symbolizing function (Green, 1986). But even as psychoanalysis sought to domesticate or contain destructive impulses, hints of their generative potential persisted. Andre Green's work on the "dead mother" complex and negative hallucination, for example, illuminates the psychic cost of unworked-through destruction: the hollowing out of aliveness, the foreclosure of symbolic possibility (Green, 1986). Yet, Green also gestures toward the ways that absence and negation can paradoxically support new psychic forms—a subtle echo of Freud's vision of "primordial loss" as both a wound and a wellspring.

In more contemporary relational and intersubjective perspectives, destruction has been rethought as a phenomenon that traverses the analytic field rather than originating solely within the patient. Jessica Benjamin (2004/2017) has argued that analytic impasses often turn on the inability to metabolize mutual destructiveness, and that creative failure—the willingness to endure psychic breakdown together—can itself be a site of generativity and transformation. Similarly, Thomas Ogden (1994) has described the analyst's encounter with psychic "non-integration" as an opportunity for creative engagement, provided the analyst can resist the compulsion to repair or resolve too quickly.

This genealogy exposes a set of recurring tensions: destruction as pathology versus destruction as generative, aggression as something to be contained versus something to be risked, and the analyst's role as healer versus witness to breakdown. If psychoanalysis is to move beyond a reparative fantasy, it must contend with these tensions directly—holding open the question of whether destruction is a force to be subdued, or a recursive ethic to be sustained. In so doing, the tradition points toward a psychoanalysis of thresholds: a discipline not only of mending, but also of bearing witness to collapse, and of recognizing the creative possibilities that arise in the wake of ruin.

Destruction as Recursive Ethic

To reframe destruction as a recursive ethic is to risk a countercultural gesture—one that resists the reassuring narrative of healing and instead foregrounds the ongoing necessity of breakdown, undoing, and refusal. In most analytic contexts, destruction is approached as an emergency: a moment to be managed, metabolized, or, ideally, repaired. Yet, to view destruction through a recursive lens is to attend not to its cessation but to its return—its capacity to recur, to unsettle, and to reorient the analytic process precisely by refusing finality. This refusal is not simply a holding pattern or a symptom of resistance, but a form of generative negative capability (Keats, 1817/1958; Bion, 1962)—a willingness to stay with what is unfinished, unintegrated, and alive in its refusal to resolve.

Recursive ethics draws its force from the recognition that destruction is never a singular event but a pattern, a movement that loops through psychic life in variable forms. It is the analytic atmosphere that gathers when old interpretations collapse, when the pressure to "know" or to "fix" breaks down, and when something irreducibly unassimilable asserts itself in the clinical field. Destruction, in this sense, is not the end of meaning, but its radical potential—the ground from which new forms may arise if only we resist the compulsion toward closure (Ogden, 1994; Eigen, 2004). This recursive stance does not glorify violence or loss, but honors the creative risk entailed in letting things fall apart.

Within the analytic dyad, recursive destruction surfaces most acutely when the frame is tested and interpretive authority fails. The analyst's interpretive interventions, which promise sense and healing, sometimes collapse into irrelevance or even injury. The patient may attack the analyst's person or method, retreat into silence, or enact breakdowns that appear to "undo" the analytic work. These moments, so often cast as impasses, are also opportunities—thresholds where the old order is suspended and the possibility of new psychic forms shimmers on the horizon (Benjamin, 2004/2017). The recursive ethic does not ask the analyst to rush into the breach with new interpretations or attempts at rescue; instead, it calls for a presence that can bear witness to the cyclicality and unpredictability of destruction, and to the truth that something vital is always at stake when things fall apart.

This vision of destruction as recursive ethic is resonant with Wilfred Bion's call for "negative capability"—the analyst's cultivated capacity to tolerate not-knowing, to resist memory and desire, and to stay with the turbulence of the analytic present (Bion, 1962). In such moments, destruction is not a problem to be solved but a weather system to be inhabited. The recursive return of breakdown—within session, across the arc of treatment, or within the wider culture—calls for an ethic of hospitality to the unknown. The analyst becomes less a technician and more a witness, less a restorer and more a fellow traveler at the edges of psychic collapse.

This stance opens a paradoxical relationship to reparation and repair. While Klein (1937) privileges reparation as the essential psychic labor following aggression, the recursive ethic suggests that premature repair can foreclose deeper forms of psychic transformation. Not every wound is ready for suture; not every loss can or should be mourned according to preexisting scripts. By attending to what resists integration, the analyst is able to mark the limits of the therapeutic frame and to keep open the possibility that breakdown is not merely a setback but an invitation—an entry point for new symbolic formations that would otherwise remain unimaginable.

Here, destruction approaches what Loewald (1978) called "the creative potential of regression"—the movement back or down that is not simply a retreat but a return to conditions of psychic plasticity, surprise, and new possibility. Ruin and breakdown become generative when they are not forced prematurely into meaning or explanation. Instead, the recursive ethic invites both analyst and patient to inhabit the intervals of collapse, to remain curious about what forms might emerge in the wake of undoing, and to honor the ethical discipline of not-knowing.

Destruction, when viewed recursively, also becomes an agent of symbolic surprise. The shattering of coherence or the eruption of aggression can make space for what Winnicott (1971) called the "potential space"—a liminal region in which new realities and new relations can be played with, experimented upon, and eventually made one's own. The refusal to resolve or integrate too quickly becomes a precondition for true creativity, for the arrival of something unanticipated and vital.

In clinical practice, this recursive ethic is often counterintuitive, even anxiety-provoking. Analysts are trained—and often temperamentally inclined—to contain, to restore order, and to shield both patient and process from psychic danger. Yet, as Eigen (2004) writes, "breakdown is a form of breakthrough"—not in a triumphalist sense, but as the slow, recursive work of living with what cannot be fixed. The analyst's stance shifts from intervention to accompaniment, from mastery to presence, and from fixing to witnessing the ongoing movement of destruction and renewal.

To close, the recursive ethic of destruction is not a renunciation of care or responsibility, but an enlargement of what care can mean. It asks the analyst to relinquish omnipotence, to make room for psychic undoing, and to risk the creative losses that make new psychic life possible. In honoring destruction's return, psychoanalysis becomes a discipline not only of repair but also of ongoing, recursive openness—a field in which ruin is not only endured but also welcomed as the necessary ground for future meaning.

Psychic Ruin and the Collapse of the Familiar

Psychoanalytic work is punctuated by moments of psychic ruin—those experiences when the old, familiar structures of meaning collapse and the analytic situation is saturated by an atmosphere of bewilderment, estrangement, or even dread. Ruin, in this sense, is not merely a catastrophic endpoint but a psychic event with its own topology and temporal logic. The collapse of the familiar is both feared and, paradoxically, necessary: it creates a space where new forms, meanings, and relations may threaten to emerge, if only one can remain with the uncertainty and loss (Bion, 1962; Eigen, 2004).

Ruin is rarely an isolated occurrence. In the clinical encounter, it often arrives as a gradual erosion rather than a sudden devastation. The patient who begins to question long-held beliefs or self-concepts, the moment an analyst's interpretation is met with incomprehension or aggression, the slow dissolution of transferential certainties—each of these can precipitate a psychic atmosphere akin to ruin (Ogden, 1994). There is a felt sense of something having come undone: the scaffolding of self, world, or relationship no longer holds as it once did. For both patient and analyst, the loss of the familiar can feel like a vertiginous fall, a disorganization that resists quick repair.

Yet, the logic of psychic ruin is not simply regressive. Ruin often operates as a recursive process—a spiraling series of collapses and partial rebuildings, where each breakdown reveals new layers of vulnerability, memory, and potential (Bion, 1962). In this sense, psychic ruin resonates with Bion's idea of "catastrophic change," where the subject faces not just a shift in content but a fundamental transformation in the psychic frame itself. The analyst's task is to tolerate, and even support, these periods of formlessness: to resist the impulse to immediately restore structure and instead to help the patient dwell in the space of the unfamiliar (Winnicott, 1958/1965; Loewald, 1978).

Clinical vignettes abound with these moments. A patient in the throes of depressive collapse, for example, may voice a sense that "nothing means anything anymore," the symbolic web that once gave order to experience now in tatters (Green, 1986). Such statements are often met by the analyst's own anxiety: a wish to reinfuse meaning, to counter despair with interpretation or reassurance. Yet, when these interventions are resisted or fail, the analytic pair may be left in a shared field of unknowing—a psychic wasteland that is, paradoxically, alive with possibility (Eigen, 2004). What if the task is not to "cheer up" the patient or to reconstruct meaning too quickly, but to recognize that this very collapse may clear ground for a new symbolic life?

Similarly, in the context of traumatic repetition, psychic ruin can manifest as haunting or recurrence. The patient who compulsively reenacts loss, betrayal, or abandonment may seem caught in a destructive cycle, unable to move forward (Freud, 1920/1961). The temptation is strong to break the cycle, to "fix" the ruin by offering explanation or redirection. But often, these repetitions mark the presence of something unformulated—a knowledge that can only announce itself through breakdown (Bollas, 1987). It is in the recurring ruin that unknowing becomes most palpable: a signal that the psyche is not ready (or not willing) to submit to a new order, that the old must remain in ruins for a time.

Ruin also has its cultural and aesthetic dimension. The fascination with ruins—architectural, historical, symbolic—permeates Western imagination (Benjamin, 1999). Ruins provoke both melancholy and awe, representing loss and the enigmatic persistence of what cannot be fully restored. In the analytic consulting room, the same affective tensions surface: the patient as haunted house, the analysis as an excavation site where remains, fragments, and echoes speak more powerfully than any single, reconstructed narrative. Analysts, like archeologists or poets, are tasked with bearing witness to what is left over—honoring both the devastation and the strangeness of what survives (Ogden, 1994).

The psychic experience of ruin is inseparable from the analyst's own capacity to dwell in breakdown. Often, the analyst's own frameworks and identities are threatened by encounters with psychic collapse (Green, 1986). The impulse to "make sense" or to restore meaning can be an act of self-preservation, a defense against the anxiety of not-knowing. Yet, as Loewald (1978) and Winnicott (1971) have argued, it is in the tolerance of formlessness—what Winnicott called "holding" and Loewald described as the "play of process"—that the seeds of psychic renewal are sown. The analyst's willingness to stand in the ruins with the patient, resisting both despair and premature reparation, becomes a central ethical and creative act.

The collapse of the familiar, then, should not be seen as merely negative or as an impasse to be quickly traversed. Ruin may be the only medium through which certain truths, affects, or forms of self-experience can be contacted (Ogden, 1994; Eigen, 2004). The field of destruction, saturated with the unknown, marks a zone of psychic intensity where the old is truly dead but the new is not yet born. In this liminal zone, analysis becomes less about restoration and more about witnessing—an act of being with, rather than fixing, the world in fragments.

In sum, psychic ruin and the collapse of the familiar call the analyst to an ethic of presence and humility. Rather than viewing breakdown as something to be avoided or repaired at all costs, it becomes possible to regard ruin as the condition for the emergence of something radically other—new meaning, new forms of relation, new possibilities for psychic life. In honoring this atmosphere, both patient and analyst may discover that ruin is not an end, but a passage; not merely loss, but the precondition for generativity and transformation.

Aggression and the Limits of Containment

Aggression is among the most anxiety-provoking phenomena to emerge in the analytic field—so often positioned as the force that threatens to rupture, contaminate, or even destroy the container itself. Within psychoanalytic history, aggression has oscillated between being seen as a drive to be tamed and a necessary component of psychic development (Freud, 1920/1961; Klein, 1937). Yet, the analytic encounter continually reveals that aggression is not simply an intrapsychic force but a relational event, surfacing in the transference and countertransference as a test of the analytic frame and the analyst's own capacities.

The urge to contain aggression—to render it manageable, interpretable, or symbolically "safe"—often reveals itself as a countertransference defense (Racker, 1968). The analyst may strive to maintain the illusion of therapeutic neutrality, avoiding direct engagement with the force of destructive feelings in the room. Yet, as Winnicott (1969/1971) insists, it is only through the actual *use* of the analyst as a real object—through destructive attacks, withdrawals, or even overt hostility—that the patient can test whether the analyst is truly capable of surviving psychic assault. The analyst's survival, in Winnicott's terms, is not achieved by denying or neutralizing aggression but by withstanding it, remaining present, and allowing the analytic frame to flex without shattering.

Aggression thus exposes the limits of containment, revealing the porous boundaries and the inevitable failures of even the most robust analytic frame (Ogden, 1994). There are moments when the analytic container—no matter how carefully maintained—cannot hold the intensity of the patient's rage, envy, or despair. These ruptures are not merely failures, but occasions that illuminate the analyst's own limits, vulnerabilities, and resistances. They invite a deeper encounter with the question: What does it mean to be the container for another's destruction, and what is risked or lost in that role?

This tension is vividly enacted in moments of analytic impasse. When aggression surges—whether as angry attack, passive withdrawal, or enactment of destructive fantasies—the analyst may feel helpless, exposed, or even retaliatory. The temptation is strong to restore order through interpretation, reassurance, or a more rigid frame. Yet, these responses often echo the patient's own historical experiences of having their aggression controlled, dismissed, or pathologized (Benjamin, 2004/2017). The analytic field, in such moments, becomes a living experiment in whether aggression can be borne, reflected, and metabolized without immediate pressure toward resolution.

Aggression, when permitted to reach the limits of containment, becomes a revelation: it undoes the fantasy of omnipotent mastery for both patient and analyst. It lays bare the reality that destruction, like creation, is foundational to psychic life (Eigen, 2004). The analyst who can bear this rupture—remaining present but not omnipotent, receptive but not annihilated—offers a different kind of holding: one marked by humility, openness, and a recursive fidelity to what cannot yet be symbolized.

Moreover, aggression is not always "negative." It can represent a movement toward truth—a breaking through of defenses, a refusal of false compliance, or a protest against suffocating interpretations (Winnicott, 1969/1971; Ogden, 1994). At its most generative, aggression asserts the patient's subjectivity, vitality, and capacity to resist psychic colonization. When aggression is received, marked, and not retaliated against or smoothed over, it can transform into a new form of contact, even a precondition for intimacy (Benjamin, 2004/2017).

The analytic task is not to neutralize aggression but to allow it to find its limit and to witness what emerges in its wake. Sometimes this means acknowledging that containment is imperfect, that there will be breakdowns, and that the analytic pair must together inhabit the anxiety, vulnerability, and surprise of what cannot be wholly controlled. The limits of containment, rather than failures to be regretted, become sites of ethical encounter—places where the truth of aggression can be recognized, survived, and, at times, transformed.

In sum, aggression in the analytic situation is not simply the force that threatens to destroy the frame; it is also the force that reveals the frame's limits, tests its ethical stance, and opens the possibility for new psychic realities. The capacity to bear aggression at the edge of containment—without retreating into interpretation or defense—marks a crucial dimension of analytic presence. In these charged atmospheres, both patient and analyst may discover that aggression is not the enemy of connection, but the very condition for the emergence of something radically new.

Clinical Vignettes—Witnessing Destruction and Refusal

1 The Refusal of Repair

David, a man in his late 40s, came to analysis at a moment of psychic collapse. His marriage had ended abruptly after a series of betrayals, and he described himself as "ruined"—incapable of trust, inhabiting a world emptied of meaning. Early sessions were marked by a hunger for repair: he asked for reassurance that he could "get better," pressed the analyst for interpretations that might restore coherence, and oscillated between hope and a furious insistence that nothing could ever change. When the analyst offered empathy or suggested the possibility of recovery, David became irritable, sometimes openly hostile. He accused the analyst of minimizing his pain or offering false hope and, in one session, said flatly, "You want to fix me, but you can't."

Over time, it became clear that David's refusal of repair was not simply resistance but a vital assertion—a defense against the premature closure of meaning. The analyst recognized that interventions designed to "restore" him risked enacting the very violence of assimilation he was mourning. By shifting away from repair toward presence, the analytic dyad found new ground: moments of shared silence, acknowledgment of ruin, and, eventually, a space where David could explore the contours of his own psychic collapse without the pressure to make it meaningful too soon. Here, destruction became a recursive process—returning in waves, each time marking both a loss and a possibility. The analyst's task was not to heal or to interpret away, but to bear witness at the edge of the ruins, allowing the full affective climate of collapse to be felt and survived (Ogden, 1994; Eigen, 2004).

The recursive atmosphere of David's analysis was defined by these cycles of hope, disappointment, and refusal. There were periods of withdrawal, in which David barely spoke at all, but the silence carried its own kind of weight—a negative presence that the analyst learned to respect. When, after many months, David remarked, "I think something happens when you just sit with me here and don't try to make it better," both recognized a subtle shift. The refusal of repair had become a new form of psychic contact, marked not by the triumph of meaning but by the slow emergence of trust amid ruins.

2 Aggression as Contact

Sara, a young woman with a history of emotional neglect, struggled with overwhelming rage in the transference. She experienced the analyst as alternately absent, suffocating, or "in the way" of her real feelings. When interpretations felt intrusive or when the analyst missed a subtle cue, Sara would abruptly withdraw, sometimes staring silently at the wall, at other times erupting in sarcasm or open attack. The analyst, at first, interpreted these moments as resistance or as regressions to an earlier developmental stage. Yet as the work progressed, it became clear that Sara's aggression was also a search for contact—a desperate test of whether the analyst could survive her anger without retreating or retaliating.

In one pivotal session, Sara yelled, "You don't get to fix me. You don't get to tell me what my feelings are!" The analyst, shaken but present, simply replied, "I won't tell you. I'm here to listen, even if you hate me for it." The atmosphere shifted: Sara's rage softened, and tears followed. In that moment, aggression was not contained by interpretation, but met as a real event—testing and revealing the limits of analytic hospitality (Winnicott, 1969/1971; Benjamin, 2004/2017). The refusal to neutralize her aggression, or to repair too quickly, created a space in which a new relational form could emerge—where destruction and contact coexisted.

This process was not linear. Periods of calm gave way to renewed storm; Sara's attacks would sometimes become more creative, even playful. At other times, her silence pressed the analyst to the edge of their own patience. Each return of aggression was an opportunity to renegotiate contact, to let destruction mark the analytic atmosphere without foreclosing surprise. Slowly, a new intimacy was forged, one capable of holding both love and hate, aggression and longing.

3 Ruin as Generative Void
A third case involved Mr. L, an older patient whose life was marked by repeated failures—broken careers, estranged children, unfinished projects. In analysis, Mr. L alternated between a narrative of victimhood and a profound sense of shame and emptiness. The analyst noted a recurring pattern: every time a hopeful interpretation was offered, Mr. L responded by amplifying his sense of ruin, sometimes with bitterness, sometimes with bleak humor. The analyst's urge to "lift" him from despair began to feel counterproductive, producing more withdrawal.

Instead, the analyst gradually shifted from intervention to accompaniment, learning to tolerate the analytic silence and psychic voids that punctuated their work. In these stretches of emptiness, something subtle began to shift. Mr. L brought dreams of ruined cities, of wandering through abandoned houses. Rather than interpreting these as symbols to be "solved," the analyst joined him in exploring the affective atmosphere of loss, uncertainty, and paradoxical freedom such ruins afforded (Loewald, 1978; Bollas, 1987). Over time, the space of destruction became less a symptom to be eradicated than a generative void—a site where meaning might, at some point, be allowed to arise anew.

As trust deepened, Mr. L began to take tentative risks—reaching out to a family member, returning to an abandoned creative project. These actions were not grand repairs but modest gestures, marked by uncertainty and fragility. The analytic atmosphere had shifted: ruin was no longer merely a site of mourning, but a place where possibility could glimmer, even if briefly, at the edge of the familiar.

4 Destruction in the Collective Field: A Group Analytic Vignette
Destruction is not confined to the analytic dyad; it reverberates within groups, institutions, and the collective spaces that analysts inhabit. During the final year of a long-standing therapy group, ruptures began to emerge as the group faced impending dissolution. What had once been a web of mutual support became a site of intensifying aggression, withdrawals, and silent refusals. One member, Anna, lashed out at another for "wasting everyone's time with the same story, week after week." Another, Mark, who had rarely spoken, abruptly announced, "I don't think any of this is real. Maybe it never was." The group's affective atmosphere turned brittle, marked by accusation, sarcasm, and a pervasive sense of disappointment.

As the group's facilitator, I felt a profound pull toward rescue. My urge was to interpret, to soothe, to "save" the group from collapse. Yet, each attempt at repair was met with further resistance or flat indifference. The group, it seemed, needed to enact its own destruction—to face the reality of ending not through reconciliation but through shared experience of breakdown. When I finally acknowledged, aloud, "It feels like we're all standing in the ruins of what this group used to be, and it's hard to know what, if anything, comes next," a hush settled. For a moment, nothing was said. Then Anna replied, quietly, "Maybe we have to let it be broken."

In the weeks that followed, the group's interactions not only grew sparse, more tentative, but also more honest. Some members chose silence, others offered memories or regrets, but the frantic search for repair gave way to a kind of shared witnessing. As the group ended, it was not restored to wholeness but marked by a new relational honesty—one forged in the refusal to deny loss or to force resolution. The destruction of the group, rather than signaling only failure, created the conditions for a deeper encounter with truth, mourning, and the potential for future relational life beyond the group itself.

This collective vignette echoes the recursive nature of destruction: breakdown returns in different registers and scales, and the refusal of premature repair opens space for new, if uncertain, forms of relational possibility.

These vignettes illustrate that destruction and refusal in the analytic field are not endpoints or failures, but ongoing, recursive phenomena that demand a shift in clinical presence. The analyst's capacity to witness—rather than "solve"—the breakdown, withdrawal, and aggression in these cases marks an ethical stance: to bear with the atmosphere of psychic ruin, to resist the pressure for premature reparation, and to sustain the possibility that, within destruction, something unexpected and vital may begin to take shape. The work of analysis thus unfolds not as a linear progression from damage to repair, but as a looping, recursive navigation of collapse, survival, and the creative risk of unknowing.

Ruin, Refusal, and the Conditions for Future Life

The aftermath of destruction in the analytic field is not a blank void, but a liminal terrain—a space marked by uncertainty, suspense, and the subtle stirring of possibility. Ruin, when not hurriedly repaired or disavowed, becomes a medium for new psychic life. The refusal to "fix" or narrate away what has collapsed is itself an ethical and creative act, honoring the truth that meaning cannot always be restored by force of will or interpretive brilliance. Instead, it is often in the holding open of ruin, in the sustained presence to psychic debris, that the conditions for genuine transformation are laid.

This psychic potential of ruin resonates powerfully with the motif of ruins in art, literature, and myth—a fascination that spans cultures and epochs. From the grandeur of Ozymandias's shattered statue in Shelley's poetry to the melancholy beauty of ancient temples or bombed-out cathedrals, ruins call forth both mourning and wonder. They are reminders not only of loss and impermanence but also of endurance: the way structures outlast their original meanings and become sites of new, unforeseen life. In myth, ruins often serve as liminal spaces where heroes confront the ghosts of the past or encounter the unknown, sites where endings and beginnings are entangled. This aesthetic and symbolic "atmosphere" is mirrored in the consulting room, where the collapse of psychic certainties exposes the possibility of new psychic forms—forms that may only become visible in the aftermath of destruction (Bollas, 1987; Benjamin, 1999).

The generativity of ruin is not simply a matter of waiting for healing to occur; rather, it involves a recursive willingness to inhabit the unknown. Both patient and analyst are called to dwell within the gaps left by destruction, resisting the fantasy of immediate synthesis. As Loewald (1978) observed, it is in these intervals of formlessness—where old structures have collapsed but new ones have yet to emerge—that the psyche regains its plasticity. The field is open, if only for a moment, to other configurations: new affective connections, creative solutions, or unexpected recognitions. The ruined landscape—psychic or cultural—is thus not just an emblem of loss, but a living, shifting ground for creative possibility.

Refusal, in this context, becomes a paradoxical form of fidelity. To refuse the closure of meaning, to resist both despair and restoration, is to remain loyal to the process itself—a recursive movement of psychic survival. Ruin, thus held, becomes the ground for resymbolization. The ruins are not erased or rebuilt according to the old blueprints; rather, they are inhabited, explored, and gradually infused with new life. The analyst who can bear witness to this process—without imposing direction or demanding coherence—becomes a co-creator in the emergence of a future not yet imaginable.

This generative function of ruin is not limited to individual analysis; it reverberates at the level of culture and collective life. Societies, too, must at times endure periods of collapse, breakdown, or creative refusal—moments when established forms lose their legitimacy and new symbolic orders are not yet in sight. We might think of the rubble-strewn aftermath of revolution, the psychic remains left by historical trauma, or the "ruins" of vanished paradigms in analytic theory itself. Psychoanalytic practice, in this sense, offers a microcosm of the broader dynamics of breakdown and renewal, showing how the refusal to prematurely mend or explain can become the crucible for collective as well as personal transformation.

Clinically, the aftermath of psychic destruction often entails long periods of confusion, emptiness, or even despair—times when neither patient nor analyst can envision a way forward. These stretches may feel interminable, and the temptation to "do something" can be overwhelming. Yet, it is precisely here, in the patient's refusal to rebuild or in the analyst's willingness to sustain the not-knowing, that the conditions for future life are being quietly laid. The ruins, far from being inert, are full of potential energy—waiting for new meaning to crystallize, for affect to shift, or for a new relation to emerge (Eigen, 2004).

A patient mourning the death of an idealized parent, for example, may pass through a period where the old narrative is impossible to sustain but no new narrative is yet available. In the absence of quick repair, the analyst's willingness to hold this vacuum allows for the slow, recursive movement of grief, fantasy, and reattachment. Similarly, when a patient's sense of self is shattered by trauma, the refusal to reconstitute identity too quickly honors the uniqueness of what has been lost and the irreducibility of the wound. Only by lingering in the ruins—by resisting the urge to rebuild on familiar foundations—can the patient begin to imagine new forms of psychic inhabitation.

This is not a call to glorify suffering or to valorize endless breakdown. Rather, it is a recognition that the process of becoming—psychically, relationally, or culturally—is neither linear nor smooth. The analytic ethic, then, is not merely to survive destruction but to cultivate the courage to dwell within its aftermath. This involves recognizing that the ruins of the familiar are not only sites of mourning but also spaces of potential. In the shadow of collapse, both patient and analyst may find themselves invited into a deeper engagement with life—a renewed willingness to risk, to imagine, and to participate in the recursive work of becoming.

In sum, ruin and refusal, when honored rather than evaded, form the conditions for future psychic life. They invite both patience and creativity, humility and openness, marking the point where destruction gives way, quietly and often unexpectedly, to the first stirrings of renewal.

The Analyst's Relationship to Destruction

If destruction and ruin are to be understood as generative elements within analytic process, then the analyst's own relationship to destruction becomes a site of special ethical and affective complexity. The analyst is never merely a neutral observer of breakdown; instead, they are called into intimate relation with the forces of aggression, collapse, and refusal that shape the analytic field. The analyst's capacity to welcome, survive, and even bear destruction—not simply in the patient but within themselves and within the analytic situation—marks a central test of analytic presence.

Classical psychoanalysis often positioned the analyst as a resilient container, able to withstand the patient's destructive projections and fantasies without retaliation or collapse (Bion, 1962; Winnicott, 1969/1971). This notion of "survival" is foundational: the analyst is to be a reliable, enduring presence, able to metabolize the patient's aggression without acting out or withdrawing. Yet, in practice, the experience of being the object of destruction is rarely straightforward or heroically neutral. Analysts may feel wounded, helpless, angry, or even tempted to retaliate—responses that challenge the myth of analytic omnipotence (Racker, 1968; Ogden, 1994).

It is in the recognition and working through of these vulnerabilities that the analyst's relationship to destruction becomes most fertile. To be affected by the patient's destructive impulses is not a failure, but a signal that real psychic work is taking place in the intersubjective field. The analyst who can acknowledge their own wounds—without succumbing to defensiveness or rescue—models an ethic of presence that is honest, porous, and generative (Benjamin, 2004/2017). This does not mean becoming passive or abdicating analytic responsibility, but rather cultivating an ongoing discipline of self-reflection and humility.

Moreover, the analyst's own aggression is inevitably implicated in the analytic process. Destruction is not the exclusive property of the patient; countertransference feelings of irritation, rejection, or even unconscious sabotage can shape the analytic atmosphere in ways both subtle and profound (Racker, 1968). When the analyst becomes aware of their own destructive currents—whether as impatience, withdrawal, or the subtle wish to "fix" the patient—these moments can be used as openings for further inquiry, self-exploration, and shared meaning-making. In this way, the analyst's ethical task is not to purge themselves of aggression, but to become more attuned to its recursive appearances and more capable of symbolizing it within the analytic relationship.

This recursive ethic also asks the analyst to risk their own "ruin" in the service of analytic honesty. There are times when the analytic frame itself is threatened—by impasse, by enactment, or by the experience of shared failure. The temptation to shore up the frame with technical expertise or theoretical certainty can be strong, especially in the face of destruction. Yet, it is precisely in these moments—when the analyst's own certainties are undone—that a more authentic analytic presence becomes possible. By acknowledging the breakdown of their own frameworks, the analyst may join the patient in the liminal space of unknowing, creating conditions for shared transformation.

This stance of hospitality to destruction is inherently paradoxical. The analyst must both survive and be willing to be affected; they must provide holding while relinquishing control; they must bear witness without foreclosing surprise. Such a position requires a tolerance for ambiguity, for repeated failure, and for the discomfort of psychic exposure. It is, ultimately, an ethic not of mastery, but of recursive, relational vulnerability—a willingness to be changed by the very forces one is tasked to contain.

In the end, the analyst's relationship to destruction is a practice of ongoing openness. The more the analyst can allow themselves to be affected, to risk presence at the threshold of collapse, and to remain available to the unknown, the more the analytic space becomes capable of hosting true psychic renewal. Destruction, in this light, is not an obstacle to be eliminated, but a resource to be welcomed—a test and an invitation, both for the patient and for the analyst, to encounter the depths of the psyche where new life begins.

Closing Reflection—Destruction, Hospitality, and Symbolic Surprise

Destruction in the analytic field is never merely an end: it is a signal, a provocation, an invitation to encounter the limits and possibilities of psychic life. When welcomed not as a pathology but as a recursive force—capable of undoing, remaking, and generating—destruction becomes both a challenge and a resource for the analytic pair. What begins as collapse may, in time, become the site where new meaning stirs, often unpredictably, beneath the ruins of the familiar.

Throughout this chapter, we have seen how ruin, aggression, and refusal create atmospheres charged with uncertainty. The analyst is asked to relinquish the fantasy of seamless repair, to bear presence at the edge of unknowing, and to find a paradoxical hospitality to what cannot be assimilated or contained. This hospitality is not passivity, nor a surrender of analytic responsibility. It is an ethic of patience, of bearing with—not against—the recursive movements of breakdown and return. To stand with destruction, to survive its onslaughts and to allow oneself to be affected, is to honor the lived complexity of psychic survival and transformation.

Destruction also reveals the surprise at the heart of symbolization. When psychic forms break down, new configurations can emerge—sometimes tentatively, sometimes explosively. The analyst's openness to surprise, to the unforeseen, becomes essential: what cannot be planned or interpreted in advance may yet unfold in the analytic atmosphere. These moments—when language falters and affect overflows—are not failures but openings: sites where the analytic field becomes alive with possibility, with the shimmer of meaning not yet realized.

If psychoanalysis is, as this project contends, a discipline of recursive hospitality, then it must continually return to the problem of destruction. It must learn not only to contain but to be changed by it; not only to survive but also to risk presence at the edge of its own undoing. This is the analytic wager: that in meeting destruction without fleeing or foreclosing, we create the only climate where something truly new can be born.

The generativity of destruction is not guaranteed, and it cannot be manufactured through will or technique. It requires the courage to let collapse take its course, to witness the withdrawal and refusal that are necessary for psychic reorganization, and to attend with humility to what emerges from the wreckage. In bearing this discipline together, patient and analyst may find that what once appeared as negation or loss is, in time, transformed into the raw material of future psychic life—a life shaped not in spite of destruction, but through it.

Chapter 8

Civilization as Remainder—Opacity, the Uncanny, and the Failure to Sublimate

This chapter reframes civilization as a psychic and collective remainder: the site of what cannot be fully symbolized, integrated, or known. Against the ideal of sublimation as the successful transformation of instinct into culture, it foregrounds the stubborn persistence of opacity, ungovernable residues, and the uncanny as the return of the repressed. Drawing on Foucault, the discussion positions civilization not as a triumph of reason but as a field of discourse, power, and unassimilable excess—haunted by what resists containment, surveillance, and legibility. The uncanny here is not merely a symptom, but the atmospheric trace of what lies beyond the symbolic, continually threatening to destabilize both psychic and social order. Failures of sublimation become generative: symptoms, estrangements, and cultural breakdowns are recast as sites where new meanings may shimmer into being. By attending to the ways in which both individual and collective life are shaped by what remains opaque, inassimilable, or uncanny, this chapter invites a psychoanalysis attuned not to closure or integration, but to the creative potential of remainder, rupture, and the persistence of the unknowable.

Introduction—The Fantasy of Sublimation and the Persistence of Remainder

Civilization, for psychoanalysis, is haunted by its own ambition. At its core lies the fantasy of sublimation: the transformation of unruly, instinctual life into the order of culture, language, and collective meaning. Freud imagined civilization as a triumph of psychic and social integration, a heroic achievement of symbolic containment that offers release from the tyranny of impulse and the threat of dissolution (Freud, 1930/1961). Klein, Winnicott, and the post-Freudian lineage extend this ambition—each, in

DOI: 10.4324/9781003747109-11

their own way, committed to the work of symbolization, reparation, and the healing of the fragmented or split psyche. Across these frameworks, the project of both the individual and the collective is often narrated as a movement toward coherence, mastery, and completion.

Yet, as psychoanalysis has always suspected, something persists at the edge of every integration—something untransformed, unyielding, and inassimilable. The **remainder**: what resists symbolization, what slips the net of meaning, what returns as symptom, haunting, or uncanny atmosphere. If sublimation is the story civilization tells itself about its own capacity for mastery, the remainder is the echo that cannot be stilled—the psychic and cultural surplus that continually undoes, complicates, or haunts that story.

In my prior writing, I tracked this logic of remainder through the language of paradox, fragmentation, and recursive unknowing. There, the fragment was not merely a wound to be healed, but a living trace of what could not be synthesized. The psychic field was figured not as a closed system, but as an atmosphere—curved, open, and permeated by the gravity of what remains outside integration. Here, the motif of remainder is made explicit: remainder as the structural necessity, the excess that gives both psyche and civilization their ongoing dynamism. Recursion is central—remainder is not static but returns, reverberates, and organizes the field as a kind of negative presence or symbolic undertow.

Psychoanalytic history is marked by an ambivalence toward this surplus. On the one hand, it is the engine of culture, the drive that powers symbolization, sublimation, and creation. On the other hand, it is a threat—a site of anxiety, uncanny estrangement, and the specter of the ungovernable. The urge to cover over the remainder, to close the gap or heal the split, is woven into the clinical and cultural history of analysis itself. Yet, the most generative analytic thinkers have always circled the gap: Freud's "navel of the dream," Klein's irreducible wounds, Winnicott's potential space, Bollas's "unthought known," Green's "dead mother," Loewald's "primordial loss," Laplanche's "enigmatic signifier," Bion's "negative capability," Lacan's Real, Derrida's *différance*, Foucault's limits of intelligibility, Gödel's incompleteness. Each in their own register refuses to treat the remainder as deficit or error; instead, remainder is figured as the very condition of psychic and social life.

This chapter repositions civilization as a field of remainder—a space where the work of integration is always partial, always haunted by the return of the inassimilable. Against the ideal of sublimation as cultural triumph, I foreground opacity, ungovernable residues, and the uncanny as recursive signatures of what civilization cannot contain. Drawing on Foucault, Derrida, Gödel, and Lacan, the discussion approaches civilization not as the achievement of reason, but as a haunted discourse, shaped by excess and its disavowals. The uncanny, introduced here in its collective form, will recur in a later chapter as a psychic and atmospheric phenomenon—demonstrating how remainder shifts scale but never disappears.

If the project of psychoanalysis is often imagined as a labor of healing or closure, this chapter insists on the creative, recursive potential of what remains unresolved. Remainder is not only a symptom but also a generative resource—a site where surprise, creativity, and new forms of meaning shimmer into being. The ethical task is not to cover over remainder, but to sustain presence at its threshold, honoring the openness, strangeness, and atmospheric charge that mark the limits of both psyche and civilization.

Psychoanalysis and the Drive to Cover Over the Remainder

From its inception, psychoanalysis has oscillated between two powerful currents: the drive to make meaning and the confrontation with what remains unresolved. The talking cure itself was founded on the conviction that what is unsymbolized, repressed, or unspoken can be brought into language—interpreted, worked through, and ultimately integrated into the psychic economy (Freud, 1900/1953). The analyst's task was to find the sense in symptoms, to decipher dreams, and to transform repetition into narrative coherence. In this founding gesture, the discipline was animated by a deep faith in the power of symbolization: that the psyche's pain and strangeness could be gathered up and rendered intelligible, healed by insight and interpretation.

This ideal of integration runs through much of psychoanalytic history. Whether in Freud's elaborations of sublimation, Klein's vision of reparation, or Winnicott's model of the holding environment, analysis has been shaped by a longing for psychic wholeness—a belief that fragments might be gathered, wounds healed, and the split psyche restored to some greater sense of unity (Freud, 1930/1961, p. 91; Klein, 1937; Winnicott, 1958/1965). Even Bion's notion of "containment" and Loewald's transformative vision of symbolization reflect a hope for psychic alchemy: that what is raw, chaotic, or unbearable might be metabolized into new forms, made available for relationship and meaning (Bion, 1962; Loewald, 1978).

Yet, woven into this quest for integration is a persistent anxiety about what resists or exceeds it—the psychic and symbolic remainders that refuse to be gathered into the nets of meaning. The **remainder**—what persists as symptom, as haunting, as the uncanny—can evoke discomfort, frustration, and a desire for analytic mastery. There is, in much psychoanalytic practice, a risk of pathologizing or disavowing the unintegrated: treating what cannot be assimilated as a deficit, a failure, or a "problem" to be solved.

This anxiety is visible in the clinical urge to interpret every silence, to make sense of every symptom, or to restore narrative order after breakdown. The analytic situation is often saturated by the pressure to "do something" with the residue—to turn what is opaque into something legible, to cover over the open wound with the suture of explanation or repair. Analysts may find themselves driven by the fantasy of closure, the temptation to erase gaps, or the wish to believe that everything can be brought into the symbolic fold.

But psychoanalysis has always harbored a countercurrent: a lineage of theorists and clinicians who refuse to treat the remainder as a mere error or shortcoming. Freud himself, for all his faith in interpretation, recognized that dreams have a "navel"—"at least one spot in every dream at which it is unplumbable—a navel, as it were, that is its point of contact with the unknown" (Freud, 1900/1953, p. 525). Klein acknowledged the persistence of wounds and splits that can never be fully repaired. Winnicott's potential space is sustained by what cannot be integrated, the play of absence and presence. Bollas described the "unthought known"—a reservoir of experience that remains outside the reach of consciousness or language (Bollas, 1987). Green, in his theory of the "dead mother," mapped the lasting atmospheric traces of psychic loss and absence (Green, 1986). Loewald identified a "primordial loss" at the heart of psychic life—a remainder that gives birth to desire, creativity, and the hunger for relationship (Loewald, 1978). Laplanche spoke of the "enigmatic signifier," an unconscious message that resists translation and persists as an excess (Laplanche, 1999). Bion's counsel to tolerate not-knowing (after Keats's "negative capability") is the discipline of bearing with, rather than erasing, what cannot be known or integrated (Keats, 1817/1958; Bion, 1962).

Lacan radicalizes this position with the concept of the Real: that which is forever outside the symbolic, the traumatic kernel that persists as remainder and which returns, again and again, to unsettle psychic and social order (Lacan, 1966/2006). Derrida's différance formalizes the endless deferral, spacing, and structural incompleteness of all meaning—remainder as necessity, not accident (Derrida, 1972/1982). Foucault, for his part, insists that every field of discourse, every exercise of power, leaves something ungoverned, opaque, or unassimilable (Foucault, 1975/1995). Gödel, through mathematical logic, demonstrates the impossibility of any system being fully closed or complete—every frame creates its own undecidable surplus, its own necessary remainder (Gödel, 1931/1986).

To honor the remainder is thus not a retreat from the analytic task, but a deepening of its ethical and creative horizon. This means recognizing the limitations of meaning, the importance of sustaining openness, and the generative power of what cannot be integrated. It means resisting the urge to pathologize or cover over the symptom, the silence, the breakdown, or the uncanny. It requires a willingness to bear with the excess, to witness what returns and persists, and to dwell at the edge of the analytic frame where the remainder is most alive.

Clinically, this stance demands humility and patience: the capacity to survive what cannot be explained, to welcome what cannot be made whole, to witness breakdown without fleeing to interpretation or repair. Analytic presence, in this frame, is not a guarantee of closure, but a practice of recursive hospitality—circling the gap, marking the atmosphere, and trusting that new meanings may shimmer into being precisely in the company of remainder.

In my own work, I have argued that the remainder is not an obstacle but a resource. The refusal to cover over the gap—whether psychic or cultural—makes possible a different kind of analytic presence, one attuned to surprise, emergence, and the ongoing reorganization of psychic and social life. If the discipline of psychoanalysis is to realize its fullest potential, it must learn not only to symbolize but also to bear the unsymbolizable, to sustain presence at the threshold, and to honor the remainder as the generative ground of both healing and creative failure.

Civilization as a Field of Remainder—From Discourse to Excess (Foucault and the Ungovernable)

Civilization is often celebrated as the achievement of order—an ongoing project of rendering the world legible, governable, and coherent through laws, language, rituals, and systems of meaning. Psychoanalysis inherited and at times reinforced this fantasy: that what is unruly or instinctual might be contained, transformed, and put to work in the service of culture and the symbolic (Freud, 1930/1961). Yet, as Foucault so forcefully demonstrated, every civilizing project—whether psychic or collective—generates its own excess: a remainder that escapes control, surveillance, and the totalizing ambitions of power (Foucault, 1975/1995).

For Foucault, civilization is not a seamless whole, but a **field of discourse**—a dynamic matrix of power, knowledge, and language that always leaves something outside its boundaries. Discipline, normalization, and surveillance never achieve perfect closure. There are always pockets of resistance, opacity, and "ungovernable" phenomena: forms of life, desire, or disorder that cannot be fully mapped or made to serve the order of things. In his studies of prisons, hospitals, and schools, Foucault shows how every system for organizing life is shadowed by what it cannot domesticate—criminality, madness, deviance, or silence itself (Foucault, 1975/1995).

Psychoanalysis itself can be understood as operating within this field: both as a technology of the self (producing new forms of subjectivity) and as a discourse attuned to what remains outside or excessive to all efforts at normalization. The analytic project is never simply the integration of the unruly into the symbolic order, but also the ongoing negotiation with what returns, resists, or escapes—what cannot be brought to speech, or what speaks in a language not recognized by civilization's code.

Remainder here becomes not a failure but a **structural feature**: every act of law or language, every new symbolic achievement, marks off new excesses. The more sophisticated civilization's machinery of meaning, the more intricate and powerful its apparatus of governance, the more complex and unassimilable its remainders become. In this sense, the remainder is the ghostly afterlife of every integration, haunting both individual and collective existence. It appears not only as deviance, subversion, the ungovernable residue but also as creativity, surprise, and the shimmer of new possibility.

We see this dynamic in the way certain affects, identities, or desires are rendered unspeakable or "illegible" within the dominant symbolic. Foucault's analysis of sexuality, for instance, reveals how discourses of confession and surveillance not only shape what can be said but also produce silences, secrets, and forbidden zones—new remainders that haunt the psychic and social field (Foucault, 1976/1990). Civilization, in this view, is not a triumph over the chaotic, but a shifting landscape continually haunted by its own discards and refusals.

The analytic consulting room is one such landscape: a bounded space that seeks to render affect, fantasy, and relation visible and meaningful, but which is always traversed by opacity and the ungovernable. The patient brings not only narrative and symptom but also a surplus of feeling, silence, or estrangement that resists analysis. Sometimes, this is felt as impasse, sometimes as atmosphere—a sense that something crucial remains unsaid, outside, or excessive to the analytic frame. The analyst's task, in these moments, is not to eradicate or "fix" the remainder, but to mark its presence, to honor the gaps and silences that exceed any given interpretation.

Foucault's insistence on the **ungovernable** becomes a resource here. Instead of seeing remainder as a failure of technique or civilization, we might begin to recognize it as the necessary ground for creativity and renewal. Remainder is the opening through which new forms of life—psychic, relational, or cultural—can emerge. If analysis is to be more than the policing of normativity or the restoration of order, it must sustain a hospitality to what cannot be governed, symbolized, or contained.

In this light, civilization itself appears as a recursive field—haunted by what escapes, shaped as much by its failures as by its successes. The discourse of reason is never complete; every advance produces new shadows, new residues, new uncanny atmospheres. Psychoanalysis, in its most generative form, is not the project of closing these gaps, but of lingering within them—recognizing that it is precisely in the space of remainder and excess that the future of both psyche and civilization is being written.

The Uncanny and the Return of the Remainder (Lacan, Freud, Derrida)

The uncanny occupies a privileged place in the landscape of remainder. It is the affective signature of what escapes integration—a sensation, atmosphere, or event that unsettles the familiar and signals the return of the unassimilable. Freud's classic essay on "The Uncanny" (*Das Unheimliche*) names it as "that class of the frightening which leads back to what is known of old and long familiar," but which has become strange through repression, return, or the breakdown of symbolic order (Freud, 1919/1955, p. 220). The uncanny is thus always recursive: it circles back, haunting the present with residues of the past and erupting where symbolic mastery falters.

The uncanny reveals the psychic cost of civilization's project—its dependence on repression, boundary-drawing, and the ongoing management of remainder. Every effort to domesticate the strange or chaotic generates new zones of opacity and repetition. The repressed does not disappear; it returns, often in unexpected forms: symptoms, dreams, cultural anomalies, or the subtle distortions of everyday life. The uncanny thus stands as evidence that the remainder is not simply a failure to be overcome, but an enduring and structuring feature of psychic and social life (Freud, 1919/1955).

Lacan radicalizes the uncanny by linking it to the Real—the unsymbolizable kernel at the heart of experience, forever beyond integration. The Real is not simply what is missing from the symbolic; it is what ruptures it, revealing the gap or "hole" that no act of signification can fill (Lacan, 1966/2006, 1977). Encounters with the Real are often experienced as traumatic, disruptive, or impossibly strange—moments when the frameworks of meaning collapse, and something irreducibly other breaks through. The uncanny, in Lacan's account, is the trace of the Real in psychic and cultural life: the place where remainder insists, disrupts, and remakes the symbolic field.

Derrida, for his part, describes this dynamic through the notion of ***différance***: the endless deferral and spacing of meaning, the structural impossibility of full presence or closure (Derrida, 1972/1982). Différance is not a failure but the very condition for the play of signification; it is what ensures that every sign, every meaning, is haunted by the shadow of what remains unsaid, unsymbolized, or deferred. In this light, the uncanny is not simply an affect but an event—a recursive irruption of difference and remainder that destabilizes the fantasy of completion.

These theoretical motifs are not abstractions; they saturate clinical and cultural experience. In the analytic room, the uncanny often surfaces as a sudden estrangement in the midst of the familiar: a slip of the tongue, a sudden shift in affect, a dream that refuses interpretation, or an atmosphere that chills the ordinary with the sense of something "not right." The analyst, attuned to these disruptions, may sense that the work has entered the territory of the remainder—the place where meaning breaks down and something excessive or enigmatic appears. The clinical task is not to dispel the uncanny or to force an interpretation, but to bear with it, to mark its presence, and to allow the recursive movement of meaning and unmeaning to continue.

The uncanny also animates the collective and cultural field. Social phenomena—cultural taboos, political symptoms, public spectacles of breakdown—frequently repeat the uncanny's logic: the return of what society cannot symbolize, the persistence of unresolved trauma or unintegrated histories, the sudden irruption of estrangement in the midst of order. The uncanny thus bears witness to civilization's remainders: its failures of sublimation, its refusals, and its haunted attempts at coherence.

The power of the uncanny lies not in its threat to meaning, but in its generative potential. When the remainder returns, it interrupts routine, opening a space for surprise, recognition, and even the possibility of new forms. The uncanny is the atmospheric sign that the symbolic field remains open—haunted, recursive, and alive. In this sense, psychoanalysis is not a technology of closure, but a discipline for marking, surviving, and inhabiting the presence of the remainder. The uncanny is the point where the limits of meaning shimmer, and the field is reorganized by what cannot be integrated.

It is important to emphasize that the uncanny, while explored here as a collective and cultural event, will return later in this book as a psychic and atmospheric motif—refracted through the singular, lived experience of subjectivity. Its capacity to shift scale, to traverse the boundary between the collective and the individual, is itself a mark of the recursive logic that animates both remainder and analytic inquiry. The reader is invited to notice how the uncanny shuttles between registers, always returning, never quite the same, structuring the rhythm of psychic and cultural life.

By foregrounding the uncanny as the return of the remainder, this chapter insists that what haunts is also what generatively disrupts. Remainder, once welcomed, becomes a resource for creativity, recursive renewal, and the continual reimagining of the possible. The analytic task is not to eliminate the uncanny, but to learn to dwell in its atmosphere—to let remainder return and to mark its presence as the living edge of both civilization and the self.

Gödel, Incompleteness, and the Structural Necessity of Remainder

If psychoanalysis and civilization are haunted by remainder—by what cannot be symbolized, governed, or fully known—this motif finds a powerful analog in the world of mathematics and logic. Kurt Gödel's incompleteness theorems, proved in the early 20th century, shattered the fantasy of completeness that had animated logic and the philosophy of mathematics since their inception. Gödel demonstrated, with irrefutable rigor, that any sufficiently complex formal system—such as arithmetic or logic—contains true statements that cannot be proven within the system itself. No matter how exhaustive the rules or how intricate the symbolic apparatus, there will always be a remainder: truths that are undecidable, propositions that persist at the edge, unassimilable and yet essential (Gödel, 1931/1986).

Gödel's remainder is not an accident or failure; it is structural and necessary. In every closed system, there exists a point where the system's own resources are inadequate to account for its truths. This incompleteness is not a deficit to be overcome, but a generative force: it keeps the system open, dynamic, and, in a sense, alive. The fantasy of total closure—of a system capable of accounting for everything, containing every anomaly—is thus revealed as a mirage. There is always a gap, a surplus, a horizon beyond which meaning escapes.

The psychoanalytic resonance is immediate. Like formal systems, psychic and cultural systems are forever confronted with their own limits. Every symbolic achievement, every act of integration or repair, leaves behind a residue—a symptom, a silence, a trace that cannot be fully accounted for within the existing frame. The more the analyst or the culture strives for completion, the more insistent and complex the remainder becomes. Just as with Gödel's theorem, there is no final mastery, no analytic frame that will resolve every enigma, explain every symptom, or heal every split.

This recognition is not cause for despair, but for humility and creative possibility. Gödel's remainder is what keeps systems from stasis and sterility; it is the condition for surprise, for new connections, for recursive return. In analysis, as in mathematics, the presence of remainder is not an obstacle to be eliminated but the very ground of generativity. The analytic frame must learn to accommodate what it cannot assimilate, to welcome the undecidable as a site of future meaning and psychic movement.

Clinically, this appears in moments of analytic impasse—those stretches when neither analyst nor patient can find sense, when interpretation fails, and the analytic pair is left circling the edge of the unknown. The temptation to resolve, to interpret, to "complete" the process is strong; yet, as Gödel teaches, it is often at these moments—at the very site of incompleteness—that the most vital psychic work is happening. The symptom, the silence, the atmosphere of not-knowing are not simply failures, but openings through which the new might enter. The analyst who can bear with the undecidable, who can hold presence at the site of remainder, models an ethic and a creativity that resists the demand for closure.

This structural incompleteness also animates cultural life. Societies, like subjects, generate ideals of wholeness, transparency, or mastery—visions of rational order that promise to contain all deviance, all excess, all unpredictability. Yet, every such vision produces its own margins, its own exceptions: the outsider, the mad, the criminal, the uncanny. These are not simply excluded, but persist as haunting presences, as reminders that no system is complete. The culture that can bear its remainder—rather than attempting to eradicate it—becomes capable of transformation, surprise, and true renewal.

The recursive signature of remainder, so central to this book's method, finds here a mathematical and philosophical anchor. Incompleteness is not only a limit but an invitation—a call to revisit, return, and reimagine what remains outside. It is the acknowledgment that every system, whether psychic, symbolic, or social, is most alive at its boundaries: where certainty falters, where new meaning is glimpsed, and where the future becomes possible.

In this light, psychoanalysis emerges not as a technology of totalization, but as a discipline for living with, and even welcoming, the necessity of remainder. Gödel's theorem, translated into the language of psychic life, teaches that the most vital truths are often those that remain undecidable—truths that can only be circled, marked, or borne. The ethic of remainder, then, is not a resignation to fragmentation, but a fidelity to the openness and surprise that incompleteness makes possible. Here, the analytic task is to dwell at the edge: to mark the remainder not as error, but as the ongoing condition for creativity, hospitality, and becoming.

Opacity, Refusal, and the Ethics of Non-Closure (Derrida, Foucault, Glissant)

If remainder and incompleteness are necessary features of psychic and collective life, what then is the ethic that arises from this condition? What stance can analysis—or any act of cultural witnessing—take toward what resists integration and closure? Here, the concept of **opacity** becomes a central resource. Derrida, Foucault, and Édouard Glissant, each in their own register, have insisted that opacity is not merely a limit to be regretted or a failure to be overcome, but a fundamental feature of the ethical and symbolic world.

Derrida's *différance* signals that the very operation of meaning requires gaps, delays, and undecidable spaces—zones where presence gives way to absence, where every assertion is haunted by what it cannot say (Derrida, 1972/1982). In this vision, the desire for full transparency or final understanding is not only doomed but potentially violent: an imposition that erases difference, ambiguity, and the play of remainder. To embrace opacity is to resist the fantasy of mastery; it is to acknowledge that what is other—whether a symptom, a person, or a fragment of culture—has a right to remain unassimilated, unreadable, or unresolved.

Foucault's analysis of power and knowledge offers a complementary ethic. Power, he writes, is always "inscribed" on the surfaces of bodies, practices, and discourses—but it is never complete, never total. There are always margins, resistances, shadows—spaces of "unreason," disorder, or refusal (Foucault, 1976/1990, 1975/1995). In Foucault's work, these margins are not mere accidents, but the very sites where new forms of life emerge: where the given order is contested, and where what has been rendered opaque or "ungovernable" becomes a seedbed for transformation. The ethic here is one of respect for what eludes capture: to hold presence at the border, to bear with what cannot be governed or explained.

Édouard Glissant, poet and theorist of relation, takes this further with his famous assertion of the "right to opacity." For Glissant, especially in the context of colonial and racial histories, the demand for transparency is a tool of domination—a means by which the powerful make the other legible, assimilable, or subordinate. Against this, Glissant insists on the ethical necessity of opacity: the right to remain untranslatable, to resist the gaze that seeks to master or possess (Glissant, 1997). Opacity, in his account, is not simply a lack but a generative refusal: the condition for relation without reduction, contact without colonization, being-with without full comprehension.

Psychoanalysis, when attuned to this ethic, becomes a discipline of non-closure. The analyst's task is not simply to interpret, repair, or resolve, but to sustain the openness of the analytic field—to welcome what resists, what remains strange, what does not "make sense." This involves a refusal to rush to explanation, to tolerate the anxiety of the undecidable, and to honor the atmosphere of opacity that pervades all genuine encounter. In the clinic, this might mean respecting the symptom that will not yield, the story that remains untold, the affect that defies language. Culturally, it might mean recognizing that some forms of suffering, difference, or refusal are not problems to be solved, but realities to be borne.

Opacity is not passivity. It is an active stance—a disciplined hospitality to remainder, an ethic of staying with the irreducible. It means refusing the violence of totalization and opening the self (and the analytic process) to the surprise of what exceeds intention or mastery. The analytic relationship becomes a microcosm of this ethic: a space where the not-yet-known, the misunderstood, and the unassimilable are treated not as threats, but as vital aspects of psychic and relational life.

This ethic reverberates through my prior writing as "recursive hospitality"—the ongoing discipline of circling the gap, returning to what remains opaque, and trusting that meaning, if it comes at all, will emerge only in relation to what cannot be fully claimed. It is the opposite of the fantasy of closure; it is a practice of presence at the edge. In honoring opacity, analysis becomes a site not just of healing or understanding, but of creative refusal, radical respect, and the cultivation of forms of life that thrive on difference, ambiguity, and the generative power of remainder.

Remainder in Clinical Practice—Vignettes and Atmospheres

The analytic consulting room is a privileged site for the encounter with remainder. Here, the drama of integration and excess, symbolization and opacity, unfolds in slow time and dense atmosphere. The work of analysis is not only about interpretation or insight but also about witnessing what persists—what will not be assimilated, explained, or closed. These are the psychic and affective remainders that resist the analyst's best efforts at meaning-making, generating climates of uncertainty, surprise, and sometimes creative impasse.

1 The Symptom That Won't Yield

Julia entered analysis with an obsessional symptom: a ritualistic need to tap the doorknob three times each morning before leaving for work. Over months, she and her analyst explored possible meanings—childhood anxieties, superstitions, the wish for control in a chaotic world. While partial insights emerged, the symptom stubbornly persisted. Julia's frustration grew; the analyst, too, felt the mounting pressure to "solve" the riddle.

Eventually, they arrived at an impasse. In the silence that followed yet another failed interpretation, Julia wept, "I just want it to stop.

I don't care why." Something shifted: instead of rushing to understand, the analyst joined her in bearing the unexplainable. The tapping became less a problem to fix and more a shared mystery—an atmosphere in the room. As they bore witness together, Julia reported feeling "less alone" with her symptom, even as its meaning remained opaque. The remainder, unyielding and undecidable, had become a site of relational contact and creative tolerance (Bollas, 1987; Ogden, 1994).

2 The Silence That Speaks
Sam's analysis was marked by long, recurring silences. Whenever emotional intensity peaked, he would withdraw into wordlessness, filling the space with a dense, charged quiet. Early in treatment, the analyst tried various strategies—gentle prompts, interpretive speculations, even patient waiting. Yet, the silences grew longer, more atmospheric, sometimes suffused with a kind of shared dread.

Over time, the analyst began to attend not only to what was missing but also to the felt quality of the silence itself. Rather than treating silence as a deficit or resistance, the analytic pair began to notice its shifts: sometimes cold, sometimes thick with anticipation, sometimes strangely peaceful. The "remainder" here was not only unsaid content but also an entire register of affective life that defied symbolization. It was in the willingness to bear this opacity—to dwell together in the unknowable—that trust deepened and a new, more subtle form of communication emerged (Green, 1986; Eigen, 2004).

3 The Uncanny Return
In another case, Amir brought dreams that unsettled both patient and analyst: dreams of familiar places that had turned strange, of loved ones who spoke in foreign tongues, of rooms that seemed to bend and collapse. Interpretation yielded little clarity. Instead, what remained was a diffuse sense of estrangement, a haunting that seemed to spill from the dreams into the waking world.

Amir began to speak of "feeling like a ghost" in his own life, unable to fully inhabit his relationships or sense of self. The analytic space became permeated with this uncanny atmosphere. Rather than attempting to explain away the disturbance, the analyst marked its presence, allowing the strangeness to linger. Over time, they came to see the uncanny as a recursive signature of Amir's psychic remainder: not a failure of integration, but a persistent invitation to stay with the unfamiliar, to risk contact with what could not be mastered or known. This stance—witnessing rather than resolving—proved crucial to Amir's eventual movement toward creative engagement with his own psychic excess (Freud, 1919/1955; Lacan, 1966/2006).

4 Cultural Remainders in the Analytic Frame

Not all remainders are strictly intrapsychic. In the context of cultural difference, social trauma, or collective rupture, remainder may appear as a dissonance that pervades the analytic field itself. Miriam, an immigrant from a war-torn country, often spoke of feeling "untranslatable." There were stories she could not tell, experiences she could not render intelligible in English or even in the analytic language. The analyst, aware of her own limits and the impossibility of full comprehension, chose not to press for narrative or clarity.

Instead, together they honored the right to opacity, borrowing from Glissant's ethic: some experiences would remain irreducibly "other," not to be assimilated or explained away (Glissant, 1997). This respect for what could not be symbolized opened space for moments of intimacy and creative exchange that were not dependent on understanding, but on a kind of mutual bearing of remainder. The analytic frame thus became a site where difference, unknowing, and the limits of symbolization were not pathologized, but acknowledged as sources of relational vitality.

5 Atmospheres of the Remainder

Across cases, what unites these moments is not their content, but their atmosphere: a recursive mood or climate that signals the presence of remainder. Sometimes, it arrives as a chill, a sense of impasse or failure. At other times, it is a shimmer—an intimation that something alive, even if unspeakable, is present. The analyst's discipline is to stay with these climates, to refrain from premature repair, to allow the analytic space to remain open to surprise, ambiguity, and new meaning.

Remainder, in clinical practice, is not a problem to be eliminated but an ongoing companion—an index of the psyche's openness to the future. By learning to bear with what cannot be assimilated, the analytic pair models a wider ethic for culture and collective life: the courage to honor what persists, the humility to dwell with opacity, and the faith that creativity emerges not from closure, but from sustained presence at the edge of what can be known.

Remainder as Creative Potential—Symptom, Surprise, and the Possibility of the New

If remainder is the haunting trace of what cannot be symbolized or integrated, it is also the ground from which surprise and newness emerge. Far from being merely a deficit or wound, remainder is what makes psychic and cultural life dynamic, recursive, and open to transformation. This creative potential of the unassimilable is one of psychoanalysis's deepest contributions: the recognition that symptom, rupture, and failure are not endpoints, but beginnings—sites where the future is quietly being negotiated.

The Symptom as Signal, Not Deficit

Psychoanalytic tradition has long taught that symptoms are not simply signs of pathology but encoded messages from the remainder—the psychic surplus that the self cannot, or will not, integrate. Freud's radical insight was that symptoms contain truth, even as they distort and conceal it (Freud, 1900/1953). The compulsion, the dream fragment, the repetition that will not yield: these are the forms in which the remainder insists, signaling both what is unmastered and what is generative. To treat the symptom solely as error or disease is to miss its vital function as a carrier of surprise and new possibility.

In clinical work, the analyst's capacity to attend to the symptom as remainder opens space for transformation. The meaning may not always become clear, and sometimes the symptom persists, yet the analytic stance of curiosity and presence makes possible new relationships to what was previously intolerable. Over time, the symptom may lose its sting, become integrated in some unexpected way, or even become a resource—a sign of creative adaptation rather than simply of failure (Bollas, 1987; Ogden, 1994). The generativity of remainder is rarely linear; it is recursive, looping, and often marked by periods of frustration and waiting. Yet, it is precisely in this waiting, in the willingness to bear with what cannot be resolved, that new psychic configurations can arise.

Surprise and the Unforeseen

Remainder is the space from which surprise emerges. In the analytic process, moments of impasse or breakdown—when meaning fails, when the familiar disintegrates—often precede eruptions of novelty. The new does not arrive as the fulfillment of a plan, but as a shimmering in the atmosphere: an unexpected word, an unfamiliar feeling, a dream that reframes the analytic field. These are not just breakthroughs in understanding, but events that shift the entire symbolic and affective landscape. The remainder, in refusing closure, keeps the psyche open to the unforeseen.

This creative function of remainder is mirrored at the level of culture. History is full of moments when breakdowns, crises, or failures of integration give rise to new forms—artistic movements born from disillusionment, social revolutions sparked by loss, cultural hybrids emerging from rupture. Remainder, as the residue of what cannot be assimilated, becomes a laboratory for invention. The symptom, the taboo, the deviant, or the unspeakable—these are not merely burdens, but reservoirs of unclaimed possibility. As Derrida and Foucault both suggest, the insistence of difference and opacity is what ensures that culture never closes upon itself but remains a living field of becoming (Derrida, 1972/1982; Foucault, 1976/1990).

Recursive Potential and the Future

The recursive atmosphere of remainder is not simply a repetition of the same, but a circulation in which the field is continuously reconfigured. What could not be symbolized yesterday may become thinkable today; what was intolerable may return, in altered form, as the ground for new connection or insight. The analytic ethic, then, is not to resolve the remainder once and for all, but to remain open to its ongoing capacity to surprise, disturb, and generate.

In my prior writing, I have described this as the work of recursive hospitality—a practice of circling the gap, trusting that what cannot be integrated may yet be the source of creative reorganization. This ethic does not glorify suffering or endless fragmentation but insists that the work of becoming—whether for individuals or collectives—requires a tolerance for remainder. The future depends not on perfect integration, but on the discipline of staying open to what exceeds our current knowledge, what persists as symptom, mystery, or uncanny trace.

By honoring the creative potential of remainder, psychoanalysis aligns itself with an ethic of openness and surprise. The symptom is not the enemy of health, but a message from the edge; impasse is not a defeat, but a portal to what has not yet been imagined. In the recursive loop of remainder, psyche and civilization remain alive to the new, perpetually invited to risk meaning, relation, and becoming.

Closing Reflection—Psychoanalysis after the Ideal of Integration

To live and work psychoanalytically after the ideal of integration is to bear witness to the remainder—not as failure, but as generative ground. The discipline's history is marked by the dream of wholeness, the fantasy that every symptom, silence, or disruption can be rendered meaningful, brought into relation, healed. Yet, what persists, returns, or resists—what remains opaque, unassimilable, or uncanny—is not a flaw in the fabric of psyche or civilization, but its ongoing condition.

The analytic task becomes one of presence at the edge: to sustain the openness of the field, to mark and circle the remainder, to honor opacity and the right to what cannot be known. This is an ethic of humility, creative patience, and disciplined refusal. Closure is not denied, but recognized as provisional; each act of symbolization produces its own excess, every healing its new edge of mystery. Remainder, in this sense, is not merely endured but welcomed—as the recursive atmosphere in which surprise, invention, and relation become possible.

If psychoanalysis, at its best, is a discipline of recursive hospitality, then it thrives precisely where the ungovernable, the unsymbolizable, and the strange press in. Civilization itself, as argued throughout this chapter, is a haunted field—open, shifting, and incomplete. It is in the presence of remainder that both psychic and social renewal take place, as new meanings and forms shimmer into being from what cannot be integrated or resolved.

The motif of the uncanny, traced here as a collective and cultural event, will recur as this book turns to the curved structures of psychic life and the lived atmospheres of the subject. In its returns—never quite the same, always altered—the remainder marks the rhythm of analytic and cultural becoming.

To honor the remainder is to recognize the life that is lived in the unfinished, the not-yet-known, and the irreducible. It is to choose, again and again, to stay at the edge—where surprise and renewal are not only possible, but necessary.

Part III

The Ethics of Unknowing

Care attends the world without seizing it.
Presence steadies at the horizon of speech.
Tenderness carries knowledge where concepts won't go.
Nothing resolved; contact made more intimate.

DOI: 10.4324/9781003747109-12

Chapter 9

Antigone's Refusal—Witnessing, Opacity, and the Ethics of Unlawful Knowing

This chapter reframes Antigone not as a static symbol of civil disobedience, but as an enduring atmosphere and analytic resource—a guide for the discipline of recursive witnessing and the defense of opacity at the borders of law, kinship, and the unknown. Through the lens of Bion's "negative capability," Antigone's refusal becomes a living ethic: the disciplined capacity to bear with what cannot be integrated, claimed, or recognized. Drawing on clinical, cultural, and political vignettes, this chapter traces how the right to opacity protects the singularity of grief, trauma, and identity against the violence of forced knowledge or assimilation. The analytic stance is reimagined not as mastery or interpretation, but as the ongoing hospitality of presence at the threshold—witnessing, defending, and sustaining what remains unclaimed or unsymbolizable. Antigone's refusal thus models a psychoanalysis oriented toward recursive hospitality, ethical non-closure, and the generativity of what endures at the limits of law and knowing.

Introduction—Antigone and the Atmosphere of Refusal

Antigone is not merely a figure of ancient tragedy, nor simply a symbol of civil disobedience. She is, in the psychoanalytic imagination, an atmosphere: a haunting mood that circulates at the border of law and life, grief and recognition, the known and the unspeakable. In every field where law meets its own limit—where witnessing is called for in the face of the ungrievable, the unsymbolizable, the unlawful—Antigone's refusal returns. It is not the dramatic gesture that gives her force, but the quality of her stance: an ethic of presence at the threshold, a fidelity to what cannot be integrated or claimed by the prevailing order.

DOI: 10.4324/9781003747109-13

This chapter opens at that threshold. Rather than rehearse Antigone as the familiar emblem of heroic defiance or doomed resistance, I invite the reader to dwell with her as the carrier of an atmosphere—one marked by opacity, ethical refusal, and the courage to sustain what cannot, or must not, be known. In my prior writing, I have traced the recursive signatures of remainder, opacity, and the uncanny as vital resources for the analytic field. Here, Antigone's refusal becomes a guide for a psychoanalysis that resists the violence of symbolic foreclosure—the pressure to render all experience knowable, legible, or contained within the law's domain.

At the heart of this ethic lies what Bion, following Keats, called **negative capability**: the disciplined capacity to bear with uncertainty, ambiguity, and not-knowing, without fleeing into explanation or repair (Bion, 1962). It is precisely this stance that distinguishes Antigone's refusal from mere rebellion. She does not demand to be recognized, nor does she submit her grief or fidelity to the protocols of legitimacy. Instead, she witnesses—she stays, she bears faithful presence to the unspeakable, the ungrievable, and the unclaimed. Hers is a refusal not only of the law's violence but also of the law's knowledge: an epistemic defiance that preserves the singularity of her relation to the dead, to trauma, and to the limits of what can be said.

This atmosphere of refusal is not only tragic; it is generative. Antigone's stance reveals the creative power of what remains opaque, the necessity of defending zones of experience that cannot be named, assimilated, or translated without loss. In the clinical situation, as in political or collective life, there are griefs that cannot be resolved, identities that must remain unacknowledged, traumas that refuse the shelter of meaning. The pressure to "bring to light," to "work through," to "heal" can itself become a form of erasure—a violence against the singular and the irreducible. Antigone teaches the discipline of holding back, of standing witness without mastery, of sustaining what remains unlawful or unknown.

To honor Antigone as an analytic guide is to cultivate negative capability within ourselves: to risk the anxiety of non-closure, to endure the discomfort of not-knowing, to resist the seduction of premature recognition. It is to recognize that the most ethical response to some wounds, some griefs, some borderlands, is not assimilation but presence—an ongoing witnessing that lets opacity remain, that shelters the right to refusal, and that sustains the future possibility of meaning without demanding its immediate arrival.

Throughout this chapter, Antigone's refusal will appear not as a single act, but as a recurring atmosphere: a climate of ethical ambiguity, tragic fidelity, and analytic resource. The myth itself will be retold not for the sake of resolution, but to illuminate the lived tensions at the borders of law and kinship, mourning and knowledge. Clinical and political scenes will show how the discipline of negative capability enables both analyst and witness to bear faithful presence at the edge of the unsymbolizable, the unacknowledged, and the unlawfully known.

In bearing with Antigone's atmosphere, psychoanalysis discovers a resource for recursive witnessing—a stance at the border that neither abandons nor assimilates but sustains the open possibility of what remains. It is here, at the very threshold of knowing, that the generativity of refusal becomes clear: not as a barrier to healing or meaning, but as the very field in which the ethics of opacity, presence, and surprise are continually renewed.

The Myth of Antigone—Law, Refusal, and the Limits of Knowledge

The myth of Antigone, most famously rendered by Sophocles, is often recited as a drama of civil disobedience: a singular woman's refusal to bow before the edicts of a sovereign king. Yet, to approach Antigone as merely a political rebel is to miss the depth of her refusal and the ethical strangeness of her fidelity. At stake is not only the conflict between individual conscience and state law but also the very question of what can—and cannot—be witnessed, recognized, or made knowable within a symbolic order.

Antigone's story unfolds in the aftermath of war. Her brothers, Eteocles and Polynices, have killed one another on opposing sides of Thebes' civil strife. Creon, the new king, decrees that Eteocles be buried with honor, while Polynices—branded a traitor—must remain unburied and left to rot beyond the city walls. This edict does not merely regulate ritual; it enacts a sovereign violence against memory, kinship, and grief. To be denied burial is to be denied recognition, mournability, and entry into the symbolic life of the city. It is a decree that reaches into the most intimate recesses of love, loss, and belonging.

Antigone's response is not a simple protest, nor is it reducible to personal loyalty. Her refusal is a **witnessing**: she honors the dead brother not by demanding his innocence, but by refusing the law's power to foreclose his meaning. She does not ask Creon to recognize Polynices, nor does she seek to justify her act. Instead, she asserts a different law—a fidelity to what cannot be brought within the domain of sovereign knowledge or legitimated by public ritual. She marks her allegiance not to a particular side, but to a logic of kinship and grief grounded in love rather than hatred.

In this stance, Antigone embodies what Édouard Glissant would later call the **right to opacity**: the ethical necessity of what remains unassimilated, untranslatable, or unwitnessed by the dominant order (Glissant, 1997). Her refusal protects not only the body of her brother, but also the atmosphere of grief and loss that defies capture by the law. Antigone's act is a defense of what psychoanalysis might call the unclaimed or unsymbolizable—those zones of experience that resist reduction to explanation, commemoration, or even speech.

The law, for its part, responds with anxiety and violence. Creon's authority cannot tolerate the border Antigone marks: her refusal threatens the fantasy of a transparent, knowable, and governable order. His insistence on burial as the limit of recognition is not just administrative, but epistemic. To let Polynices be grieved would be to acknowledge what escapes the law, to admit the presence of what cannot be contained. The tragic structure of Antigone lies precisely in this stalemate: the mutual incapacity of law and refusal to witness, recognize, or resolve the excess that persists at the border.

This drama is not confined to myth or ancient society. Psychoanalytic theory has long mapped the tension between law and what escapes it. Freud's own struggles with mourning, loss, and the limits of symbolization echo through the story: what cannot be mourned returns as symptom or haunting, shaping the psychic field with residues that resist integration (Freud, 1917/1957). Klein's vision of the depressive position—the endless work of mourning and reparation, always incomplete—finds its tragic twin in Antigone's fidelity to the ungrievable (Klein, 1940/1975). Winnicott's incommunicado core and unintegrated states point to the necessity of preserving spaces that cannot, and perhaps must not, be known or represented (Winnicott, 1958/1965). Laplanche's enigmatic signifier, the message that stings without resolution, vibrates in Antigone's act: an address to the dead, to absence, to what resists symbolization (Laplanche, 1999).

In each of these registers, Antigone's refusal emerges as an epistemic stance—a form of negative capability that resists the demand for explanation, recognition, or closure. Hers is an ethic of remaining with the unspeakable, of sustaining presence at the threshold where law and kinship, grief and governance, collide. She does not rush to fill the gap with meaning, nor does she surrender to the violence of forgetting. Instead, she keeps the border open—a zone of mourning, memory, and relation that cannot be foreclosed by decree.

This is not a static refusal. Antigone's act circulates as atmosphere—structuring the mood of those who live at the edge of law, who bear the charge of unrecognized loss, or who defend the right to opacity against the violence of assimilation. Her refusal is neither heroic nor nihilistic; it is tragic in the deepest sense, marked by a discipline of bearing with what cannot be known or resolved. In the analytic situation, as in cultural and political life, this atmosphere returns: the pressure to explain, to witness, to name—and the counterpressure to remain with what escapes knowledge.

By foregrounding Antigone's myth as an emblem of the limits of law and the ethics of refusal, this chapter invites a reimagining of witnessing—not as a project of making everything visible, but as a recursive discipline of negative capability. The analyst, like Antigone, is called to bear presence at the border, to defend the right to opacity, and to honor the generativity of what remains unlawful or unknown. The myth endures not as a call to resolution, but as an invitation to inhabit the borderland where law, love, and knowledge continually fail to coincide—and where, in that failure, a new ethic of psychoanalytic hospitality might be found.

Opacity as Ethical Stance—The Right to Remain Unassimilated

Opacity, in its deepest sense, is not a failure of understanding but a resource—a vital shield for the singular, the wounded, the unintegrated. In Antigone's refusal, the ethic of opacity is made manifest: a commitment to the right to remain unassimilated, to keep certain relations, griefs, and knowings outside the reach of the law's gaze and the violence of interpretation. This stance is not simply a reaction to the brutality of power, but a principle in its own right: a disciplined practice of negative capability, defending the necessity of what must not be rendered transparent or resolved.

Édouard Glissant's "right to opacity" is often cited in postcolonial and political thought, but its relevance for psychoanalysis—and for Antigone's myth—is profound. Édouard Glissant articulates the ethical necessity of a "right to opacity," arguing that neither understanding nor transparency should be demanded of the other (Glissant, 1997). In insisting on opacity, he is not advocating for indifference, but for the ethical refusal to assimilate the other's difference, suffering, or experience into the grids of one's own knowledge or mastery. Opacity is the condition of respect—an acknowledgment that what is most vital or wounded in another may need, and indeed deserve, to remain shielded from exposure.

Antigone's fidelity to her brother is not an insistence that his story be told, his innocence proved, or his name redeemed in the city's archives. Rather, her refusal is a defense of his unknowability—a stance that honors his right to remain ungrieved by the law, untranslatable within its terms. Her act becomes an emblem for all those forms of suffering, love, and memory that must not be made fully visible, lest they lose their singularity or become subject to the erasures of assimilation.

In psychoanalysis, the ethic of opacity is often at odds with the field's foundational faith in insight, interpretation, and the healing power of making the unconscious conscious. The analytic tradition is shaped by the drive to "lift repression," to bring into speech what is hidden, to transform the unthought known into symbol and narrative (Bollas, 1987; Freud, 1900/1953). Yet, the discipline is equally haunted by those experiences that resist symbolization, that cannot be worked through without loss, that require a different kind of holding—one grounded in negative capability rather than in explanatory zeal.

Laplanche's concept of the "enigmatic signifier" is instructive here. The enigmatic signifier is an address from the other that cannot be translated, a message that stings but remains undecidable, marking the place where meaning fails and the subject is left exposed to the unclaimed (Laplanche, 1999). In analysis, these enigmatic residues persist as symptoms, silences, or affective climates that refuse reduction to familiar categories. The analyst's discipline becomes one of bearing with the enigma, of defending its right to opacity, rather than forcing it into premature legibility.

Opacity also functions as a shield for the self. Winnicott's "incommunicado core"—the protected center of being that remains outside relational exposure—reminds us that some parts of experience must be held back, kept in reserve, or simply left unsaid (Winnicott, 1958/1965). Antigone's stance can be read as a defense of this core: her grief and fidelity are not open to the city's rituals or to Creon's forms of public knowledge. They are reserved and kept in a sacred zone of secrecy and singular relation. This is not withdrawal, but the maintenance of a boundary—an assertion that some wounds must be shielded from the gaze of the law, and that some acts of love must remain beyond its grasp.

In the clinic, this ethic often appears in the analyst's willingness to resist the lure of interpretation when faced with silences, repetitions, or refusals that feel opaque. To rush into meaning can be to violate the patient's right to unassimilated experience, to override the logic of refusal that may be essential for psychic survival. The practice of negative capability means learning to stay with the not-yet-known, to let opacity function as a form of care, and to recognize that not all suffering is made more bearable by being rendered intelligible.

Consider the patient who withholds, who keeps secrets, or whose suffering seems unnameable. The analyst, trained to notice the urge to explain or "break through," may find that true hospitality lies in sustaining the gap—in respecting the patient's refusal as a form of psychic self-preservation, or even dignity. The right to opacity is not a retreat from relation, but an ethic that permits the patient to approach the analytic space at their own pace, to reveal or conceal, to risk or withhold as needed. This ethic aligns with Bion's negative capability: the capacity to tolerate confusion, ambiguity, and the suspension of judgment, rather than collapsing difference into the familiar.

Opacity is also a resource for collective life. Social traumas, marginalized identities, and histories of violence often require that certain stories remain unclaimed or unfinished, not to evade reckoning, but to avoid the second violence of assimilation. Antigone's refusal echoes in the refusals of those who will not be rendered legible by the state, who will not surrender their pain to public consumption, or whose kinship cannot be mapped onto prevailing codes. In these atmospheres, opacity becomes both a shield and a necessity—a condition for ethical relation in the presence of irreducible difference.

Antigone's example, then, is not only tragic; it is visionary. She models the possibility of bearing faithful presence to what cannot be reconciled or resolved. The ethic of opacity, defended by her refusal, becomes an analytic resource: it permits the singularity of grief, trauma, or identity to survive the pressure of assimilation, to remain a site of future potential, and to resist the violence of explanation. This stance is both analytic and political, personal and collective. It is a refusal to translate every loss into a story, every trauma into a diagnosis, every difference into sameness.

To defend opacity is to defend the right to unassimilated life—to honor the borders and silences that give shape to subjectivity, community, and mourning. It is to recognize, with Bion and Antigone alike, that some forms of knowledge are best left in suspense, that the courage to witness sometimes means not knowing, not recognizing, not integrating. In this, opacity is not an absence but a gift: the atmosphere in which surprise, new relation, and recursive meaning may yet arise.

Witnessing beyond Law—Unlawful Knowing and Radical Presence

Witnessing, as figured in Antigone's myth, is not a matter of seeing, interpreting, or even testifying in the conventional sense. Rather, it is a radical presence at the border—an act of being-with what is unspeakable, unlawful, or unacknowledged by the prevailing order. Antigone's refusal is not only to act against Creon's decree but also to bear presence at the scene of exclusion, to remain with her brother's ungrievable body, to honor what cannot be brought within the circle of law, ritual, or public mourning. Her witnessing is at once an act of defiance and an embrace of opacity: she refuses not only to comply but also to translate, justify, or assimilate what she knows. In so doing, she embodies the analytic discipline of negative capability—the willingness to sustain presence at the limit of symbolization, to witness without mastery, and to remain faithful to the unknown.

This kind of witnessing has profound resonances in the psychoanalytic situation. In the clinic, the analyst is often confronted with experiences, affects, or histories that cannot be integrated or symbolized without loss. The pressure to interpret, to "know," or to render experience legible is strong—shaped by the clinical imperative to make the unconscious conscious, to provide meaning, or to facilitate narrative closure. Yet, the most transformative moments in analysis are often those in which the analyst sustains presence at the threshold, bearing witness to what cannot be assimilated or resolved.

Consider a patient who carries the weight of a traumatic event that defies speech—a loss, a violence, or a betrayal that remains unspeakable. The analyst, moved by empathy and training alike, may feel compelled to offer interpretation, narrative, or explanation. But the deeper work may be to simply remain present, to "be with" the wound in its opacity, to honor the patient's refusal of integration as a form of psychic dignity. In such moments, negative capability becomes both an ethic and a technique: the analyst resists the urge to explain, instead sustaining a disciplined openness to the unknown, the unsymbolizable, the unlawful knowing that shapes the analytic field (Bion, 1962).

This form of witnessing is not passive. It is an active stance of respect, curiosity, and courage. To witness beyond law is to risk the anxiety of uncertainty, to endure the discomfort of non-closure, and to trust that the most vital forms of psychic and relational movement often arise from what remains unsaid. The analyst who can bear this threshold creates a space in which the patient's refusal is not pathologized, but recognized as a necessary defense of the self's most vulnerable zones. The right to opacity, in the clinic, is a shield against the violence of assimilation, a safeguard for the singular and the wounded.

Antigone's refusal of symbolic foreclosure also models a stance for collective and political life. In a world where certain stories are forced into the open, where recognition is made a precondition for dignity or inclusion, the act of witnessing what cannot—or should not—be claimed becomes an urgent ethical task. This is evident in the politics of grief and protest, where mourners refuse to assimilate their dead into the narratives of the state or where communities insist on the right to remember, mourn, or protest in ways that cannot be codified or sanctioned by law. The refusal to recognize, the insistence on opacity, becomes itself a form of witnessing—a way of keeping faith with the unclaimed, the excluded, the abject.

This ethic of unlawful knowing finds resonance in the analytic frame whenever the analyst resists the demand to "fix," "heal," or "make sense of" what must remain open. Clinical vignettes abound: a patient whose pain is met not with interpretation, but with presence; a trauma that is witnessed in silence rather than narrated in speech; a secret that is held, not as a problem to be solved, but as a climate to be sustained. In each case, the refusal to force knowledge or recognition is not a failure, but an analytic resource—a way of protecting what must remain outside the circle of law and closure.

The discipline of recursive witnessing—returning again and again to the threshold, marking the atmosphere of refusal, sustaining the field of opacity—transforms both analyst and patient. Over time, the space of non-closure becomes generative: what was unspeakable may become shareable, what was unwitnessed may acquire its own dignity, what was unlawful may find an unexpected hospitality in the analytic atmosphere. The analyst's capacity for negative capability, for bearing with the unknown, is mirrored in the patient's own capacity to risk presence at the edge of what can be known or claimed.

This ethic extends beyond the analytic dyad. In social movements, acts of protest, or the defense of minority experience, the courage to witness without assimilating, to sustain relation without demanding translation, is a form of political and ethical fidelity. Antigone's stance recurs wherever the right to opacity is asserted against the demands of surveillance, recognition, or public legibility. To bear witness in these fields is not to resolve, but to sustain presence at the border—honoring refusal as a necessary act of care and hospitality.

In sum, witnessing beyond law is a practice of radical presence. It is grounded in negative capability, disciplined by the courage to endure what cannot be made knowable, and animated by the generativity of refusal. The analytic task, in this frame, is not to "solve" or "heal" every wound, but to cultivate the atmosphere in which the unassimilated, the unlawful, and the opaque can be witnessed, protected, and, in time, given the dignity of ongoing presence. This is Antigone's gift to psychoanalysis: the courage to sustain the unknown, and the recognition that true witnessing may require not knowledge, but faithful presence at the threshold of the unsymbolizable.

Tragic Refusal as Analytic Resource—Generativity of the Unsymbolizable

To dwell with Antigone's refusal is not only to accept the limits of knowing but also to recognize the strange, generative potential of what cannot be assimilated. In both the clinical situation and collective life, the refusal to symbolize, translate, or resolve every fragment of experience is not merely a tragic impasse—it is a resource, a discipline, and an atmosphere that gives rise to new possibilities. The unsymbolizable does not simply signify lack or defeat; it is the condition for surprise, transformation, and the birth of forms not yet imagined.

Antigone's act is tragic in the deepest psychoanalytic sense, but it is not sterile. The tragic refusal creates a charged border zone—a space in which the meanings sanctioned by law, kinship, or collective narrative are suspended and in which something new might shimmer into being. In her fidelity to the dead and the ungrievable, Antigone models a capacity for negative capability that does not resolve grief or contradiction but sustains them as living atmospheres. This is the climate in which new modes of relation, imagination, and subjectivity may emerge.

In the analytic encounter, the generativity of the unsymbolizable is most evident when both analyst and patient can resist the pressure to repair or interpret and instead allow the symptom, the silence, or the refusal to circulate. Clinical work is punctuated by moments when a patient's suffering seems resistant to every interpretive effort: the trauma that remains unspeakable, the loss that cannot be worked through, the desire that refuses to find its place in language. These moments are not analytic failures; they are invitations to dwell in the field of tragic refusal—to practice negative capability in the service of generativity.

Consider the case of a patient, Mara, whose sessions were marked by recurring dreams of locked doors and shadowed rooms. Every attempt to "open" the dream—through associations, history, or interpretive conjecture—produced anxiety, withdrawal, or even somatic symptoms. Only when the analyst named the atmosphere of the room—a climate of secrecy and suspended possibility—did Mara begin to shift. Together, they learned to "stay with" the locked doors, letting them signify nothing but themselves and honoring the opacity and strangeness of the dream as a form of psychic protection. Over time, the dreams changed: the rooms brightened, the locks softened, but not everything was revealed. Some doors remained closed, and that, they discovered, was necessary. The refusal to force entry became, paradoxically, the ground for new forms of safety and trust. The unsymbolizable was not a site of lack, but of ongoing creative tension—a source of recursive surprise, waiting to be re-encountered in different keys.

In this way, tragic refusal and negative capability reframe analytic progress. Healing is no longer measured by the degree to which everything is rendered conscious or legible, but by the capacity to bear, together, what resists closure. The unsymbolizable does not block growth; it ensures that the analytic space remains open to transformation. The analyst's fidelity to the unknown becomes a living resource, sustaining the possibility that what cannot be said now may find another form or voice in the future.

This ethic has clear cultural and political implications. Collective traumas—wars, migrations, exclusions, histories of violence—are often sites where the demand for narrative, recognition, or restitution risks doing new harm. To insist that every wound be named, every history be integrated, is to risk violating the right to opacity, the dignity of refusal. Antigone's stance offers an alternative: an ethic of witnessing that allows certain losses, kinships, and memories to remain outside the official archive.

In these atmospheric zones, unsymbolizable experience becomes the seedbed for new alliances, forms of solidarity, and creative eruptions that do not depend on legibility.

This is not to romanticize silence or secrecy, nor to deny the urgency of working through when possible. Rather, it is to recognize that the analytic and collective fields alike require climates of ambiguity and unfinishedness—zones in which mourning, difference, and refusal can be sustained without being resolved. The generativity of the unsymbolizable is precisely that it keeps the future open, allowing surprise, invention, and relation to arise in forms that cannot be predicted or forced.

Recursive witnessing is essential to this process. It is the practice of returning, again and again, to the threshold, marking the presence of refusal and honoring the "not yet" of meaning. In psychoanalysis, as in tragedy, the return is never simply a repetition; it is a circling that produces new resonances, new atmospheres, new openings. The analyst's presence at the border—the willingness to witness, not resolve, to dwell with, not explain—creates a climate in which patients may discover possibilities for living with loss, uncertainty, and the unknown.

Antigone's refusal thus becomes a living resource, not a static ideal. It animates the analytic encounter, the political movement, the collective ritual, wherever there is need to defend the right to remain unassimilated. The unsymbolizable is not what psychoanalysis must overcome, but what it must learn to sustain—an atmosphere in which ethics, creativity, and subjectivity are continually refigured.

To remain faithful to tragic refusal is to honor the ongoing, unfinished work of living at the border. It is to accept that the most vital forms of healing and relation arise not from closure, but from the discipline of negative capability: the courage to sustain what cannot be symbolized, and to trust that, in this openness, something new—however fragile or unclaimed—may come to life.

Clinical and Political Fields of Opacity—Defending the Unclaimed

The right to opacity, as modeled by Antigone's refusal, is most vividly encountered in the borderlands where individual suffering and collective history meet. In both the clinical setting and the political world, there are experiences, identities, and losses that demand protection from premature assimilation—zones of life that must remain unclaimed, unrecognized, or even unspeakable if their singularity and vitality are to be preserved. The defense of the unclaimed is not only a political or ethical act but a foundational task of psychoanalytic witnessing. Here, the analyst and citizen alike are called to bear with opacity, to defend the threshold where meaning cannot—and perhaps should not—be fully articulated.

Clinical Vignette: Grief without Witness

Elena comes to analysis after the sudden death of her estranged mother. Her grief is complicated, marked not only by loss but also by a history of unresolved hurt and ambivalence. Well-meaning friends and family urge her to "find closure," to speak or write about her loss, to join rituals of mourning. But Elena resists: her mourning is silent, private, difficult even for her to name. In the analytic room, she offers only fragments—a sigh, a memory, a phrase spoken half in jest. The analyst feels the pull to interpret, to name, to help her "work through" the loss. But something in Elena's refusal feels necessary, even sacred.

Over time, analyst and patient come to recognize the dignity of what remains unspoken. The analytic space holds Elena's right to opacity, allowing her grief to remain partly unclaimed, unsymbolized, unexposed to the demand for narrative or public recognition. This stance does not prolong suffering but gently preserves the particularity of Elena's loss—a climate in which mourning is allowed to circulate without being assimilated or resolved. In this atmosphere, negative capability becomes an act of respect: the analyst's presence affirms that not all wounds require words, not all griefs need to be witnessed in the register of knowledge.

Clinical Vignette: Identity and the Refusal of Forced Recognition

Isaac, a nonbinary patient, struggles with pressures to "come out" and name their identity for family, friends, and colleagues. The analytic work is marked by cycles of self-disclosure and withdrawal, by ambivalence about naming or claiming any fixed label. At times, Isaac's refusal to "choose" or "declare" a single identity frustrates both themselves and the analyst. Yet, as the work deepens, it becomes clear that the right to opacity—the right to inhabit ambiguity, fluidity, or even silence—is vital to Isaac's sense of psychic freedom.

Here, psychoanalytic hospitality means defending not only the right to be known but also the right not to be known, not to be assimilated into the prevailing codes of gender or selfhood. The analyst's negative capability—bearing with uncertainty, not forcing identity into a narrative—models a practice that is both therapeutic and political. The analytic space becomes a field where refusal is not resistance to growth but an act of care: a defense against the violence of recognition when recognition would entail foreclosure, simplification, or erasure.

Collective Vignette: Mourning in the Shadow of Political Violence

In the aftermath of state violence or mass trauma, communities often confront the pressure to narrate suffering and to memorialize loss in public rituals or official histories. Yet, some wounds remain unclaimable—not because they are denied, but because to expose them is to risk retraumatization, misrecognition, or the cooptation of memory by the state. The mothers of the Plaza de Mayo in Argentina, for instance, refused to name all the disappeared, holding open a space of silence and ambiguity that became a site of resistance and survival (Taylor, 1997). Their collective refusal was an act of radical opacity—a strategy that protected the unclaimed dead from being assimilated into the language of reconciliation or closure.

This ethic is echoed in smaller ways wherever communities, families, or individuals hold onto secrets, silences, or unfinished griefs. The right to opacity, in these cases, becomes a way of defending the unclaimed—the residue that cannot be absorbed by the collective narrative, the identity that cannot be contained within the logic of the state, the trauma that will not be smoothed into official memory.

Political Protest and the Refusal of Forced Legibility

Antigone's refusal also reverberates in acts of protest where the demand for legibility, for explanation, or for public performance is itself a form of violence. In movements for racial, sexual, or cultural justice, there is often a pressure to "speak out," to testify, to render suffering and identity visible to the dominant order. Yet, there are times when refusal is the more radical act: the choice not to name, not to translate, not to submit to the logic of recognition.

This stance is neither nihilistic nor antisocial. Rather, it is a way of protecting the unclaimed as a living resource for future possibilities. In such atmospheres, protest is less about making oneself visible than about defending the right to remain opaque—to maintain borders, silences, or zones of indeterminacy in which new alliances, languages, and forms of resistance can gestate.

The Analyst as Defender of the Unclaimed

In both clinical and political fields, the analyst's role is not to drag every silence into speech, nor to force every secret into recognition. Instead, the ethic of negative capability demands the courage to defend the unclaimed: to let some aspects of the self, some wounds, some identities, remain protected by opacity. This is not a refusal of engagement, but a disciplined hospitality—a practice of witnessing that honors the patient's (or community's) right to set the terms of what can be known, spoken, or claimed.

This discipline is not always easy. The analyst (like the citizen) must bear the anxiety of not knowing, the discomfort of ambiguity, the frustration of non-closure. Yet in doing so, the analytic frame becomes a resource for the preservation of difference, singularity, and the possibility of the new. The field of opacity is not a wasteland but a generative border—an atmosphere in which meaning, relation, and resistance remain possible.

Recursive Witnessing and the Future of Psychoanalysis

To defend the unclaimed is to trust in the ongoingness of experience, the generativity of what has not yet found its form. Recursive witnessing—returning again and again to the threshold, honoring what cannot be resolved—makes space for the possibility that what remains silent today may speak tomorrow, or that what is unclaimed now may become the seed for future transformation. Antigone's refusal, in this sense, is an enduring analytic resource: it teaches us that the most vital forms of healing, relation, and political resistance arise not from forced closure, but from the courage to sustain the atmosphere of opacity.

In the end, the right to opacity is the right to become—slowly, unpredictably, and on one's own terms. It is the defense of the unclaimed not as a deficit, but as the ongoing field in which subjectivity, relation, and freedom may continually be refigured.

The Analyst as Witness to Unlawful Knowing

If Antigone models the refusal of imposed knowledge and the defense of opacity, the analyst is called upon daily to enact a similar ethic in the analytic space—a stance of bearing witness to what cannot, or should not, be claimed as lawful knowing. This role is neither natural nor easy; it is a recursive discipline that demands both humility and courage. To become a witness to unlawful knowing is to stand at the threshold where meaning falters, to hold presence at the border of what resists integration, and to sustain a field in which opacity is not merely tolerated, but honored as a living necessity.

The psychoanalytic tradition has often celebrated the analyst as an interpreter, a translator of the unconscious, or a guide through the labyrinth of the symptom. Yet, this image, for all its utility, cannot account for the profound uncertainties that shape the lived analytic encounter. In reality, the analyst is as often a witness to silence, ambiguity, or failure as a maker of sense. The most ethically charged moments in analysis are rarely those in which the analyst "knows" but those in which they can admit not-knowing—those moments of negative capability where the urge to interpret is held in suspension, and presence itself becomes the primary act of care.

This stance is fraught with difficulty. Analysts are trained to value knowledge, mastery, and technical skill. The discomfort of opacity can stir anxiety—both the analyst's and the patient's. Silence, resistance, or refusal may be experienced as threats to progress, or even as indictments of the analytic frame. There is a temptation to rush into explanation, to patch over the unknown with theory, or to encourage the patient toward "breakthrough" when what is needed is the discipline of waiting. It is precisely here, at this threshold, that the analyst must bear the burden of negative capability: the willingness to hold open the space of the unlawful, the unsymbolizable, and the unclaimed.

Countertransference, too, becomes a crucial guide. The analyst's own feelings of inadequacy, restlessness, or frustration are not simply obstacles but signals—affective reminders of the stakes of opacity and refusal. When the analyst feels the urge to "do something," to break the silence, to press for confession or insight, it may be a sign that what is most alive in the analytic field is precisely what resists such interventions. The discipline of recursive witnessing requires the analyst to stay with these affective currents, to track their own desire for mastery, and to risk remaining in the discomfort of not-knowing.

A clinical example: David, a survivor of early neglect, spends months in analysis circling the same handful of stories—narratives marked by missing pieces, contradictions, or unexplained absences. He offers no new material, resists the analyst's invitations to explore certain memories, and sometimes retreats into long, watchful silence. The analyst, at first, worries about stagnation, feeling responsible for "moving things forward." But with time, it becomes apparent that David's refusals are not passive resistance but active self-protection—a defense of experiences that cannot, and should not, be exposed before their time. By learning to bear the tension, to listen without demand, and to refrain from forcing entry, the analyst creates a climate in which David's right to opacity is respected. Gradually, the analytic atmosphere shifts: silences grow less tense, new associations emerge, and the work acquires a different rhythm. The analyst's capacity for negative capability—her willingness to witness what remains unlawful—proves more healing than any particular interpretation.

This ethic reverberates through all analytic practice. Analysts encounter secrets that are never told, traumas that remain unnamed, identities that are tested but never declared. Some patients will never recount their most formative experiences or may reveal them only in partial, coded ways. The analyst, rather than seeking to "uncover" at any cost, becomes a custodian of atmosphere—one who protects the unclaimed, even from themselves. To witness to unlawful knowing is to affirm that what is most vital in psychic life may be what cannot be captured, narrated, or integrated. It is to trust that meaning can circulate in silence, in gesture, in the atmospheric mood of the analytic hour.

Negative capability, in this frame, is not only a tolerance for ambiguity but also an ethical commitment: a choice to defend the borderlands of psychic life against the colonizing impulses of knowledge, recognition, and integration. The analyst's humility is not a sign of defeat but a resource—an invitation to the patient to explore the edge of the unknown without fear of being claimed, named, or assimilated. The recursive nature of this stance—returning again and again to the threshold, marking the presence of refusal, honoring what cannot be resolved—creates an analytic field where transformation is possible precisely because it is not forced.

The analyst's experience is mirrored in political and cultural life. The courage to bear with the unclaimed, to protect the opacity of difference, is as necessary in the public sphere as in the analytic one. Just as Antigone's refusal is not simply for herself but for the dead, for memory, for what exceeds the law, so the analyst's refusal to assimilate, translate, or expose serves a wider ethic. It defends the future possibility of relation, healing, and surprise.

Ultimately, the analyst as witness to unlawful knowing is not a passive observer but an active participant in the ongoing negotiation of presence, absence, and opacity. To stand at the border, to bear with what cannot be claimed, is to align oneself with the recursive, unfinished rhythms of psychic and collective life. It is to make room for the possibility that what remains outside the law's grasp may yet be the ground from which something new—something freer, more vital—can emerge.

Closing Reflection—Antigone as Guide to Recursive Psychoanalysis

To close with Antigone is, paradoxically, to resist closure. Her refusal lingers as atmosphere: an invitation to dwell in the borderlands of law and kinship, knowing and opacity, grief and the generativity of what remains unclaimed. Antigone's stance, so often misread as merely tragic or heroic, is in fact a lesson in recursive psychoanalysis—a model of bearing with, returning to, and circling the limits of what can be symbolized, claimed, or healed.

Throughout this chapter, Antigone's refusal has illuminated the necessity and generativity of opacity in both psychic and collective life. She bears faithful presence not only to her brother but also to all that is unspeakable, unlawful, or unrecognized within the symbolic order. Her discipline is not that of the legislator or interpreter, but of the witness: she marks the threshold, defends the right to unclaimed suffering, and protects the fragile possibility of meaning that has not yet arrived. In this, Antigone becomes a guide for an analytic ethic grounded in negative capability—a commitment to the unfinished, the unknowable, and the recursive work of sustaining presence at the border.

The analytic field is most alive not in the moments of explanation or narrative resolution, but in those atmospheres of ambiguity, refusal, and waiting. Negative capability—the courage to remain with the unknown, to resist the rush to integrate, to dwell with what cannot be named—becomes the hallmark of psychoanalytic hospitality. The analyst's presence is not measured by the knowledge they confer, but by the climate they create: a field in which the patient's right to opacity is sheltered, and the future is allowed to remain open.

In clinical life, this ethic demands a humility and patience that can be difficult to sustain. The pressure to "help," to "know," to "repair" is ever-present, fueled by the culture's faith in mastery and by the analyst's own longing for efficacy. Yet, the most radical forms of healing emerge not from the successful assimilation of trauma or difference, but from the willingness to sustain presence at the edge, to mark what remains outside, and to affirm the value of refusal. Antigone's lesson is not simply to mourn the impossibility of synthesis, but to recognize its ethical necessity. The atmosphere of refusal is not a dead end, but a generative climate in which surprise, relation, and creative refiguring can take root.

Politically and culturally, the ethic of opacity and the defense of the unclaimed offer a template for living with difference, for resisting the violence of forced recognition, and for creating spaces where new forms of life can emerge. Antigone's refusal is not just for herself or for her brother—it is a stance for all who live at the margins, whose griefs, identities, or histories are too singular, too painful, or too unfinished to be claimed by the law or public ritual. In defending the right to opacity, she keeps alive the field in which subjectivity, memory, and community may be continually refigured.

Recursive psychoanalysis, as envisioned here, is not a method for resolving contradiction, but a discipline of bearing with it—of returning again and again to the border, the silence, the refusal, and finding there the conditions for transformation. The analyst, like Antigone, is called to be a witness at the edge: to honor the law's limits, to protect what remains unlawful, and to shelter the unknown as the ongoing source of analytic and collective renewal.

As this chapter draws to its own provisional close, the reader is invited to keep Antigone's atmosphere alive—to let her refusal echo through the recursive movements of analytic practice, political engagement, and relational life. What remains unsymbolizable is not a deficit, but a field of future possibility. The courage to sustain the unknown is the wellspring of both ethical relation and creative becoming.

The chapters that follow will deepen this recursive ethic, tracing how the uncanny, the curved structure of the self, and the atmospheres of collapse and surprise all depend upon this foundational capacity: to bear with what cannot be claimed, to honor what resists integration, and to welcome the generativity of refusal. Antigone, guide to opacity and negative capability, remains with us at the threshold—opening the analytic field to whatever new forms, meanings, and relations might yet emerge from the atmosphere of the unlawful and the unknown.

Chapter 10

The Uncanny as Curved Structure—Estrangement, Surprise, and Recursive Affect

This chapter reconceives the uncanny not as a fixed symptom or simple return of the repressed, but as a recursive and generative structure—an atmospheric field in which surprise, estrangement, and the unclassifiable mark the very edge of psychic and symbolic life. Drawing on surrealist art, psychoanalytic theory, and clinical material, the discussion foregrounds the uncanny as a curved terrain: a domain of collapse, condensation, and remainder where boundaries bend, meanings echo, and affect circulates in recursive loops. Rather than striving for mastery or resolution, psychoanalysis is reframed as a discipline of recursive hospitality—an analytic openness to the surprises that arise when the familiar turns strange and when collapse becomes a portal for emergence. Through clinical vignettes and cultural motifs, this chapter traces how the uncanny disrupts fixed identities and categories, inviting both analyst and patient to dwell at the rim of knowing. In this climate of ongoing becoming, the unclassifiable is not a deficit but a generative signature: the mark of a psychic and cultural field alive with recursive affect, surprise, and the creative possibility of transformation.

Introduction—Curved Structure and the Atmosphere of the Uncanny

Consider the surrealist painting: a staircase that folds into itself, doors opening onto impossible spaces, a clock draped like fabric over the edge of a table, or a familiar room where gravity bends and objects float. In the world of surrealism—Magritte's endless corridors, Dalí's melting clocks, Tanguy's landscapes of dream logic—the viewer is invited not merely to "see" but to *feel* the uncanny: a mood in which the ordinary turns strange, and the boundaries between self and world, sense and nonsense, seem to

DOI: 10.4324/9781003747109-14

waver. The psychic field, too, harbors such atmospheres—zones where categories collapse, certainty dissolves, and the familiar curves unexpectedly into the alien.

This chapter takes up the uncanny not as a static symptom or the mere return of the repressed, but as a recursive event: an *epistemic climate* in which surprise, estrangement, and affective excess become the conditions for psychic transformation. The uncanny, in this sense, is a curved structure—neither a linear narrative nor a closed system, but a field in which boundaries bend, meanings echo, and the self is both recognized and rendered strange. Just as in surrealist art, where the ordinary is unsettled by improbable conjunctions and shifting perspectives, the analytic situation is often shaped by recursive atmospheres—moments when the patient, the analyst, or the analytic frame itself seems to warp under the pressure of unclassifiable affect.

The surrealists understood that the unconscious does not simply "speak" in symbols, but organizes reality as a field of surprise, condensation, and discontinuity. Dreams, slips, and everyday misrecognitions were not failures of perception, but invitations to inhabit a different mode of knowing—one marked by play, anxiety, wonder, and the uncanny return of the repressed. In Magritte's famous painting, "Not to Be Reproduced," a man gazes into a mirror only to see the back of his own head—a visual paradox that evokes the recursive loop of self-reflection, misrecognition, and the impossibility of full self-possession. Such images do not resolve; they provoke an ongoing, unfinished relation to the scene, just as the analytic encounter circles the rim of the unsymbolizable.

The curved structure of the uncanny is thus not merely conceptual, but lived. Patients describe entering the analytic space and suddenly feeling as if the world is "tilted"—as if time, memory, or even the sound of their own voice has become uncanny, doubled, or strangely unmoored. The analyst, too, encounters these moments: a sudden sense of déjà vu, a patient's story that echoes a dream or memory from another life, a mood that condenses histories and futures into a single, shimmering moment of surprise. These are not mere clinical curiosities; they are the atmospheres in which analytic work becomes possible and in which transformation takes place through recursive passage rather than direct interpretation.

To dwell with the uncanny as curved structure is to cultivate a form of analytic hospitality—a discipline of bearing with surprise, uncertainty, and the recursive loops that shape psychic life. Rather than seeking to master or resolve uncanny experience, this stance invites the analyst and patient alike to inhabit the borderlands of knowing: to stay present at the rim, where the familiar becomes strange and the strange becomes a resource for new forms of meaning. The recursive movement of the uncanny—its looping affect, its condensation of past and present, its refusal of easy recognition—demands an openness to what cannot be planned or contained.

Throughout this chapter, the surrealist motif will serve as a guiding thread: a reminder that the analytic field, like the painted dreamscape, is organized by curved spaces, impossible objects, and atmospheres of strangeness that resist reduction. The uncanny is not an error to be eliminated, but a climate to be inhabited—a psychic weather system that signals both danger and possibility. In the recursive hospitality of psychoanalysis, surprise and estrangement become sites of emergence, where new relations, forms, and futures shimmer at the curved edge of experience.

As the discussion unfolds, we will see how the uncanny unsettles the presumed integrity of self, object, and world—opening analytic and cultural life to recursive affect, symbolic collapse, and the generativity of the unclassifiable. In this way, this chapter itself will enact the curved structure it describes: circling motifs, bending boundaries, and inviting the reader to risk surprise at the rim of what can be known.

What Is the Uncanny?—Estrangement, Ambiguity, and the Limits of Recognition

The uncanny (*unheimlich*) is one of psychoanalysis's most evocative and elusive concepts, perennially resisting definition even as it leaves its mark on theory, art, and lived experience. Freud's 1919 essay, "The Uncanny," famously pursues the phenomenon through etymology, literature, and clinical observation, tracing its origin to the "heimlich"—that which is homely, familiar, intimate—and then to its shadow, the *unheimlich*, the strange, concealed, or repressed. The uncanny, for Freud, is not the radically unfamiliar, but rather "that class of the frightening which leads back to what is known of old and long familiar" (Freud, 1919/1955, p. 220). The return of the repressed, the double, the automaton, the animated object—all are symptoms of this paradox: the strange that is at the heart of the known.

Yet, Freud's text itself is haunted by ambiguity. He confesses that "the uncanny is in reality nothing new or alien, but something which is familiar and old-established in the mind and which has become alienated from it only through the process of repression" (p. 241). The split between heimlich and unheimlich is never absolute; it is a folding, a recursive bending of the familiar into the strange and vice versa. This ambiguity becomes the uncanny's very structure: a looping affective and symbolic field in which recognition and disrecognition, comfort and anxiety, cannot be cleanly separated. The uncanny unsettles the boundaries of category, making what is most intimate suddenly foreign and what is most foreign uncomfortably close.

Surrealist art offers a living laboratory for this ambiguity. In works like Dalí's "The Persistence of Memory," the landscape is recognizably earthly, yet the melting clocks and bending forms defy the logic of space and time. The viewer experiences a simultaneous pull toward and away from the scene: the comfort of recognition is always already undermined by an undercurrent of estrangement. Magritte's "Time Transfixed"—a train emerging from a fireplace in a perfectly ordinary room—evokes the same looping structure. These images are not merely odd; they produce an atmosphere of psychic vertigo, a momentary suspension of the viewer's habitual sense of reality. The uncanniness is affective before it is intellectual; it is felt in the body as a kind of shudder, wonder, or sense of danger. The analytic field, likewise, is often shaped by these atmospheres: moments when a patient's story, dream, or gesture produces a ripple of the strange within the ordinary.

Contemporary theorists have deepened Freud's insight by attending to the uncanny's recursive and atmospheric dimensions. Ogden (1994) describes the analytic third as a field in which the familiar becomes strange, and the strange is discovered to be a vital part of the self. For Ogden, the uncanny is not just an event but a climate—an emergent mood that signals the breakdown or reformation of psychic boundaries. Derrida (1994), in his meditations on hauntology, echoes this: the present is always shadowed by traces of what is absent, unclaimed, or yet-to-come. Every act of recognition is haunted by the possibility of misrecognition, every declaration of identity shadowed by the unclassifiable. The uncanny, in this sense, is not an exception but a recursive condition of psychic and symbolic life.

In clinical experience, the uncanny may emerge as a sudden estrangement from one's own body, voice, or history. A patient recounts walking into their childhood home and feeling it "wasn't theirs," despite every object being in its place. Another dream of being pursued by a double or wakes in the night unable to remember their own name. These are not always dramatic events; sometimes the uncanny is a subtle, persistent background noise—the analytic room "tilts," the familiar rituals of the hour seem to stutter, or the analyst experiences an inexplicable déjà vu. Surrealist art renders these moments visible: the glove that moves on its own, the mannequin that gazes back, the staircase that never quite arrives. The uncanniness is not only in the image or story, but in the recursive atmosphere it produces.

Estrangement, then, is both a symptom and a resource. The uncanny breaks open the illusion of seamless selfhood, stable object relations, and the transparent world. It exposes the limits of recognition—those thresholds where the known curves into the unknown, and where meaning begins to shimmer with the possibility of surprise or collapse. For the analyst, these moments are invitations rather than errors: occasions to bear with ambiguity, to remain open to what cannot be quickly named or resolved, and to trust that transformation often emerges from the field of the unclassifiable.

In the era of artificial intelligence and digital mediation, the uncanny proliferates in new forms. Deepfakes, uncanny valley robots, and the eerie sense that our phones are "listening"—all are cultural iterations of Freud's insight. The boundaries of human and machine, animate and inanimate, self and other, become curved, recursive, and porous. Surrealist art anticipated this: its automatons and dream-machines dramatize the anxieties and exhilarations of a world where the familiar is always on the verge of becoming strange.

To ask, "What is the uncanny?" is thus to open a recursive inquiry—a question that, like the curved structure itself, resists final answer. It is to dwell in the atmosphere of estrangement, ambiguity, and the limits of recognition, and to recognize these as the very conditions for psychic and symbolic becoming. The uncanny is not a problem to be solved, but a field to be inhabited—a climate in which surprise, collapse, and creative emergence are always possible.

Curved Structure—From Symptom to Psychic Terrain

If the uncanny is not simply a static symptom but an atmosphere, then what is its structure? In this chapter, I propose the uncanny as a **curved structure** within psychic life—a field in which boundaries bend, time loops, and the familiar doubles back upon itself. The "curved" in this context is not only spatial but also temporal, aesthetic, and affective. It marks the places in analytic and everyday life where psychic experience resists the linear, refuses final synthesis, and instead generates recursive forms of meaning, estrangement, and surprise.

The motif of curved space has long animated surrealist and kindred illusionist art. Consider Escher's impossible staircases, Magritte's endless corridors, or Dalí's melting clocks that refuse to "keep time" in the ordinary sense. These images capture a felt sense of psychic terrain where the rules of reality are bent or suspended, where repetition and difference echo in the same field, and where every return brings both recognition and disturbance. In psychoanalytic experience, the curved structure is not an external architecture but a mode of psychic organization: a recursive topology in which symptom, memory, and affect move in loops, never quite settling, always on the verge of the strange.

Freud's account of repetition compulsion explicitly anticipates this curved, looping organization of psychic life, where returns are not mere stasis but conditions for emergent meaning (1920/1955, pp. 7–64). The symptom is never simply an error to be eliminated; it is a signpost marking the places where psychic reality cannot be fully "straightened out." Symptoms loop back, returning in new guises, as if the psyche were searching not for resolution but for the conditions under which meaning might begin to shimmer at the edge of experience. The uncanny, as curved structure, is the psychic field where these returns are both feared and desired—a space of recursive risk and creative potential.

Clinical Vignette: Circling the Rim of Knowing

Anna, a patient in her mid-30s, entered analysis in the aftermath of a destabilizing breakup. Her presenting complaints were familiar—anxiety, intrusive memories, a sense of loss—but what emerged in the analytic hour was something less easily named. Sessions were marked by an atmosphere of repetition: Anna would describe dreams in which she wandered familiar streets that suddenly bent into alleys she didn't recognize, or where doors opened onto rooms both known and utterly strange. She often described a sensation of "walking in circles," unable to escape a feeling that something crucial was just out of reach.

Early in the work, both Anna and her analyst felt the pull to "straighten out" her stories—to map the dreams onto past trauma, to find the hidden meaning that would render the strange familiar. Yet, the more they pursued this, the more the analytic field itself seemed to curve. Interpretations failed to "take"; the sessions became recursive, looping back to the same dream images, the same affective weather. There was a growing sense that something in Anna's experience refused integration, that the symptom was not a sign of psychic failure, but a lived climate—a curved structure organizing her relation to memory, loss, and the limits of knowing.

Gradually, a different analytic posture emerged: one of curiosity and hospitality toward the atmosphere itself. Rather than demanding resolution, the analyst began to circle with Anna, returning again and again to the threshold moments in her dreams—the doors, the corridors, the sense of estrangement. In this field, surprise began to surface: new memories arrived, not as straightforward disclosures, but as fragments that shimmered with both recognition and unfamiliarity. Anna spoke of feeling both more "at home" and more alive in the analytic space, even as much remained unresolved. The curved structure had become not a problem to be solved, but a terrain to be inhabited.

Temporal Curvature: Echoes and Doublings

The curved structure of the uncanny is also a temporal phenomenon. Time in the analytic hour is rarely linear; it bends, echoes, and folds back on itself. Anna's stories were often punctuated by déjà vu—moments when past and present seemed to collapse or when the analyst felt as if they had already lived through a given scene. The recursive return of dream images, symptoms, or affects is not mere stasis; it is the psyche's way of marking the places where meaning is in flux, where the future shimmers at the edge of the not-yet-known.

This temporal curvature is mirrored in surrealist cinema: Buñuel's films, with their looping narratives and scenes that repeat with subtle variations, evoke the experience of time as curved rather than straight. In these works, and in analytic process, every repetition is also a mutation—a recursive chance for the new to emerge from the strange.

Curved Structure as Analytic Resource

To name the uncanny as curved structure is to shift the analytic ethic from mastery to hospitality, from diagnosis to presence. The symptom is no longer just a signal of repression or return, but a doorway into a field of recursive affect and surprise. The analyst's task becomes one of bearing with the atmosphere—circling, doubling back, risking the discomfort of not-knowing, and trusting that meaning will arise not through linear explanation but through recursive presence.

This approach is not a retreat from rigor, but an expansion of what counts as analytic work. The curved structure is both a constraint and a resource: it limits the reach of interpretation but opens the field to creative emergence. Just as surrealist art invites the viewer to inhabit impossible spaces, the analytic encounter asks both patient and analyst to dwell at the rim of knowing, where the strange and the familiar are always entwined.

Curved structure, in this sense, is the psychic terrain in which surprise, estrangement, and new relation become possible. The uncanny ceases to be a symptom to be eliminated and becomes the very climate in which analytic and psychic life unfold—circling, returning, and shimmering with the recursive possibility of the new.

Recursive Affect—Loops, Surprises, and the Shifting Rim of Knowing

If the uncanny is a curved psychic structure, then **affect**—feeling, mood, emotional weather—is the medium through which its recursive logic is most intimately lived. In the analytic situation, as in surrealist art, affect does not flow in a straight line; it moves in loops, ripples, and sudden swerves, often refusing to resolve into coherent story or stable meaning. The recursive movement of affect is the signature of the uncanny: a climate of surprise, repetition, and emergence that shapes the field as much as any interpretation or insight.

Bion's (1962, 1965, 1970a) writings on reverie and *O* are instructive in this context. Reverie is not simply the analyst's empathy or "understanding," but an openness to the full complexity and ambiguity of the analytic atmosphere. The analyst listens with the whole body and mind, allowing affect to circulate, recur, and surprise. What returns in the analytic hour is rarely just content or memory; it is an atmosphere, a recursive affective loop in which the familiar can suddenly become strange, and the strange can become uncannily intimate. Bion's *O*—that which cannot be known in advance, but must be experienced—hovers at the rim of every analytic encounter, an invitation to dwell with the unclassifiable.

Surrealist Atmospheres and Affective Weather

Surrealist art is filled with recursive affects—emotions that do not rest but circulate, intensify, or double back on themselves. In Tanguy's "Indefinite Divisibility," the dream landscape is both serene and unsettling, a mood that cannot be fixed in a single word. Dalí's "The Persistence of Memory" conjures an atmosphere at once nostalgic and threatening, as if time itself were caught in a recursive loop of decay and reformation. These atmospheres are not about any one thing; they are recursive fields in which affective possibilities shimmer, collide, and multiply.

The analytic hour, too, is marked by shifting affective weather. Consider the patient who arrives cheerful, only for sadness or irritation to surface in a wave. Or the analytic dyad which notices that the same mood returns at the same point in every session, as if the field itself were governed by hidden tides. These loops are not pathologies to be eliminated, but recursive signatures of the psyche's ongoing attempts to metabolize, symbolize, or transform what cannot be known in advance.

Clinical Vignette: Affect as Recursive Surprise

Jasper, a patient struggling with chronic shame and self-critique, describes a recurring dream in which he is lost in a city that is at once his childhood neighborhood and an unknown metropolis. The atmosphere is suffused with longing and dread; every street seems both familiar and alien. In session, Jasper's feelings circle: pride turns to shame, relief to anxiety, hope to resignation, often in loops that neither he nor the analyst can predict or fully explain.

The analytic task is not to "solve" these loops, but to bear with them—to attend to the shifting rim of knowing, the climate of affective surprise that organizes Jasper's psychic world. The analyst's reverie here is recursive: she feels herself swept into the loops, notices her own emotional echoes, and becomes a participant in the field's recursive movement. At times, she experiences sudden surges of hope or despair, as if Jasper's affects were reverberating through the analytic atmosphere itself.

Over months, the field changes. The loops persist, but new affects begin to appear: curiosity, even playfulness, enter the hour. Jasper and the analyst discover that they can "surf" the recursive currents together, using the surprises that emerge as opportunities for new relation rather than evidence of stuckness. The affective climate remains unpredictable, but it is no longer merely threatening; it becomes a space in which surprise and transformation can shimmer at the rim of the analytic encounter.

Loops as Creative Resource

Recursive affect is not simply a repetition of trauma or symptom; it is a resource for creative emergence. In surrealist art, repetition is always mutation: the same motif recurs but is never identical, each loop creating new meaning and affective resonance. In analysis, the affective loops of shame, anxiety, or desire may at first feel oppressive, but when witnessed and inhabited recursively, they begin to open—allowing space for the unexpected, the joyful, the strange.

This creative potential is also evident in the analytic process itself. Moments of impasse—when patient and analyst feel caught in an endless loop—can become portals for surprise if approached with negative capability and recursive presence. The courage to stay with the loop, to "wait and see" rather than force resolution, often gives rise to new insight, connection, or affective climate. It is at these curved edges of knowing that the analytic field is most alive.

Surprise, Atmosphere, and Analytic Hospitality

Recursive affect produces not only repetition but surprise—the signature of the uncanny. The analytic frame is haunted by these surprises: a slip of the tongue that changes everything, a sudden mood that reconfigures the field, a dream or memory that arrives "out of nowhere" but feels charged with meaning. The analyst's hospitality to surprise—to the recursive loop, the unclassifiable affect, the strange echo—is what makes transformation possible. The field of knowing is not flat but curved; every return is also an opening, every loop a site for potential change.

Surrealist motifs—clocks that melt, doors that open onto impossible rooms, landscapes that fold back on themselves—mirror the recursive affects of psychic life. They remind us that the analytic field is not a space for linear progress, but a climate for surprise, estrangement, and the ongoing negotiation of meaning. The uncanny is the rim at which analytic hospitality is most needed and most generative.

Recursive Affect as Field for Becoming

In the end, recursive affect is the lived dimension of the uncanny's curved structure. It is the atmosphere in which knowing, feeling, and relating are never fixed but always circling, doubling back, and shimmering with the promise of surprise. The analyst's task is to bear with this climate—not to straighten it out, but to remain present at the rim, where the familiar curves into the strange and where new forms of relation and meaning may begin to emerge.

The Atmosphere of Recognition and Unrecognizability

If the uncanny's signature is recursive affect, its habitat is the shifting atmosphere of recognition and unrecognizability—a field in which subject, object, and world never quite settle into stable form. In both analytic and everyday life, recognition is never a simple act of naming or knowing; it is an ongoing, precarious achievement, haunted by the possibility of the strange, the unclassifiable, the unrecognized. This atmosphere is where the familiar suddenly slips, the self-doubles or dissolves, and what had seemed known is exposed as partial, provisional, or porous.

Psychoanalysis has long grappled with the instability of recognition. Freud's own account of the uncanny is rooted in the sudden turn: the heimlich that becomes unheimlich, the reassuring object that reveals a shadow, the ordinary space that begins to shimmer with threat or possibility. In the clinic, this atmosphere can appear as a subtle shift—an analyst's face momentarily unfamiliar, a patient's story that "rings false," or a shared silence that suddenly grows dense with meaning. These moments are not simply interruptions; they are recursive events that open the field to surprise, uncertainty, and the emergence of the new.

Surrealist Atmospheres: Recognition on the Brink

Surrealist art specializes in this destabilization of recognition. In Magritte's "The Lovers," two figures embrace, their faces veiled by cloth. The gesture is unmistakably intimate, yet their identities are withheld, creating a tension between recognition and opacity. In Ernst's collages, familiar objects are recombined into impossible assemblages—a chair grows wings, a landscape is populated by unrecognizable forms. The viewer is invited to search for meaning, to "make sense" of the scene, but the satisfaction of recognition is always deferred. The artwork holds the viewer in a field of unclassifiable relation, a climate in which what is seen cannot quite be named.

The analytic situation, too, is marked by these atmospheres of partial recognition. Consider a patient, Miriam, who speaks of "not recognizing herself" in the aftermath of a significant life change. She describes moments when her own face in the mirror feels strange or when her familiar routines seem to belong to someone else. The analyst notices a shift: Miriam's usual affect is muted, her stories lack their usual narrative thread. As the work deepens, the analytic frame itself becomes a site of estrangement—the room feels unfamiliar, the analyst's voice echoes oddly. These are not moments of dissociation or pathology, but recursive passages through the atmosphere of unrecognizability.

Recognition as Ongoing Negotiation

In psychoanalytic theory, recognition is always partial, always shadowed by the unrecognizable. Winnicott (1965, 1971) reminds us that even the most intimate relational achievements preserve an incommunicado core, and Benjamin (1995) reframes mutual recognition as an "encounter between subjects who are never fully known to each other" (p. 30), a relational achievement that depends on the acceptance of irreducible difference. Derrida's hauntology furthers this: every act of recognition is haunted by what cannot be claimed, every identification shadowed by traces of the other, by echoes of the strange.

Clinically, this negotiation is lived in micro-moments. The analyst finds themselves wondering, "Do I know this patient? Do I know myself in this hour?" The atmosphere may shift suddenly—a word misheard, a silence stretched too long, a memory that arrives unexpectedly and reframes the field. Recognition, here, is never final; it is an ongoing, recursive labor. The patient's sense of self is similarly porous: the uncanny mood may arrive as an inexplicable sadness, a laughter that feels alien, a gesture that seems to "belong to someone else." The analytic task is not to restore stable recognition, but to inhabit the field where knowing and unknowing circulate, where surprise and estrangement remain possible.

Clinical Vignette: The Patient Who Doubled

Consider Robert, a patient whose analysis was marked by recurring dreams of doubles: a stranger with his face, a voice that mimicked his own, a shadow that followed him through familiar spaces. In waking life, Robert described periods when his own thoughts felt "not quite mine," when his relationships took on an eerie, impersonal cast. The analytic hours became charged with these atmospheres—moments when the analyst felt as if Robert were both present and absent, both recognizable and somehow foreign. Interpretations fell flat; the usual narrative coherence dissolved into a series of images, feelings, and recursive loops.

Gradually, the work shifted. Instead of seeking to "integrate" the doubles or resolve the uncanny, analyst and patient began to explore the field of unrecognizability together. They marked the passages where recognition failed, naming them as climates rather than problems. In this shared field, new forms of relation emerged: a mutual curiosity, a playful openness to the possibility that not all of self or other could be known, named, or claimed. The atmosphere became less threatening, more generative—a climate in which surprise, new feeling, and creative relation could shimmer at the edge of recognition.

The Ethics of Analytic Hospitality

The shifting rim between recognition and unrecognizability is not a problem to be solved, but a terrain for analytic hospitality. The analyst's task is not to force closure, but to shelter the atmosphere in which difference, strangeness, and surprise can circulate. This is an ethic of presence at the curved edge—a willingness to dwell with what cannot be fully recognized or assimilated, and to trust that relation does not depend on mastery.

Surrealist art and psychoanalytic practice both teach that subjectivity is a recursive achievement, not a given. The atmosphere of unrecognizability is a resource, not a deficit: it is the field in which new forms of self, other, and world can emerge, where meaning is always in motion, and where analytic work becomes a practice of ongoing, creative becoming.

Collapse, Condensation, and Symbolic Remainder

To fully inhabit the uncanny's curved structure is to encounter the phenomenon of collapse—not merely as breakdown or failure, but as a creative event in psychic and symbolic life. In the analytic situation, as in surrealist art, collapse does not simply mean a loss of form or coherence; it is often the very condition that allows for new assemblages, meanings, and forms to emerge. Psychic collapse, condensation of meanings, and the residue of symbolic remainder all belong to this terrain where the strange, the unclassifiable, and the "leftover" become vital resources for becoming.

Collapse as Portal, Not Just Breakdown

Collapse, in its analytic sense, is rarely absolute. It marks moments when a previously stable structure—of identity, narrative, or relational meaning—can no longer be sustained. In clinical work, collapse may present as a period of confusion, affective flooding, or even dissociation. But beneath the anxiety lies an opportunity: as old forms fail, the field opens to new possibilities that could not be conceived within the prior arrangement.

Surrealist art embodies this logic. In Dalí's "The Great Masturbator," facial features, objects, and landscapes melt into each other, collapsing boundaries between categories. There is no stable figure/ground distinction; objects condense, meanings collide, and the scene is saturated with symbolic remainders—those psychic fragments that do not fit into any narrative but nevertheless shape the atmosphere. The painting does not invite simple interpretation but demands a recursive seeing, a willingness to inhabit collapse as the precondition for creative emergence.

The analytic hour can be similarly structured. When a patient's self-narrative collapses—through loss, trauma, or the sheer pressure of recursive affect—the result may at first feel unbearable. Yet, when the analyst is able to bear with the collapse, resisting the urge to "rescue" or prematurely reassemble meaning, a different kind of psychic work becomes possible. In the shattered atmosphere, new images, affects, and associations can surface, often with a surprising sense of relief or even playfulness. Collapse reveals not only what is lost but what remains: the symbolic fragments, leftovers, and potentialities that persist in the wake of disintegration.

Condensation: The Uncanny's Creative Principle

Condensation is Freud's term for the dream's ability to fuse multiple meanings, images, or affects into a single composite. The uncanny is saturated with such condensations—doubles, echoes, objects that hold more than one identity. In surrealist collage and montage, the principle of condensation is central: the familiar is joined to the strange, the object is always "more than itself," and meaning arises through the recursive layering of form.

Clinical vignettes echo this dynamic. Take Clara, a patient who arrives at analysis in the wake of a romantic breakup and the death of her grandmother, both occurring within weeks. Her dreams become dense, even bewildering: a single image of a key morphs into a childhood toy, a door, a heart, a cemetery gate. The analytic hours are charged with condensed affects—grief and desire, longing and guilt, memory and fantasy, all woven into the same scene. At times, the atmosphere in the room feels thick, as if multiple times and selves were present. This is not a sign of pathology, but of psychic creativity: the capacity to condense, to hold multiple meanings in play, to allow the analytic field to curve and thicken with the weight of symbolic remainder.

Symbolic Remainder: The Generative Leftover

Every act of collapse or condensation produces remainder: those fragments that cannot be fully resolved, translated, or assimilated. The uncanny's curved structure is a climate in which these symbolic remainders are not discarded, but held in suspense—a recursive resource for new forms of knowing and relating.

Surrealist art dramatizes this by foregrounding the leftover: the broken clock, the half-seen figure, the object whose use is unclear. These remainders evoke both loss and potential, the sense that meaning is never exhausted, that every scene harbors the possibility of surprise. In analysis, the symbolic remainder might be a story left unfinished, a gesture whose significance is never explained, a recurring image that resists interpretation but gathers emotional gravity over time. The analytic task is not to "tidy up" these fragments, but to sustain their presence—to recognize that the field's generativity depends precisely on what cannot be finally known.

Collapse and the Ethics of Analytic Presence

To bear witness to collapse, condensation, and remainder is to cultivate a discipline of presence at the edge. The analyst's willingness to stay with the residue—rather than forcing coherence—enacts an ethic of hospitality to the strange and the unclassifiable. Collapse, in this frame, becomes a portal: not simply a crisis to be resolved, but an opening to recursive creativity, surprise, and the emergence of new psychic configurations.

A clinical example: Mark, a patient whose career and marriage both unravel within a short period, enters a period of profound psychic collapse. For months, sessions are marked by confusion, broken sentences, a sense of "not knowing who I am anymore." At first, both patient and analyst struggle with anxiety, tempted by the wish to "rebuild" the lost structures as quickly as possible. But over time, a different climate takes hold. Mark begins to notice small, unexpected joys—a new song, a forgotten hobby, an odd, recurring image from childhood. The analytic hour becomes a space to dwell with these remainders, to let them accumulate and resonate. Slowly, a new sense of self emerges—not a return to the old, but a curved, recursive identity capable of holding contradiction, loss, and possibility together.

From Collapse to Emergence: Surrealism and the Uncanny

The psychoanalytic field shares with surrealism a faith in the generativity of collapse and remainder. When the world "falls apart"—in dream, analysis, or cultural life—the result is not only anxiety but also the possibility of transformation. The symbolic remainders, condensations, and fragments are not just evidence of loss, but seeds for new meaning and relation.

This is the creative promise of the uncanny's curved structure: that collapse and condensation, when witnessed and held with analytic hospitality, become climates in which the future shimmers—not as a return to order, but as an opening to surprise, invention, and the recursive becoming of the self.

Surprise and the Unclassifiable—Becoming at the Curved Edge

If collapse and condensation create the atmosphere of the uncanny's curved structure, then surprise is its signature—a felt punctuation in psychic life where the unclassifiable emerges and new forms of becoming become possible. In both surrealist art and psychoanalytic process, surprise is not simply an affect but an epistemic event, marking the rupture of expectation, the arrival of the not-yet-imagined, and the generativity that inheres in zones of ambiguity and non-knowledge.

Surprise as Analytic Event

In the analytic field, surprise arrives in many guises. It can be a slip of the tongue, an unexpected association, a laugh that erupts in the midst of sorrow. It is the moment when both analyst and patient recognize that something has shifted: a symptom reveals a new face, a silence acquires unexpected weight, a recurring dream image suddenly links two seemingly disparate memories. The surprise is rarely one of content alone—it is a structural event, signaling the presence of the unclassifiable, the intrusion of something that does not fit, yet cannot be denied.

Surrealist art dramatizes this logic of surprise. In Man Ray's "The Gift," an ordinary iron is transformed by the addition of a row of metal tacks, rendering the object both useless and arresting. The viewer experiences a jolt of unclassifiability: what is this object now? What is it for? The familiar is made strange, and the act of seeing becomes recursive—a looping attempt to integrate the new form into existing categories, only to find the categories themselves have bent. The analytic field, too, is a site where the familiar becomes strange, and the strange becomes a resource for new relation and meaning.

Bion's "O" and the Ethics of Surprise

Bion's concept of *O*—the ultimate unknowable that must be experienced rather than mastered—sits alongside Bollas's *unthought known*, lived forms of experience that surface as surprise-events before they can be symbolized (Bion, 1962; Bollas, 1987). To approach O is to risk the discomfort of the unclassifiable, to forego the shelter of certainty and open oneself to what cannot be anticipated or controlled. Analytic hospitality to surprise is thus an ethic: a willingness to allow the field to be punctuated by the unexpected, to treat these ruptures not as errors but as events of becoming.

The analyst's task is not to explain surprise away, but to dwell with it—to circle back, to ask what new possibilities the rupture has made available, to allow the patient (and oneself) to be changed by what arrives. In this sense, the analytic hour enacts a discipline of becoming at the curved edge: the border where meaning is not fixed and where the future shimmers with the possibility of transformation.

Clinical Vignette: The Emergence of the Unclassifiable

A patient, Eve, comes to analysis after years of feeling "stuck"—caught in repetitive relational patterns, haunted by dreams of ambiguous landscapes and hybrid creatures. She is wary of surprise, preferring the comfort of the known, and often expresses a desire for clear answers or diagnoses. Yet, as the analytic work unfolds, Eve finds herself drawn to moments that escape classification: a joke that "doesn't make sense but feels right," a story that loops back on itself, a painting she can't stop thinking about—a surrealist composition in which a woman's face is composed of fruit, flowers, and clouds.

In session, these unclassifiable moments initially create anxiety. Eve worries she is "making no progress," that the work is not "going anywhere." The analyst, too, feels the pull to organize, to interpret, to impose coherence. But as both learn to dwell at the curved edge—to bear with the surprise of what cannot be named—something shifts. The analytic field becomes a space where laughter and sadness mingle, where new associations spring up unexpectedly, where Eve's dreams become less frightening and more inviting. Surprise, once a threat, becomes a resource: the curved edge of the uncanny is revealed as a site of becoming, where new forms of self and relation can take shape.

Surrealism and the Unclassifiable

The surrealists made a practice of courting the unclassifiable. Their "exquisite corpse" games—collaborative drawings in which each participant adds to an image without knowing what has come before—are exercises in analytic surprise. The resulting figures are often strange, funny, or unsettling, but always irreducible to a single meaning. The surrealist object is a curved structure, impossible to assimilate yet generative in its very resistance to category.

In psychoanalysis, the unclassifiable is not a deficit but a portal. It is the terrain in which the analytic dyad becomes capable of transformation—not by resolving difference or ambiguity, but by welcoming surprise as a teacher. The field of analytic hospitality is not flat; it curves at the edge, inviting both patient and analyst to risk new forms of becoming.

The Ethics of Welcoming Surprise

Welcoming surprise is not a passive openness but an active stance—a discipline that refuses premature closure and that makes room for the future to arrive in forms that cannot be planned or even imagined. It requires courage, patience, and humility from both analyst and patient. Surprise destabilizes identity, challenges the supremacy of knowledge, and confronts the analytic frame with the limits of control. Yet, it is precisely at these moments that the work of analysis becomes most alive.

To bear with surprise is to honor the generativity of the unclassifiable. It is to dwell at the curved edge, where psychic life is always in the process of becoming—where the uncanny is not a symptom to be eradicated, but an atmosphere in which transformation shimmers. The analytic field becomes a living laboratory for this ethic: a space in which surprise is not only tolerated but also celebrated, in which the unclassifiable becomes the signature of new psychic and relational forms.

Curved Structure and the Art of Becoming

As this section closes, it is clear that the curved structure of the uncanny is not simply an analytic metaphor, but a way of inhabiting life itself. The surprise of the unclassifiable is the mark of living on the rim—where the familiar curves into the strange and where the future remains radically open. In both art and analysis, the discipline of welcoming surprise is the foundation for becoming: an ongoing, recursive process that enacts the very ethic of hospitality, transformation, and relation at the heart of psychoanalytic work.

Closing Reflection—Recursive Psychoanalysis at the Rim

To linger at the rim of the uncanny is to inhabit the very spirit of recursive psychoanalysis—a discipline that circles the edge of knowing, welcoming the strangeness that shimmers where the familiar turns. This chapter has traced the uncanny as a curved structure: a psychic and symbolic terrain where surprise, estrangement, collapse, and the unclassifiable emerge as the raw material for becoming. Here, analysis is not a project of straightening out the psyche, but of learning to bear with its loops, doublings, condensations, and atmospheric weather.

Surrealist art, from Dalí's melting clocks to Magritte's impossible mirrors and Ernst's hybrid forms, has accompanied us as both metaphor and method. The surrealist invitation is not merely to tolerate the uncanny but to *dwell within it*: to let the collapse of categories, the condensation of meanings, and the eruption of surprise become the condition for seeing and becoming anew. Psychoanalysis, in this frame, is less an art of explanation than of recursive hospitality—a willingness to meet the world, the patient, and oneself at the curved edge, with openness to what cannot be anticipated or resolved.

This ethic requires a particular discipline from the analyst. It asks for patience, humility, and the courage to risk non-closure. The field of knowing is curved, not flat; every approach to the center is also a circling of the rim, a recursive return to sites of uncertainty, unrecognizability, and surprise. The analyst's presence is not that of the master or the expert, but of the companion at the threshold—bearing witness to collapse and remainder, condensation and unclassifiability, and making space for the future to emerge in forms that cannot yet be known.

For the patient, too, the curved structure of the uncanny offers relief from the demand to explain, integrate, or fit experience into predetermined forms. The analytic hour becomes a climate in which surprise is possible, in which the self may shimmer into new relation, and in which even collapse is revealed as a portal rather than a defeat. Transformation arises not from mastery but from the ongoing, recursive practice of returning to the rim—of letting the atmosphere of the strange become a field for play, invention, and new forms of psychic and relational life.

Culturally, this ethic is urgent. In a world that prizes explanation, certainty, and the flattening of difference, the discipline of recursive psychoanalysis stands as a defense of what remains curved, unclassifiable, and alive. The uncanny is not an anomaly to be eradicated, but a signature of the world's ongoing generativity—a climate in which surprise, estrangement, and becoming are always possible. Surrealism, in both art and analytic practice, becomes a guide to this recursive work: a method for cultivating presence at the edge, a celebration of the atmosphere where knowing fails and new forms shimmer at the rim.

As we close, the invitation is to carry forward this ethic of curved presence—to welcome surprise, to honor collapse and remainder, to trust in the generativity of what cannot be planned. Recursive psychoanalysis, like the best of surrealist art, does not promise the comfort of closure but the possibility of transformation at the rim. To dwell with the uncanny is to embrace life as recursive, emergent, and curved—to inhabit the atmosphere where the self, the world, and the analytic relation are always becoming something more than what can be named.

Chapter 11

The Ethics of Failure—Witnessing, Not-Knowing, and Containment

This chapter reconceives failure not as a therapeutic shortcoming or deficit, but as a vital and ethical dimension of psychoanalytic work. Rather than pursuing mastery, repair, or perfect containment, it centers the analyst's task as one of recursive witnessing—returning, again and again, to the limits of knowing, breakdown, and the remainder that resists symbolization. Drawing on clinical vignettes, theoretical reflections, and mythic motifs, this chapter explores how analytic presence becomes most generative when it can sustain the climate of non-integration, opacity, and the unformulated. Failure emerges as an opening: a recursive atmosphere where both analyst and patient are called to humility, curiosity, and the discipline of not-knowing. By tracing the collapse of interpretive authority, the enduring residue of remainder, and the ethical invitation to "fail better," this chapter reframes analytic work as a living laboratory for surprise and transformation. Ultimately, the future of psychoanalytic ethics is found not in omniscient guidance or perfect repair, but in the courage to dwell at the edge of understanding—where new forms of relation and becoming shimmer precisely because both participants are willing to risk, return, and remain with what cannot be resolved.

Introduction—The Necessity of Failure

Failure is the specter that haunts every analytic hour, the climate in which both patient and analyst are called to dwell, and the terrain that most resists the grand narratives of mastery or cure. In the contemporary culture of psychoanalysis—so often preoccupied with interpretive agility, repair, and the successful containment of affect—the very notion of failure is shadowed by anxiety, discomfort, and the suspicion that something essential has gone wrong. Yet, beneath this unease lies another possibility: that failure

DOI: 10.4324/9781003747109-15

is not a deficit or error, but a necessary, even ethical, dimension of analytic life—a field where the limits of knowing and the remainder of the unintegrated become openings rather than ends.

I begin with a scene that is at once ordinary and hauntingly atmospheric: a seasoned analyst sits with a patient in the aftermath of a heated rupture. Words, which have once served as bridges, now fail. Every interpretation falls flat; even the analyst's silence feels intrusive. The patient looks away, shoulders curled inward, as if folding herself around something unspeakable. The room thickens with the presence of something unresolved—a psychic remainder that neither participant can metabolize, explain, or soothe. There is no tidy repair, no elegant moment of mutual recognition. The analyst feels exposed, powerless, even ashamed: a witness to breakdown, not its repair.

What is the task in such moments? If failure is inevitable, even constitutive, of analytic work, how might the analyst learn to inhabit its atmosphere not as a defeat, but as a resource—a zone in which the recursive discipline of witnessing, the ethic of presence, and the humility of not-knowing can take root?

The project of this chapter is to reframe failure not as the opposite of therapeutic success, but as the crucible in which the ethics of psychoanalysis are most potently forged. Failure, in this view, is not simply the collapse of technique, containment, or interpretive prowess. It is the field in which both patient and analyst are required to bear with what cannot be resolved, symbolized, or healed. It is the climate of remainder—the residue of psychic life that resists integration, that insists on its opacity, that remains unformulated despite every analytic effort. And it is the recursive atmosphere in which both participants are invited, again and again, to return to the threshold of what cannot be known.

This reframing is not simply a plea for humility, nor a philosophical gesture toward the limits of language or knowledge. It is, above all, a call to presence: a demand that the analyst learn to dwell in the climate of failure as a site of ethical attunement. In the recursive arc of this book, failure is revealed as a motif that recurs in multiple keys: the remainder that cannot be symbolized (as in the earlier chapters on projection and the uncanny), the opacity that must be honored (as in the stance of Antigone), the collapse of interpretive authority (as in the ethics of curved structure), and the discipline of presence in the face of the unformulated (as in every analytic impasse).

This approach draws on the lineage of analysts and theorists who have made space for the unintegrated, the unformulated, and the unknowable: Bion's "negative capability," Winnicott's incommunicado core, Laplanche's enigmatic signifier, and contemporary reflections on the ethics of not-knowing (Ogden, 2005; Benjamin, 2018; Harris, 2021). Each in their own way insists that analytic presence is most vital when it can remain with what cannot be metabolized or resolved—when the analyst is willing to fail as a way of sustaining the climate in which something new might emerge.

To witness failure is to risk humility, exposure, and discomfort. It is to renounce the fantasy of omniscience or seamless containment, to allow for breakdown as well as breakthrough, and to sustain presence at the very edge of what can be symbolized. Failure, in this sense, is not the end of analytic work, but its horizon—a recursive border that must be revisited, inhabited, and borne. It is the site where the limits of mastery are made visible and where the ethics of psychoanalysis become most palpable.

In the chapters that precede, the motifs of remainder, collapse, opacity, and recursive witnessing have circulated as atmospheric conditions—climates in which analytic life unfolds. In this chapter, these motifs converge in the ethics of failure: the recognition that analytic presence is not a function of what can be known or achieved, but of the willingness to bear with what remains unfinished, unresolved, or unknown.

What follows, then, is not a manual for overcoming or repairing failure, but a meditation on its necessity. Through clinical vignettes and theoretical reflection, this chapter will trace the ways in which analytic failure becomes an opening: a site where both patient and analyst are called to a deeper form of attunement, curiosity, and humility. It is here, at the very edge of understanding, that the discipline of not-knowing becomes a form of ethical witness—and where the future of psychoanalytic work might shimmer, precisely because we are willing to fail.

Witnessing at the Edge—Analytic Presence in the Face of Non-Integration

To witness is not to master, resolve, or even fully understand, but to remain present at the threshold of what cannot be integrated. Psychoanalysis, in its most radical form, is an invitation to stand with another at the edge—where language falters, affect swells, and the psyche resists the demand to make sense. Witnessing at this edge requires a discipline of presence: a recursive willingness to return, again and again, to the sites of impasse, breakdown, or non-integration. It is in these climates that analytic presence finds its most ethical and generative expression.

What does it mean, then, for the analyst to witness failure—not as a shortcoming of technique, but as a constitutive dimension of the analytic field? The temptation is always toward repair, interpretation, or narrative closure. Yet, it is often in the moments where nothing "works"—where the container is breached, meaning collapses, or the patient's suffering remains unformulated—that the analyst's presence becomes most vital. The analyst becomes, in these moments, a witness not to the triumph of the analytic method but to the enduring residue of what cannot be metabolized. This is the climate of remainder: a field where the unclaimed, the unrecognized, and the unsymbolized gather density and weight.

Clinical Vignette: The Session That Failed

Consider the case of Ben, a patient whose early life was marked by loss, silence, and the chronic absence of reliable caregivers. Ben comes to analysis not with a story to tell, but with a climate to inhabit: his hours are punctuated by long silences, sudden affective storms, and moments of deep withdrawal. The analyst, experienced and attuned, nevertheless finds herself repeatedly unable to "reach" him. Interpretations fall flat, empathy seems to miss the mark, and even silence—so often a holding space—feels hollow, rejected, or overwhelming. After one particularly difficult session, in which Ben leaves abruptly and with palpable frustration, the analyst is left with a sense of failure that is more atmospheric than eventful. The room is thick with remainder: the residue of what could not be held, symbolized, or metabolized.

In supervision, the analyst's first impulse is to seek technical solutions: Should she have spoken more? Less? Interpreted differently? Yet as the supervision unfolds, it becomes clear that what is being witnessed is not a "failure" in the ordinary sense, but an encounter with the limits of analytic containment and knowing. The analyst did not abandon her presence; she did not retreat from the climate of breakdown. Rather, she bore witness to the fact that some wounds cannot be quickly repaired, some silences cannot be filled, and some psychic climates must be endured rather than explained.

This is not resignation, but a form of ethical attunement. To remain present at the edge of non-integration is to recognize the remainder not as a deficit, but as a living field of possibility. The analyst's presence becomes an anchor—not for certainty, but for the discipline of not-knowing, the recursive willingness to return to what remains unresolved. It is here, in the willingness to witness failure, that new forms of relation may begin to glimmer: not as sudden breakthrough, but as the slow accumulation of trust, safety, and the sense that even the unintegrated can be endured together.

Witnessing as Recursive Discipline

The ethic of witnessing at the edge is, above all, recursive. The analyst is not asked to solve, fix, or even understand in a final way. Instead, the work is to return—to revisit the climate of failure, to mark the sites of remainder, and to remain open to what may shift, surprise, or change across time. This recursive stance transforms failure from an endpoint to an ongoing process: a climate in which both analyst and patient can risk new forms of presence and meaning.

Theoretical traditions have long grappled with this task. Bion's "negative capability" urges the analyst to remain in the state of "not knowing," to bear the turbulence of unintegrated experience without rushing to contain or explain. Winnicott writes of the capacity to be alone in the presence of another (Winnicott, 1958/1965), suggesting that true containment is not the elimination of absence or breakdown, but the creation of a climate in which the unintegrated can be witnessed without being erased. Laplanche's enigmatic signifier is another version of this discipline: the analyst is a witness to the message that cannot be fully decoded, the remainder that is constitutive of psychic life.

These traditions converge on a crucial point: analytic presence at the edge of non-integration is not a failure of technique, but a condition for ethical relation. The analyst who can bear with failure—who can sustain presence in the climate of remainder—is not abandoning the patient, but offering the most radical form of hospitality. This is the hospitality of the curved edge: a willingness to remain at the border, to risk not-knowing, and to allow new forms of symbolization or relation to shimmer, however tentatively, at the rim of experience.

Atmosphere, Humility, and the Limits of Knowing

The atmosphere of failure is also the atmosphere of humility. The analyst is called to relinquish the fantasy of omniscience, to let go of the hope that every wound can be named, every silence made meaningful. Instead, analytic humility becomes a climate in which both patient and analyst can dwell with what remains unresolved. This is not a climate of despair, but of possibility: an invitation to curiosity, to the recursive discipline of returning to the threshold, and to the ongoing work of bearing with what cannot be integrated.

In Ben's case, as in so many others, the analyst's presence at the edge of non-integration became the ground for future possibility. Over time, the climate shifted: silences became less brittle, frustration softened, and moments of shared presence emerged—not as sudden breakthroughs, but as the slow, recursive accumulation of trust. Failure, in this frame, was not an endpoint but an opening—a field in which both patient and analyst learned to witness the unintegrated, the remainder, and the possibility of something new.

Recursive Unknowing—Impasse, Rupture, and the Limits of Interpretation

In the psychic economy of analytic work, impasse and rupture are not accidental derailments but elemental features of the recursive field. Psychoanalysis begins in the fantasy of interpretation—the hope that the symptom, the silence, or the repetition can be deciphered, translated, or rendered transparent. Yet, every seasoned analyst discovers, sooner or later, the profound limits of interpretation: moments when understanding fails, the familiar tools turn blunt, and the analytic hour drifts into the uncharted weather of not-knowing. It is here, in the recursive encounter with impasse, that the ethic of failure acquires its most generative force.

Impasse is not a static obstacle but a dynamic threshold—a climate that returns in multiple keys, demanding to be endured, revisited, and reframed rather than simply overcome. For both analyst and patient, impasse is often accompanied by anxiety, frustration, and the wish for forward movement. Yet, paradoxically, it is the willingness to remain within the atmosphere of impasse—to circle its edges, to risk not-knowing—that allows the analytic field to become hospitable to surprise, symbolization, and the emergence of new relation.

Theory: Negative Capability, Enigmatic Message, and the "Incommunicado Core"

Bion's notion of negative capability—an openness to psychic reality that resists premature understanding—asks the analyst to bear turbulence "without memory or desire" and to inhabit the field of not-knowing long enough for something new to take form (Bion, 1962). For Bion, the analyst's most important discipline is the capacity to remain "without memory or desire," open to the turbulence of psychic reality as it unfolds, unclouded by premature understanding or technical ambition. In practice, this means learning to dwell in the field of not-knowing, to bear the anxiety of impasse, and to trust that something vital may arise in the absence of interpretive mastery.

Winnicott's "incommunicado core" and his account of the capacity to be alone make the same claim in another key: analytic relatedness depends on safeguarding what cannot be made transparent, on a shared ability to be alone in the other's presence (1958/1965, pp. 29–36; 1965). The analytic relationship, in this frame, is not a conduit for seamless understanding but a recursive negotiation with the limits of communication. Each analytic hour is a return to this threshold: the space between what can be spoken and what must remain unformulated, the place where the patient's and analyst's subjectivities meet, overlap, or resist each other.

Laplanche's enigmatic message captures yet another aspect of this recursive field. Every utterance, every silence, every analytic gesture carries with it a residue of the untranslatable—a remainder that resists assimilation into conscious meaning. For Laplanche, the "otherness" of the message is not a problem to be solved but a constitutive feature of psychic life. The analyst's task is to bear with the enigma, to return again and again to the message that cannot be deciphered, and to hold open the possibility that meaning may arrive, if at all, in unpredictable ways.

Clinical Vignette: Impasse as Generative Field

Consider the case of Naomi, a patient whose analytic journey is punctuated by repeated ruptures and the feeling of "going nowhere." Naomi speaks of childhood trauma but finds herself circling the same stories, unable to move beyond a certain threshold. The analyst, at first, strives to interpret—to offer reframings, connections, or empathic understanding. Yet, these interventions fall flat; at times, they are met with irritation or even withdrawal. Sessions settle into a recursive rhythm: the same image recurs, the same silence stretches, the same frustration bubbles up. Both participants begin to sense the atmosphere of failure.

It is in this field of impasse that something unexpected occurs. The analyst, relinquishing the drive to interpret, begins to narrate the impasse itself: "We keep returning here. It feels as if we are circling something that can't be reached, and maybe that's part of what needs to be felt." Rather than a breakthrough, what emerges is a subtle shift in the climate. Naomi sighs, acknowledging the relief of not being pressed to "move forward." The recursive discipline of returning—of witnessing the impasse without the demand for resolution—creates a field in which trust, curiosity, and even playfulness begin to take root.

Over time, Naomi and the analyst find themselves able to mark and revisit the impasse without shame or defeat. New memories surface; affect shifts; moments of humor punctuate the gloom. The recursive movement through impasse becomes a living resource—a space where surprise and symbolization can shimmer, if only fleetingly, at the rim of the analytic hour.

The Limits of Interpretation: Humility, Creativity, and Atmospheric Change

Recursive unknowing is not a passive waiting, but a creative discipline—a stance that values humility, curiosity, and the willingness to be changed by what remains outside the reach of knowledge. The analyst who can witness impasse without anxiety or defensiveness makes the field available for new forms of meaning, relation, and subjectivity. Impasse is no longer a "failure" but a climate of possibility.

This approach invites both analyst and patient to loosen their grip on mastery. The hour may end in uncertainty; the session may conclude with no clear resolution. Yet, the recursive willingness to return—to dwell at the threshold of the unformulated—becomes itself a mode of transformation. Over time, the analytic climate shifts. What once felt like sterile repetition is revealed as a slow, spiraling movement toward new possibility: an atmosphere in which surprise, symbolization, and relational truth can take form.

In this way, impasse and rupture are reimagined not as dead ends, but as vital elements of the recursive field. The limits of interpretation are not failures to be overcome, but the very ground in which the ethics of psychoanalysis are renewed.

The Analyst's Collapse—Containment, Humility, and the Ethics of Not-Knowing

If the analytic field is structured by recursive returns to impasse and failure, it is also marked by moments when the analyst's own position collapses: when containment breaks down, interpretive authority falters, and the analyst is forced to confront the limits of expertise. Far from being a rare crisis, these moments of collapse are woven into the ordinary fabric of analytic life. They form the very ground on which the ethics of psychoanalysis—humility, presence, and the willingness to bear with what cannot be known—are continually renewed.

Collapse is often felt first as an affect: a sudden loss of confidence, a wave of uncertainty, a sense of disorientation or exposure. The analyst may feel at sea, unmoored from the usual anchor points of theory, technique, or self-assurance. This can be experienced as anxiety, shame, or even a fleeting wish to escape the analytic hour altogether. Yet, beneath this discomfort lies an opening: a portal to a different mode of presence, one that is grounded not in mastery, but in humility, attunement, and the ethics of not-knowing.

Clinical Vignette: Letting Go of Expertise

Consider the experience of Dr. S, an analyst working with Thomas, a patient haunted by intractable guilt and shame. Sessions are fraught with repetition—Thomas circles the same episodes of self-blame, while Dr. S tries, again and again, to offer reframing, interpretation, or empathy. Each effort seems to make things worse; Thomas grows more entrenched, and Dr. S feels herself sinking into frustration, then hopelessness. The analytic hour becomes thick with tension, the field curdled by a shared sense of stuckness. One afternoon, after yet another failed intervention, Dr. S finds herself admitting aloud, "I don't know what to do here. I feel lost with you."

The effect is immediate: Thomas is startled, then unexpectedly relieved. He admits he, too, is tired of "trying" and "failing." The collapse of Dr. S's authority—her willingness to let go of expertise and bear with not-knowing—shifts the analytic climate. In the following sessions, both participants are able to acknowledge their mutual vulnerability; the analytic field becomes less rigid, more spacious, even open to moments of humor or play. The collapse is not a catastrophe, but a recursive opening: a site where a new ethic of relation and presence can take root.

Collapse of Containment: From Failure to Generative Field

Containment, in psychoanalytic terms, is often imagined as a technical skill—the analyst's ability to hold, metabolize, or transform the patient's unmanageable affect. But containment, too, has its limits. There are moments when the analytic frame is breached, when the analyst cannot absorb the patient's pain, or when the encounter with suffering is simply too much to bear. Rather than a mark of analytic inadequacy, these breaches are inevitable events in the life of the analytic relationship. They signal the boundaries of the self, the reality of difference, and the persistent presence of the remainder—what cannot be integrated or contained.

The ethics of the analyst's collapse reside not in denial or compensation, but in the capacity to witness and endure these limits. To admit one's own inability to contain, to survive the collapse of omnipotence, is to offer the patient a model of humility and recursive presence. The analytic relationship is transformed from a project of rescue or repair into a climate where failure, breakdown, and not-knowing are lived, witnessed, and even honored.

Theoretical Resonances: Humility as Ethical Atmosphere

Contemporary psychoanalytic writers have begun to explore humility as a core ethical stance. Jessica Benjamin (2018) insists that analytic presence is not about perfect attunement, but about the willingness to acknowledge difference, rupture, and the impossibility of total understanding. Bion's negative capability reappears here as an ethic of humility: the analyst who can remain present in the climate of collapse—who can resist the impulse to repair or explain—offers a hospitality to the unknown that is more generative than any technical intervention.

Winnicott's image of the "good enough" mother—one who inevitably fails but survives her failures and remains present—serves as a further guide. Analytic failure, in this light, is not a deficit but a climate of becoming: a recursive field in which patient and analyst can risk new forms of relation, subjectivity, and symbolization.

Atmosphere, Collapse, and Recursive Presence

The collapse of the analyst's authority or containment is never merely an individual failure; it is an atmospheric event, a recursive movement within the analytic field. Its power lies not in the drama of breakdown, but in the possibility that new climates—of trust, curiosity, or relational truth—may arise in its wake. The analyst's willingness to bear with collapse, to name it, and to remain present within it becomes the ground for future analytic work.

In Thomas's case, as in so many others, the analyst's collapse was not the end of the relationship, but the beginning of a new ethic. The recursive return to the edge—where knowing fails, where containment breaks down—became a shared practice. Over time, the analytic field grew more robust, more able to accommodate both the pain of failure and the possibility of emergence.

The Ethics of Not-Knowing: Ongoing Discipline

The analyst's collapse is not a one-time event, but a recurring feature of analytic life. Each return to the limits of containment, each admission of not-knowing, deepens the field in which ethical relation and transformation become possible. The discipline is ongoing: to resist the fantasy of mastery, to risk presence in the climate of uncertainty, and to welcome collapse as a condition for recursive becoming.

Analytic humility, in this frame, is not weakness, but strength—a capacity to bear with the discomfort of not-knowing, to survive the collapse of authority, and to make space for the future as the horizon of what cannot yet be symbolized or resolved.

This experience of collapse is not unique to the analytic dyad; it is echoed in myth, literature, and cultural imagination across time. The broken vessel, the tower struck by lightning, the "dark night of the soul"—all are symbols of the necessity and inevitability of breakdown on the path to transformation. In many traditions, collapse is not simply disaster, but the precondition for a new order: the shattering of the old that makes space for emergent forms, unexpected gifts, or deeper truth.

By framing analytic collapse within this broader mythic atmosphere, both analyst and patient are invited to see their failures not as isolated or shameful, but as moments in a larger, recursive cycle of becoming. The humility required to endure collapse is not an end, but a passage: a climate in which the remainder and the unformulated may shimmer, and where both participants are called to bear witness to the uncertain, the unfinished, and the possibility of something radically new.

Across myth and literature, the necessity of failure and collapse is a recurring motif. In the Greek myth of Sisyphus, condemned to eternally push his stone up the mountain only to see it fall again, the point is not the stone's arrival but the enduring presence with the task itself. In the Odyssey, Penelope's endless weaving and unweaving each night is less a failure to finish than a discipline of ongoing relation—a recursive act that preserves both her autonomy and her connection to what cannot be resolved. Beckett's insistence on trying again, on failing again and failing better, captures the atmosphere of recursive becoming: failure is not an end, but the very field in which the future remains open.

Psychoanalysis, read in this mythic key, is less a science of solutions than a climate for endless return—a willingness to dwell with what fails, collapses, or resists closure. To fail better is not to succeed, but to deepen one's presence at the edge, to honor the recursive cycles of loss and becoming, and to keep the field open for what may yet emerge.

Failure as Remainder—Opacity, the Unformulated, and the Discipline of Presence

If the analyst's collapse reveals the limits of containment and the necessity of humility, failure itself emerges as a psychic and relational remainder—a persistent residue that marks the edge of what can be symbolized, healed, or even recognized. In the recursive climate of analytic work, failure is not a single event to be overcome, but an ongoing presence: an atmosphere in which what cannot be metabolized or resolved circulates, accumulates, and quietly shapes the field of relation.

Remainder as the Lived Trace of Failure

What is left after every effort has been made, every interpretation offered, every silence inhabited? The remainder is that which cannot be claimed or transformed—what lingers as excess, opacity, or the unformulated. It is the echo of failed connection, the fragment that resists assembly, the affect or image that hovers just beyond the reach of narrative or conscious thought. In this sense, failure is not absence but presence: the mark of what persists, endures, and recurs in the analytic field despite all attempts at mastery.

This remainder may be felt as a psychic "weather system"—a subtle thickening of atmosphere when a patient returns, again and again, to the same threshold without crossing it; when a dream or symptom refuses to yield its secret; or when a moment of connection slips away before it can be held. For both patient and analyst, the experience is at once frustrating and oddly generative. The remainder cannot be named, but it can be marked; it cannot be resolved, but it can be sustained as a climate in which relation continues to unfold.

Opacity as an Ethical Resource

Opacity—Édouard Glissant's concept of the right to remain unknowable—becomes a crucial resource in the ethics of analytic failure. Where psychoanalysis is so often committed to making the unconscious conscious, to transforming opacity into transparency, Glissant's ethics insist on the generativity of what cannot be fully seen, grasped, or rendered clear. In the analytic relationship, this means that both participants are invited to respect the right of the other to remain partially opaque: to recognize that some elements of psychic life cannot—and perhaps should not—be named, translated, or assimilated.

This stance is not a retreat from engagement, but a discipline of presence. The analyst does not turn away from the patient's suffering or from the field of failure, but remains with it, honoring the climate of opacity as a field of ongoing potential. The patient, too, may discover relief and dignity in having their unformulated experience recognized and borne, rather than prematurely integrated or explained.

Glissant's philosophy of opacity offers not just an ethical permission, but a radical inversion of the Western project of knowledge. Where so much psychoanalytic thought has assumed that the aim is to bring the obscure to light—to translate all opacity into transparency—Glissant's "right to opacity" insists that not everything need be rendered knowable or assimilable. He extends ethical relation beyond the recognition of difference itself, arguing for a right to opacity—an insistence that relation does not require transparency, comprehension, or the reduction of the other to what can be made legible (Glissant, 1997). For Glissant, opacity is not a barrier to relation but its very ground: "We clamor for the right to opacity for everyone." This means that genuine relation depends on allowing otherness to remain irreducible, on respecting the zones of psychic and cultural life that cannot be grasped, named, or possessed.

For the analyst, this is more than a theoretical stance—it is a discipline enacted in the hour: to refrain from forcing understanding, to risk presence with the unknowable, and to honor the singularity of the patient's suffering, desire, or withdrawal. Opacity becomes a climate in which the patient's difference is not a problem to be solved, but the very field where relation is possible. The recursive ethic of analytic failure is thus doubled by the ethic of opacity: together, they mark the discipline of remaining with what cannot, and perhaps should not, be known.

Clinical Vignette: The Unformulated as Atmosphere

Consider Julia, a patient whose trauma is less a story than an atmosphere—a background radiation that infuses her life with vague dread, restlessness, and an unnameable sense of threat. In analysis, Julia struggles to articulate her pain, and the analyst, despite every effort, finds herself unable to "help" in the traditional sense. The hours are marked by long silences, failed interpretations, and moments when both feel adrift. Yet over time, a new discipline emerges: the analyst learns to mark the presence of the unformulated, to say, "It feels like there's something here we can't quite find words for, but I'm with you in it." Julia, in turn, feels less alone, less pressured to perform or produce meaning. The failure to symbolize becomes, paradoxically, the ground for trust and safety.

This climate is not static. At times, the atmosphere shifts—Julia is able to bring forward an image, a sensation, a memory fragment that surprises both participants. The remainder has not disappeared, but it now becomes a resource: the space in which relation can deepen, and where the possibility of transformation is kept alive by the very refusal to force resolution.

The Discipline of Presence

To "stay with" the remainder—what cannot be integrated or resolved—is perhaps the central discipline of analytic ethics. This is not a passive endurance, but an active form of attention: a recursive willingness to revisit the threshold, to bear with the opacity of the other (and of oneself), and to remain present to the ongoing field of unformulated experience.

The analyst's discipline is double: to resist both the lure of technical intervention and the temptation to withdraw into resignation or cynicism. Presence at the rim of failure is a practice that demands humility, patience, and the courage to bear with what cannot be known. In this sense, analytic failure becomes a climate of possibility—a recursive atmosphere in which both patient and analyst can continue to risk new forms of relation, meaning, and selfhood.

Remainder, Recursion, and the Climate of Becoming

The remainder—failure as persistent residue—is not a dead end but a climate for ongoing becoming. Each analytic hour is a recursive return to the site of what cannot be metabolized; each session is an opportunity to witness, mark, and sustain the climate of opacity and unformulated life. The ethics of presence here is not one of omnipotent care, but of willingness to be changed by what resists change, to be moved by what cannot be fully known or claimed.

In Julia's case, the discipline of analytic presence—of honoring the remainder, sustaining opacity, and marking the unformulated—becomes the foundation for trust, curiosity, and the slow, recursive work of healing. Failure, in this context, is not a deficit to be erased but the very signature of a living, ethical relationship: the climate in which both patient and analyst learn to bear with the unfinished, the opaque, and the promise of what may yet emerge.

Surprise and the Ethics of Relational Truth

In analytic work, surprise is not simply an event or affect—it is a signature of the recursive ethic, the unexpected flowering that arises precisely from the discipline of remaining with failure, opacity, and not-knowing. Where psychoanalysis begins with the hope of making the unconscious conscious, it often achieves its greatest potency not in the anticipated revelation but in those moments that break the frame, disrupt the narrative, and open the field to something wholly unplanned. Surprise, in this sense, is not the opposite of failure, but its most generative offspring: the sign that presence at the edge of knowing has created the conditions for new relational truth.

Surprise as a Recursive Event

To be surprised is to have one's expectations punctured, one's scripts upended, and one's sense of mastery temporarily suspended. In analytic terms, surprise often arrives in the wake of sustained impasse: after patient and analyst have circled the same terrain, endured repeated breakdowns, and risked presence in the atmosphere of remainder and not-knowing. The recursive return to failure is not a passive endurance but an active discipline—it is precisely this willingness to revisit what cannot be resolved that makes the field available for surprise.

Surrealist art has long understood this logic: the sudden juxtapositions, the eruption of the unclassifiable, the invitation to see the familiar through strange new eyes. In analysis, surprise can emerge as an unexpected image in a dream, a shift in affective tone, a moment of shared laughter in the midst of sorrow, or the sudden recognition of something vital in what was previously overlooked. These surprises are not imposed from outside; they arise from the recursive movement of the analytic field itself, the slow accumulation of presence at the rim of knowing.

Clinical Vignette: Surprise at the Threshold

Consider the analytic work with Amir, a patient who has spent years circling the experience of abandonment and distrust. Session after session, he brings stories of betrayal, disappointment, and failed connection. Both patient and analyst become accustomed to the rhythm of despair, the atmosphere of chronic failure. Yet one day, in the midst of another account of loss, Amir pauses, looks up, and says, "But you're still here. No matter how much I push, you haven't left." The analyst, herself startled, feels a surge of emotion—surprise, relief, even joy.

This is not the surprise of interpretation, nor the triumph of technique. It is the surprise of relational truth: the sudden recognition that something new has emerged from the recursive climate of failure and remainder. Neither participant could have planned or forced this moment; it is the product of their shared willingness to return, again and again, to the place where nothing worked, and to risk presence in the atmosphere of the unformulated.

Amir's surprise is double-edged. It not only brings hope but also anxiety: if connection is possible, so too is loss. The analyst's surprise is likewise ambivalent; it destabilizes her sense of role and expertise, reminding her that transformation is not a function of mastery but of shared risk. The analytic field is changed: both now know that surprise is possible, that the recursive return to failure is not a dead end but the portal to emergent relation.

Clinical Vignette: The Unclassifiable Laughter

Another example comes from the analysis of Mara, a patient whose analytic hours are often marked by heaviness, grief, and a near-ritual solemnity. Mara rarely laughs and tends to approach every subject with careful gravity. After months of working through cycles of disappointment, rupture, and periods of analytic silence, an unexpected moment occurs. During a session in which the analyst, momentarily flustered, mispronounces the name of a theorist, Mara bursts into laughter—a bright, spontaneous eruption that surprises them both. The laughter is not mocking; it is oddly joyous, breaking the prevailing atmosphere of seriousness and inviting a new current of play into the room.

At first, both are startled. Mara covers her mouth, as if she has violated an unspoken rule; the analyst, too, feels a moment of self-consciousness, unsure whether to join in or steer the session "back on track." But instead of returning to the solemn script, they pause together—allowing the surprise to expand, to become something shared. Mara later remarks, "I didn't know I could laugh here. I didn't know you would laugh with me." The analytic field shifts: the possibility of joy, play, and even hope emerges, not because suffering has been resolved, but because something unclassifiable has been welcomed.

This vignette, like Amir's, demonstrates that surprise is often relational—a climate event, not an individual achievement. It signals a change in what can be felt, shared, or endured together, emerging only after both have risked presence in the uncertain terrain of failure and not-knowing.

Relational Truth as Emergent, Not Pre-Ordained

Jessica Benjamin has argued that relational truth is never given in advance; it emerges in the space between subjectivities, in the shared negotiation of difference, opacity, and uncertainty. In analysis, relational truth is not a static fact to be discovered, but an ongoing event—a recursive process of mutual recognition, surprise, and ethical attunement.

The discipline of analytic presence is thus a discipline of risk: the willingness to stay at the edge, to remain open to surprise, and to welcome the emergent rather than the pre-ordained. This ethic is at odds with much of contemporary culture, which prizes certainty, mastery, and the fantasy of omniscience. In the analytic field, however, it is precisely the willingness to fail—to bear with the remainder, the unformulated, and the unknown—that creates the climate in which new truth can arise.

Cultural Motif: Surprise as Generative Force

Surprise is not only a clinical event; it is an ethical and cultural force. In literature and myth, the most profound transformations are often heralded by surprise—by the trickster's intervention, the sudden appearance of the unexpected, or the moment when the protagonist encounters something that cannot be assimilated into the old order. Surprise not only disrupts, unsettles, and destabilizes, but also makes possible the birth of the new, the reconciliation of difference, and the emergence of forms that could not have been predicted or willed.

The analytic field is a microcosm of this larger recursive logic. By returning, again and again, to the threshold of failure, both patient and analyst create a climate in which surprise is possible, even inevitable. The discipline is not to force surprise, but to make the field available for its arrival: to bear with the discomfort of not-knowing, to honor the opacity of the other, and to trust in the generativity of what cannot be planned.

The Ethics of Surprise: Humility, Curiosity, and the Open Future

To welcome surprise is to embrace humility, to relinquish the fantasy of control, and to recognize that the most vital forms of truth are those that emerge in the space of shared risk and presence. Curiosity becomes not the search for mastery, but the willingness to be changed by what arrives. The future, in this climate, is not an extension of the past but a field of possibility—a recursive horizon where failure, opacity, and surprise continually reshape what is possible.

In Amir's case, as in so many analytic journeys, surprise marks the place where relational truth is born—not as an achieved insight, but as an event that transforms both patient and analyst. The recursive discipline of staying with failure, bearing with remainder, and welcoming the unformulated is not simply a technical strategy; it is an ethical commitment, a climate in which new forms of relation, meaning, and selfhood can continually emerge.

Closing Reflection—The Future of Psychoanalytic Ethics

As this chapter closes, the horizon of psychoanalytic ethics reveals itself as less a destination than a climate—a recursive field shaped by humility, presence, and the discipline of not-knowing. Failure, remainder, opacity, surprise: these are not impediments to analytic work, but the very conditions that allow the future to shimmer, inviting both patient and analyst to risk new forms of relation and becoming.

Throughout this chapter, we have witnessed how failure is transformed from a source of shame or defeat into an opening—a space where the analyst's collapse, the limits of containment, and the atmosphere of impasse are not only endured but marked, held, and even honored. To dwell at the rim of knowing, to bear with what cannot be metabolized or named, is to cultivate a form of recursive hospitality: a willingness to revisit sites of breakdown, to mark the residue of what resists integration, and to recognize that the work of psychoanalysis is as much about what cannot be known as what can.

This ethic is not a prescription for analytic passivity or stoic resignation. Rather, it is a discipline—an ongoing practice of humility and curiosity in the face of the unformulated. The analyst, like the patient, is called again and again to risk the discomfort of not-knowing, to survive the collapse of expertise, and to inhabit the atmosphere of remainder without rushing to repair or resolve. In this recursive movement, the analytic field becomes a living laboratory for new forms of relational truth—emergent, surprising, and always provisional.

Humility, in this sense, is not simply a virtue but an atmospheric condition—a climate that pervades the analytic hour, shaping what is possible for both participants. It is the soil in which trust, safety, and creative becoming can take root. The willingness to fail, to acknowledge the limits of mastery, and to welcome the unclassifiable is not a mark of weakness, but a sign of analytic strength—a testament to the courage it takes to dwell at the edge of what can be known.

The future of psychoanalytic ethics, then, lies not in the pursuit of omniscient guidance, perfect containment, or flawless technique, but in the cultivation of recursive witnessing—the discipline of returning, again and again, to the threshold where something remains unfinished, unresolved, or opaque. It is in these climates that the possibility of surprise is kept alive, and where both analyst and patient can participate in the slow, recursive process of transformation.

In a world increasingly preoccupied with certainty, mastery, and the elimination of error, the ethic of analytic failure stands as a quiet refusal: an insistence that the most vital truths are those that emerge in the climate of not-knowing, those that shimmer in the atmosphere of remainder and surprise. The task of psychoanalysis is not to overcome failure but to bear with it—to make it hospitable, to let it become the ground for the future as something truly unknown.

As we move forward, this ethic offers both a challenge and an invitation. It calls on analysts—and indeed, all who care for others—to embrace the humility of presence, the discipline of recursive return, and the courage to witness what cannot be healed. In doing so, psychoanalysis enacts its most radical promise: to remain with the other, at the edge of understanding, where new forms of life may yet emerge, not despite failure, but because of it.

Chapter 12

The Other Side of Knowing—Secrecy, Surprise, and the Symbolic

This chapter explores the ambiguous edges of analytic knowing, where secrecy and surprise disrupt the drive toward mastery and invite new forms of symbolic life. Rather than treating secrecy as pathology or surprise as analytic failure, the discussion reframes both as generative climates—vital zones that protect the psyche's capacity for renewal, recursive transformation, and symbolic emergence. Drawing on an epistemic-affective matrix, this chapter maps how knowledge, acknowledgment, and affective resonance combine and shift, producing ever-changing psychic weather. The matrix is offered not as a rigid taxonomy, but as a living map—an invitation to trace the recursive crossings, ambiguous states, and atmospheric shifts that animate analytic presence. Through clinical vignettes and theoretical reflection, secrecy becomes not a barrier but a generative resource, surprise a sign of analytic vitality, and the symbolic a medium for ongoing negotiation at the rim of knowing. This chapter closes by inviting the reader to dwell in these unmastered zones, where secrecy, surprise, and the symbolic field continually renew the possibility of transformation.

Introduction—Margins and Thresholds

Psychoanalysis has always been drawn to the margins—to the places where words falter, where knowledge breaks down, where the drive toward mastery is interrupted by something withheld, ambiguous, or unspeakable. It is here, in these thresholds, that the climate of analytic work is most alive. The field becomes charged not by certainty, but by a tension between what can be said and what must remain secret; between what is revealed and what continues to elude symbolization. It is this very tension, this recursive oscillation at the rim of knowing, that animates the analytic hour and gives rise to surprise, renewal, and the possibility of transformation.

DOI: 10.4324/9781003747109-16

Consider the atmosphere of a session in which the presence of a secret is palpable. The analyst sits with a patient, both aware—though perhaps never explicitly—that something important has been withheld. The words that are spoken circle around a gap; laughter feels brittle, silence thickens, the air is charged with unformulated possibility. Nothing is confessed, and yet everything in the room is touched by the climate of secrecy. The secret is not simply a fact to be discovered or an event to be confessed; it is an atmosphere, a zone of recursive potential that shapes everything that can be felt, imagined, or thought. In this atmosphere, both analyst and patient find themselves hovering at the edge—alert to surprise, haunted by the unspoken, drawn toward a symbolic logic that curves away from certainty.

In much of classical theory, secrecy is framed as a problem to be solved or a symptom to be interpreted—an obstruction to the analytic project of making the unconscious conscious. Surprise, too, is often met with suspicion: an index of the analyst's failure to anticipate, a rupture to be repaired, a sign that something has escaped the net of interpretive mastery. But what if, instead, we begin from the premise that secrecy and surprise are not merely obstacles or failures, but vital climates—generative zones at the threshold of knowing, where the symbolic is always in motion and the psyche is protected from premature closure?

The analytic field, viewed from this angle, is less a space of final revelations than of recursive crossings—places where what is hidden, unacknowledged, or withheld becomes the very soil for symbolization, play, and renewal. The symbolic is not a static structure but a living medium, through which unknowing moves: a weather system that allows for the unexpected, the emergent, and the unfinished to circulate. The secret, in this climate, is not only something kept; it is something that keeps the field alive, guarding the possibility of surprise, inviting new forms of meaning to take shape at the rim of language.

To dwell at these margins is to give up the fantasy of analytic omniscience. Here, knowledge is never complete; the analyst is continually returned to a recursive humility, an acknowledgment of what remains unformulated or opaque. The climate of secrecy and surprise is one of creative limitation—a reminder that what escapes mastery is not only what cannot be known, but what must not be too quickly named. It is this zone of recursive not-knowing that generates the conditions for genuine analytic presence: the discipline of remaining, again and again, at the ambiguous edge, where both analyst and patient are shaped by the weather of what is hidden or unspoken.

In this chapter, we turn explicitly to these liminal states—the climates and crossings where secrecy, surprise, and the symbolic subvert the drive toward mastery and certainty. We will trace how what is withheld or unformulated does not merely obstruct knowing but protects and renews the psyche's capacity for transformation. Our inquiry moves beyond the question of "what is the secret?" or "what was the surprise?" Instead, we ask: What kind of climate is produced when knowing is suspended? What recursive possibilities emerge at the threshold of the unspoken? How does the symbolic field shift when we attend not just to what is said, but to the atmospheres of secrecy and surprise that shape every analytic hour?

To explore these questions, I will introduce a provisional epistemic-affective matrix—a "weather map" rather than a taxonomy—designed to help us trace the shifting psychic climates produced by different combinations of knowledge, acknowledgment, and affective resonance. Yet, even this chart, as we will see, is offered not as a tool for final mastery but as a recursive resource—a way of mapping what moves, what escapes, and what continually returns at the rim of analytic experience.

Through clinical vignettes, theoretical reflection, and recursive movement between zones of knowing and unknowing, this chapter invites you to inhabit the ambiguous edge of analytic life. Here, secrecy and surprise are not pathologies to be cured, but vital resources for thought, presence, and symbolization. The task is not to master the secret or to anticipate the surprise, but to sustain an analytic hospitality to what escapes mastery—to dwell in the weather of the unknown, where the symbolic is always becoming.

The Matrix as Weather Map—Mapping Psychic Climates

To navigate the recursive landscapes of secrecy, surprise, and the symbolic, we need more than a set of interpretive rules or static categories. The analytic field is not composed of discrete points, but of shifting climates—zones of knowing, unknowing, acknowledgment, disavowal, affective resonance, and the strange crossings between them. Rather than fixing these states in place, we might use a matrix as a kind of weather map: a way of charting psychic atmospheres and movements, of tracking how knowledge, ownership, and feeling combine and recombine to create new conditions for thought, relation, and surprise.

Below is the epistemic-affective matrix that will anchor our inquiry in this section:

Cognitive (X)	*Ownership (Y)*	*Affective (Z)*	*Resulting Zone*	*Psychoanalytic Correlate*
Known	Acknowledged	Felt	Articulated Knowing	Integrated self-knowledge, truth in speech
Known	Disavowed	Felt	Defensive Knowing	Rationalization, intellectualization
Unknown	Disavowed	Felt	Haunting	Repetition compulsion, dream atmosphere
Unknown	Acknowledged	Felt	Negative Capability	Holding unformulated experience
Unknown	Disavowed	Unfelt	The Unthought Known	Bollas, deep structure
Known	Acknowledged	Unfelt	Dead Knowledge	Dogmatized self-knowledge; ritualized speech cf. Bollas (1987)
Unknown	Acknowledged	Unfelt	Pre-symbolic Readiness	Winnicott's potential space
Known	Disavowed	Unfelt	Symbolic Foreclosure	Perverse denial, ideology

A Living Map, Not a Taxonomy

It is crucial to foreground: this matrix is not a taxonomy of psychic types or a rigid diagnostic tool. Rather, it is a living map—its cells are not boxes in which one remains, but climates to be entered, exited, circled, or revisited. Analytic work is marked by recursive movement between these states. The same patient (and analyst) may traverse several zones in a single hour or may find themselves haunted by one climate for years before the weather shifts. The matrix is a means of tracking these movements, of making the atmospheres of secrecy and surprise visible—if only for a moment—before they once again dissolve or transform.

Walking the Matrix: Micro-Vignettes and Analytic Resonance

Let us move through several of these zones, not as fixed locations, but as shifting climates—each illustrated by a brief clinical or cultural micro-vignette and anchored in psychoanalytic theory.

Articulated Knowing

Known, Acknowledged, Felt

The analytic field is clearest here: the patient voices a truth, claims it, and feels its reality. "I am angry at you for missing my call," a patient says, eyes bright, body alive with affect. The analyst responds not with interpretation, but with acknowledgment. In this zone, self-knowledge is integrated, speech is true, and the room feels transparent. Yet, this clarity is always precarious; even as it emerges, other climates hover at the rim.

Defensive Knowing

Known, Disavowed, Felt

The patient explains their behavior in careful, rational terms but never allows these explanations to touch their core. "I know my father was abusive, but it doesn't bother me," says the patient, lips tight, eyes glistening. The affect is there, but the acknowledgment is withheld. The atmosphere is one of rationalization, intellectualization—a defensive climate that protects by splitting knowledge from ownership.

Haunting

Unknown, Disavowed, Felt

A secret not yet articulated, but present as atmosphere. The patient dreams of a locked room, wakes feeling unease, cannot say why. Repetition compulsion returns to the same failed relationship or scene. In the analytic field, haunting is felt as a chill, an inexplicable heaviness, or a tension in the air. Both participants are aware of "something" that cannot be named but insist on its presence.

Negative Capability

Unknown, Acknowledged, Felt

Here, the analytic dyad is able to hold the unformulated: the analyst says, "I don't know what this is, but I can feel it with you." The patient responds, not with relief, but with the sense that their confusion or pain is finally shared. Winnicott, Bion, and Laplanche all valorize this climate—where the unknown is held, not rushed toward meaning, and where both analyst and patient allow for what is not yet symbolized.

The Unthought Known

Unknown, Disavowed, Unfelt

The analytic weather is dense with something unformulated—Bollas's "unthought known." The patient cannot speak it, does not feel it, but it shapes their world nonetheless: a style of attachment, a repetitive act, a persistent dream. The analyst senses a "field effect," a pattern that recurs across sessions, yet remains below the threshold of feeling or acknowledgment.

Dead Knowledge

Known, Acknowledged, Unfelt

Here, the patient recites truths that have lost vitality—"dead knowledge." Speech is correct but affectless; the hour feels flattened, with little room for play or surprise (Bollas, 1987).

Pre-Symbolic Readiness

Unknown, Acknowledged, Unfelt

Winnicott's "potential space" lives here (1958/1965, 1971): the patient (or child) is open to what may emerge, not yet feeling or naming it, but able to tolerate the unknown as a space for play. The analytic climate is light, tentative, hopeful. The analyst may sense a "pregnancy" in the field—a readiness for new form.

Symbolic Foreclosure

Known, Disavowed, Unfelt

In this zone, knowledge is present but forcibly excluded from symbolic play or feeling. Perverse denial, rigid ideology, or moments of manic certainty may structure the hour. The analyst senses a violent edge, the refusal of ambiguity or contradiction. This is not simply absence, but the enforcement of a closed climate.

Movement and Crossing: The Weather of Analytic Life

The power of this matrix is not in its individual cells, but in the movements between them. A secret may begin as haunting, pass through defensive knowing, erupt into surprise, and—if the analytic climate permits—eventually become articulated, integrated, or symbolically transformed. Yet, as often, the process is not linear: old climates recur, the unthought returns, new secrets are generated in the very process of working through the old.

The analyst's task is not to shepherd the patient from "defensive knowing" to "articulated knowing" by force, but to accompany the recursive movements through these psychic weathers. At times, the most generative stance is to dwell together in haunting, to acknowledge dead knowledge, or to cultivate negative capability—the discipline of not-knowing—rather than to force meaning or confession.

The Matrix as Recursive Resource

As we move through this chapter, the matrix will serve not as a map for mastery but as a recursive tool: a way of tracking how secrecy and surprise, the hidden and the emergent, animate the symbolic field. Its greatest value lies in its refusal to promise finality. Analytic life is lived in crossing, return, and recursive weather; the climates of secrecy and surprise do not end but continually renew the possibility of presence, symbolization, and creative relation.

The Generativity of Secrecy—Recursive Protection and Emergence

Secrecy is often cast in psychoanalytic theory as a problem: the source of pathology, the cause of symptom, the sign of what has been split off or repressed. Yet, secrecy is never so simple. In the analytic field, secrecy is as much a creative and protective act as it is a defense. To keep a secret is to carve out a psychic space—a hidden room, a pocket of opacity, a weather system within the self or between self and other—where something can live without being prematurely named, exposed, or integrated. The very climate of secrecy can be the condition for future emergence, renewal, and symbolic transformation.

Secrecy as Atmosphere, Not Only Content

We are accustomed to thinking of a secret as a discrete bit of knowledge, a fact withheld from view. But the atmosphere of secrecy is something else: it is a psychic climate that saturates the analytic hour, sometimes without any "content" being clear. A child sits at a dinner table, head down, certain that everyone knows something she cannot name. An adult patient enters analysis feeling as if a "secret" is present, but can only offer fragments—a smell, a sensation, an image that hovers on the edge of words. In these atmospheres, secrecy is less an act than a condition, less an object than a climate of possibility.

Winnicott recognized the vital necessity of such hidden spaces. His concept of the "potential space" was built on the idea that the psyche needs protected zones—regions of privacy, fantasy, and play—where new meanings and forms of selfhood can take shape, free from the intrusions of the outside world or the premature gaze of the other. In this sense, secrecy is not the enemy of symbolization but its soil: what is kept back, withheld, or left unsaid becomes the generative ground for play, creation, and emergence.

Bollas and the Aesthetic Moment of Secrecy

Christopher Bollas takes this even further, linking secrecy to the "aesthetic moment"—those sudden openings in which the unthought known becomes experientially available without premature explanation (1992; 1987). In his exploration of the "unthought known," Bollas describes how psychic life is shaped by atmospheric, pre-conceptual experiences—those which cannot be easily thought or narrated yet organize feeling and perception at the deepest level. The "unthought known" is not simply a buried fact but an entire aesthetic, an unconscious resonance that animates subjectivity from within. Secrecy, for Bollas, often operates not as a wall but as a vessel: a container in which the unspeakable is preserved and cultivated until the psyche is ready to encounter it anew.

Bollas's idea of the "aesthetic moment" is crucial here. Sometimes, when secrecy is respected—when the analytic hour is able to contain the unspeakable without forcing its revelation—there is a sudden opening: a moment in which what was hidden becomes available not as a confession, but as an experience of beauty, recognition, or depth. These moments are rarely direct; they arrive as a shift in the symbolic atmosphere—tone, image, pace—more than as content, and they work by depth of resonance rather than by disclosure (Bollas, 1992). The analyst who can dwell with secrecy is able to foster these moments of emergence, making the analytic field available to new forms of psychic life.

Clinical Vignette: What Is withheld as Soil for Symbolization

Consider the analytic work with "Eli," a patient haunted by a pervasive sense of shame and vigilance. For months, Eli arrives at sessions restless, unable to settle, shifting between topics but always circling something unspoken. The analyst senses a secret in the room, though nothing has been revealed or confessed. The hours are punctuated by cryptic jokes, self-interruptions, or sudden laughter that quickly dies away. Eli sometimes glances toward the analyst as if expecting something to be discovered or uncovered, but when questions are posed directly, he retreats into silence.

Rather than pushing for disclosure, the analyst chooses to "dwell in the climate": she marks the presence of secrecy, respects the atmosphere of withholding, and lets it be the background for the work. "It feels as if something important is here with us—something we can't quite name yet," she remarks, more as an invitation than an interrogation.

Over time, the secret does not dissolve, but it transforms. Eli's sense of shame begins to soften; the vigilance lessens. Without ever fully naming "the secret," new stories, dreams, and affects begin to surface—some related to the original atmosphere, others unexpected. The analytic field grows more spacious; both patient and analyst become able to play, imagine, and symbolize in ways that had previously felt dangerous or impossible. The secret, far from being an obstacle, has functioned as a recursive protection—a climate that guarded Eli's capacity for emergence until he was ready to risk new forms of presence.

Bollas and the Unthought Known in Analytic Atmosphere

Throughout Eli's analysis, the secret is never fully articulated; it hovers, alive, like a field effect. This is precisely the kind of atmospheric secrecy Bollas describes: the "unthought known" that, if forced too soon, would collapse into a defensive lie or a deadened story. But in analysis, it is permitted to shape the weather. Sometimes, an image or mood passes between Eli and his analyst—an uncanny familiarity, an echo of loss or hope—that is more meaningful than any content. These are Bollas's "aesthetic moments," the fleeting experience of presence and recognition when the secret is honored as generative, not simply withheld.

Music and Analytic Weather

Music offers a powerful metaphor for secrecy and surprise in the analytic field. Every musical phrase is shaped not only by what is heard but also by the silences, rests, and unresolved tensions that precede and follow it. A sustained chord, the pause before a cadence, the unresolved dissonance held just a moment longer—these musical secrets invite the listener into a climate of anticipation, a space of not-knowing that is often more powerful than resolution itself. In the analytic hour, secrecy functions similarly: what is withheld or unspoken shapes the atmosphere, calling forth curiosity, affect, and the recursive possibility of transformation.

Surprise in music is both structural and affective: a sudden modulation, an unexpected theme, a syncopated rhythm that disrupts the expected flow. These moments do not just break the surface; they invite the listener to experience the familiar anew, to participate in a recursive encounter with meaning. The analytic surprise, too, is rarely a matter of pure novelty; it is often the return of something half-known, now transformed by context, feeling, or the weather of relation.

Recursion is the grammar of music and of analysis. Themes repeat, shift, are hidden, and rediscovered; silences are as charged as sound. Just as a piece of music comes alive in its movement through tension and release, the analytic field is animated by the recursive crossings of secrecy, surprise, and the symbolic. Both are living mediums—always unfinished, always open to new forms, inviting analyst and patient (and listener) to dwell at the edge, where unmastered knowing becomes the climate for transformation.

Secrecy and the Recursive Logic of Symbolic Birth

The generativity of secrecy lies in its recursive temporality: the secret protects what is not yet ready to be known and, in doing so, preserves the possibility of creative transformation. Psychoanalysis is filled with stories of patients who could not bear the direct light of interpretation, whose secrets, once prematurely exposed, became lifeless or brittle. The recursive stance—returning again and again to the edge of the secret, honoring its timing, and allowing its climate to shift—enables the symbolic to be born not as forced confession, but as emergent form.

In this way, secrecy is not simply "the opposite of knowing," but a necessary partner in recursive becoming. The symbolic field is always inhabited by secrets: some that may be spoken, some that remain atmospheric, and others that are never fully known. The analyst's hospitality to secrecy is not a failure to "get to the bottom of things," but a discipline of presence—a willingness to let what is hidden remains so, for as long as it must, in order to generate new life.

Symbolic Atmosphere vs. Fixed Meaning: Art as Analogy

What is true for secrecy in the analytic field is also true for art and poetry. Great works often withhold as much as they reveal. In a painting by René Magritte, the meaning is never quite on the surface; the visible image alludes to an unseen logic, a secret atmosphere that draws the viewer into recursive interpretation. The poet Emily Dickinson, in her elliptical lines, teaches us how the unsaid and the nearly-said can be more generative than explicit statement. Like the analyst, the artist protects a space for the "unthought known," inviting the audience to dwell with ambiguity, to risk surprise, and to participate in the birth of meaning.

Secrecy in art, as in analysis, is never only a lack or failure; it is a field of generativity, a medium in which new forms may take shape. The weather of secrecy is the climate of possibility.

The Analyst's Discipline: Dwelling with the Unspoken

To dwell with secrecy is to accept the limits of mastery. The analyst must cultivate patience, humility, and a recursive willingness to let the secret keep its time. There is an ethics here: not to force what is hidden into the open, not to violate the atmosphere of protection, but to remain with the possibility that what is withheld may someday become what is shared or may remain forever in the climate of not-knowing.

Secrecy thus becomes a generative resource for both patient and analyst. It is the recursive ground in which surprise, transformation, and symbolic birth continually arise—not despite what is withheld, but because of it. The task of analytic presence is not to master the secret, but to sustain the climate in which it might someday emerge, shift, or surprise us.

Supervision as Recursive Climate

These dynamics are not confined to the analytic hour; they reverberate in the climate of supervision, where secrecy, surprise, and symbolic ambiguity are replayed in a new register. In supervision, the supervisee's secrecy—their unspoken uncertainties, defensive omissions, and moments of not-yet-formulated understanding—becomes the generative ground for learning, growth, and recursive reflection. The supervisor, for their part, is not an omniscient authority but a fellow traveler, subject to their own zones of not-knowing, surprise, and atmospheric resonance.

Consider the case of "Laura," a new analyst struggling with a patient whose silence feels suffocating. In supervision, Laura hesitates to share her sense of frustration, fearing it will be judged as a failure of technique. The supervisory hour is thick with a shared secret—an unspoken worry that hovers between them, shaping the dialogue in subtle ways. When the supervisor finally names the atmosphere ("It seems there's something we're both feeling but haven't said—maybe a sense of being stuck, or not knowing how to move forward?"), the climate shifts. Laura exhales, laughs, and admits to her own fear of being inadequate. This small disclosure is less a solution than an opening; it permits new meanings, affects, and strategies to emerge. The secret, protected by supervisory hospitality, becomes the soil for symbolic renewal.

Supervision, then, is less the transmission of technical knowledge than the cultivation of a recursive climate—a place where secrecy guards vulnerability, where surprise is welcomed as a resource, and where both participants learn to dwell at the edge of the unformulated. Just as in analysis, the discipline is not to master the secret, but to honor its generativity and remain companions in the weather of the unknown.

Surprise and the Symbolic Field—Ambiguity as Resource

If secrecy is the climate that shelters what is not yet ready to emerge, surprise is the eruption that transforms the analytic field—an event that cannot be willed, planned, or anticipated. In psychoanalysis, surprise is not merely a byproduct of failed mastery or a rupture to be overcome; it is a resource, a recursive invitation to recognize the limits of knowing and the generative ambiguity at the heart of symbolic life.

Surprise as Psychic Climate and Recursive Event

Surprise is often treated in analytic literature as an anomaly—a disruption in the smooth surface of the hour, an index of unconscious forces breaking through. But if we approach surprise recursively, we see it not as a flaw but as an essential rhythm in analytic life. The analytic field is structured less by the steady progression of insight than by the sudden, recursive appearance of the unexpected. Surprise signals a shift in psychic weather, a breach in the atmosphere of secrecy, and the birth of something unanticipated at the edge of symbolization.

It is important to note: surprise is not always pleasant. Sometimes it arrives as a shock, a rupture, or an unsettling ambiguity. At other times, it is marked by play, laughter, or the gentle opening of new possibilities. In every case, surprise exposes the limits of mastery and the porous boundary between what is known and what remains concealed. The symbolic field becomes a space where ambiguity is not a deficit but a resource—a climate in which both patient and analyst are free to be changed by what arrives.

Laplanche: The Enigmatic Signifier and Surprise

Jean Laplanche's concept of the "enigmatic signifier" provides a powerful theoretical anchor for the generativity of surprise. For Laplanche, the psychic field is always inhabited by messages that cannot be fully decoded—enigmatic transmissions from the other that arrive without context, demanding a work of translation that is never complete. Surprise, in this sense, is the signature of the enigmatic: the analytic encounter is always punctuated by moments in which something is said, dreamed, or enacted that cannot be assimilated into existing knowledge. The analyst's task is less decoding than sustaining a recursive space of translation and play—an openness to "unknowing" aligned with Bion's negative capability and Ogden's account of analytic reverie (Bion, 1962; Ogden, 1997, 2005).

This is the heart of surprise: it reveals the analytic field as unfinished, always open to the arrival of new meanings. The recursive movement between secrecy and surprise is not a linear trajectory but a looping path, in which the climate of the hour is changed, not by solving the enigma, but by remaining available to its unpredictable effects.

Winnicott: Transitional Phenomena and Surprise in Play

Winnicott's theory of transitional phenomena deepens this climate of ambiguity. In his view, the "potential space" between mother and child—later, between analyst and patient—is a field in which surprise is both risked and welcomed. Play is not simply a means to mastery, but a recursive negotiation with what cannot be fully controlled. The analyst who can join the patient in play is not offering safety from the unknown, but a shared climate in which surprise is possible and the rules can be bent, broken, or reinvented.

Surprise, then, is less about the analytic act of "surprising the patient" than about creating the conditions in which both participants can be surprised together. This is a recursive achievement: a climate of trust, ambiguity, and symbolic freedom in which new forms of relation and meaning can take root.

Clinical Vignette: Surprise as Turning Point

Consider the analytic work with "Sara," a patient whose sessions have long been characterized by careful self-control and a reluctance to feel strong affect. Sara arrives each week with detailed accounts of her daily life, always anticipating the analyst's questions, rarely leaving room for the unexpected. The analytic climate is one of ritualized knowing—dead knowledge, to borrow from the matrix—a zone in which both parties feel safe but slightly bored.

One afternoon, in the midst of a session about her childhood, Sara pauses. There is a silence, and then she laughs—sudden, bright, irrepressible. "I just realized I've never told you about the night I ran away," she says, astonished at herself. The analyst, surprised as well, laughs too, feeling the weather in the room shift. For the first time, Sara allows herself to speak of her anger and fear, to risk the ambiguity of not-knowing what will happen next.

The surprise does not resolve the old climate overnight. There are returns to caution, moments of defensiveness, even minor ruptures. But the analytic field has been transformed: ambiguity is no longer only threatening, but creative. The recursive work of symbolization—the movement between secrecy and surprise—has become a resource for both patient and analyst.

Ambiguity, Recursion, and the Creative Edge

What sustains this climate of surprise is the recursive willingness to return to the ambiguous, the unfinished, and the unpredictable. Both patient and analyst must be able to dwell in the atmosphere of "not yet"—to accept that meaning emerges through crossings, reversals, and sudden openings. The symbolic field is kept alive not by mastery, but by a continual movement between the known and the unknown, secrecy and surprise, structure and play.

Here, ambiguity is not the enemy of analytic work but its precondition. The analytic hour is most alive when it becomes a living laboratory for surprise—a space where secrecy protects what must be hidden, but also where the hidden can, at any moment, break through. The recursive ethic is one of return, risk, and renewal: to stay at the edge where surprise remains possible, where the symbolic field is not fixed, and where both analyst and patient can be transformed by what neither anticipated.

Conclusion: The Symbolic as Ongoing Invitation

Surprise reveals the symbolic field as a living, emergent climate—a medium in which ambiguity, secrecy, and the unexpected continually shape what is possible. The analyst's discipline is not to manage or eliminate surprise, but to welcome it as a resource: a sign that the analytic process is alive, recursive, and open to transformation. In this climate, surprise is not an accident to be controlled, but the very signature of a living relation, a recursive invitation to the ongoing work of symbolization, and a testament to the generativity of what escapes mastery.

Ethics at the Edge—Opacity, Acknowledgment, and the Analyst's Secret

If the climate of secrecy and surprise is vital for analytic transformation, the question of ethics hovers at the very edge of this terrain. What is the ethical responsibility of the analyst in a field marked by secrecy, opacity, and the inevitability of the unspoken? How can psychoanalysis remain a generative practice when both participants are shaped by what cannot be confessed, named, or even fully known?

The Analyst's Secret: Field Effects and Unconscious Withholding

Psychoanalysis has long been preoccupied with the patient's secrets—the things not said, the memories split off, the traumas hidden in shadow. Yet, the analyst, too, is never fully transparent, even to themselves. There are the obvious secrets: aspects of the analyst's own life, desires, or history that are consciously withheld for reasons of boundary, privacy, or technical neutrality. But there are also unconscious secrets—unknowable residues of the analyst's subjectivity, affect, or history that shape the field in ways that cannot be named in the moment. Every analyst brings to the encounter their own matrix of knowing and not-knowing, their own climate of disavowal, dead knowledge, or haunting.

At times, what is withheld by the analyst becomes as structuring as the patient's own secrets. An analyst who cannot allow themselves to feel anger may collude unconsciously in keeping certain affects out of the room. Another, unable to acknowledge their own envy or uncertainty, may unconsciously encourage the patient's disavowal or defensiveness. These are not merely technical failures; they are atmospheric realities, recursive effects that shape what can be spoken, felt, or symbolized. In this way, the analyst's secrets—conscious and unconscious—become part of the climate in which analytic life unfolds.

Vignette: The Analyst's Unspoken

Consider the work of Dr. R, an analyst who, after a personal loss, finds herself less able to tolerate certain affects in the analytic hour. Her patient, Marc, begins to bring dreams of loss and grief but consistently interrupts himself, downplaying his feelings. Dr. R notices her own tendency to steer sessions toward more intellectual topics, feeling a vague discomfort whenever the conversation edges toward mourning. Over months, the analytic field is marked by a climate of unspoken sadness—present but never articulated, haunting both analyst and patient.

Eventually, Dr. R chooses to mark the weather: "I wonder if there's something we both haven't been able to say here—something about loss that feels too much, or too close." The room grows quiet. Marc nods, and tears well up, but he does not need to explain. The acknowledgment of the analyst's own opacity, her capacity to be affected by what she cannot fully name, shifts the climate. The secret has not been confessed, but its atmosphere has been honored. This recursive move—bringing the analyst's own limits into the field without demanding disclosure—opens new space for symbolization, mourning, and surprise.

Opacity as Ethical Resource: Glissant's Right Not to Be Known

Édouard Glissant's notion of opacity offers a radical lens for the ethics of secrecy in analysis: "the right to opacity" is constitutive of relation, not a barrier to it (1997). Glissant insists that the right "not to be known" is as fundamental as the right to difference or individuality. Opacity is not a barrier to relation, but the very condition for its possibility. In the analytic field, this ethic means respecting that both analyst and patient will always remain, to some degree, untranslatable—zones of self and other that cannot be fully mastered, appropriated, or understood.

Opacity is an ethical climate: it permits each participant to remain partially obscure, to retain secrets that are generative rather than threatening. This is especially crucial for patients whose histories are marked by violation or the loss of boundaries. Hospitality to opacity—the refusal to demand total transparency—creates the psychic space in which patients can risk disclosure and play in their own time, without foreclosure of difference (Glissant, 1997; Benjamin, 2018).

Benjamin's Acknowledgment and the Recursive Ethics of Presence

Jessica Benjamin has written extensively about acknowledgment—the act of recognizing the other's subjectivity, difference, and limits, rather than demanding assimilation or mutuality at all costs. In analytic ethics, acknowledgment means marking the weather of what cannot be shared, without forcing it into the light. It is the discipline of saying: I see there is something here I do not know, and I am willing to be with you in that uncertainty.

In the analytic hour, acknowledgment is not always about bringing secrets into speech, but about sustaining presence at the edge—holding the climate of the unspoken, honoring opacity, and allowing both parties the dignity of their own recursive processes. When surprise or secrecy interrupts the familiar rhythm of knowing, acknowledgment offers a recursive invitation: to remain in relation, to revisit the edge, and to risk the creative possibilities of what cannot be owned or explained.

Recursive Hospitality: Containing What Cannot Be Known

The analyst's task, then, is not to extract secrets or dissolve all opacity, but to cultivate a recursive hospitality—to create a field in which both parties can return, again and again, to the edge of what is hidden, ambiguous, or unspeakable. This hospitality is not a passive waiting; it is an active discipline, an atmospheric stance that makes room for secrecy, surprise, and the ongoing birth of symbolization. In this climate, not-knowing becomes an ethical resource: the analyst's willingness to fail, to remain uncertain, to honor what escapes mastery, sustains the generative tension at the core of analytic work.

Ethics, Ambiguity, and the Future

The ethics of secrecy is never fully resolved. Even as new forms of symbolization emerge, new secrets are born; each recursive movement through knowing and not-knowing reshapes the climate of the analytic field. The future remains open—not because everything has been confessed, but because the recursive interplay of secrecy, acknowledgment, and opacity continues to generate new possibilities for relation, surprise, and renewal.

In this way, the analyst's secret is not merely a problem or an error; it is a weather system in the field, a recursive force that can foster or foreclose creativity, play, and transformation. The discipline is to attend, not only to the content of secrets but also to the climates they generate—and to the ongoing ethics of presence at the edge of what cannot be owned or known.

Recursive Movement—Transformations at the Rim

If the analytic field is structured not by static knowing but by atmospheric crossings—if secrecy and surprise are less objects than climates—then the true life of psychoanalysis is found in movement. The recursive movement among states of knowing, unknowing, acknowledgment, and affect is the living weather of the analytic relationship. It is through these recursive crossings—rather than through any final revelation—that symbolization, relation, and psychic renewal continually emerge.

The Matrix as Dynamic Map

As we have seen, the matrix is not a taxonomy but a weather map—a guide to the climates and shifts that mark analytic experience. No analytic hour remains within a single zone; the recursive movement from dead knowledge to haunting, from defensive knowing to negative capability, is continual. Sometimes this movement is sudden and dramatic—a secret breaks through, a surprise erupts, and the field is changed. More often, it is subtle: an affect softens, a silence grows less heavy, a climate shifts without anyone quite knowing why.

The recursive life of the matrix is less about progress than about looping: what was unformulated yesterday may become articulated tomorrow; what is acknowledged now may slip into disavowal or deadness in the future. The analyst's presence is most vital not as a guide to destination, but as a companion in these weather changes—a presence attuned to the recursive nature of becoming.

Bollas: The Fascination and the Dreamlike

Bollas's work on "fascination" and dream states expands our sense of the recursive. Fascination, he writes, is a form of psychic absorption, a moment when the mind is captured by the presence of something unknown, alive, and evocative. In analysis, fascination often signals a shift in weather—a moment when patient and analyst are gripped by a shared sense of mystery, beauty, or dread. The analytic field becomes "dreamlike," Bollas suggests, not because it escapes reality, but because it allows what is secret, strange, or surprising to become the generative matrix for new symbolic life.

These are the moments when time seems to double back, when meaning is incubated rather than produced, when both analyst and patient are held in suspense. Recursion here is not repetition as stasis, but a living, creative engagement with the edges of knowing.

Recursive Crossing: The Analyst and Patient in Motion

Consider the recursive journey of "Leah," a patient who entered analysis with a secret she could not name. Early sessions were haunted by a vague dread—an unthought known, dense and silent. As the work unfolded, Leah began to intellectualize her experience, moving into a climate of defensive knowing: "I know what my problem is, I just can't feel it." The analyst recognized the shift, but did not force affect. Instead, she mirrored Leah's uncertainty, saying, "It feels as if there's something here we can talk about, but maybe we don't quite want to feel it yet."

Over time, this recursive stance allowed new climates to emerge. In one session, Leah found herself weeping without knowing why—haunting had become negative capability, the affect acknowledged even as the meaning remained unknown. Later, a memory surfaced unexpectedly, transforming the climate again: for the first time, Leah could name what had been secret. The analytic field was alive with surprise; both analyst and patient felt the relief of articulated knowing, if only briefly.

Yet, the movement did not end there. In the months that followed, the old weather returned: the newly articulated secret grew flat, losing its charge—dead knowledge. But because the analytic relationship had cultivated a recursive hospitality, Leah and her analyst could notice this shift without panic or frustration. "It seems like what once felt so urgent is now hard to feel," the analyst remarked. The recursive movement among matrix zones had become familiar, even welcomed. The weather would change again.

Art, Poetry, and Analytic Weather

Like poetry or surrealist painting, analytic work makes a life of these weather shifts. Rilke's ethic of openness—to beauty and terror alike—captures the stance required here: no single feeling is final (Rilke, 1905/1996). In the analytic hour, this means staying attuned to the climate of the unspoken, letting images, affects, and associations recur and transform. The poet's discipline is mirrored by the analyst's: to wait, to return, to let the weather shift, to trust the generative value of what is unfinished.

The artist Magritte, in works like "The Lovers," paints figures whose faces are shrouded—revealing that even in intimacy, secrets remain, and that what is hidden is not simply lost but full of creative possibility. Analytic weather is like this: what is not seen or spoken becomes part of the field, a medium for emergence, surprise, and the unpredictable work of symbolization.

From Secrecy to Surprise to Renewal

This clinical journey illustrates the recursive crossings that mark analytic life. Secrets do not simply move from hidden to revealed; they cycle through climates of affect, acknowledgment, and unknowing. Surprise does not only break through as a one-time event, but may recur, sometimes in minor ways—a new dream, a slip of the tongue, a moment of shared laughter that interrupts the old pattern.

Renewal in analysis is rarely a matter of permanent insight or closure. It is more often the slow, looping process of returning, again and again, to the rim—where what is known and what is hidden circle one another and where the possibility of transformation is always alive. The analyst's discipline is to stay in motion, to cultivate the flexibility to move with the changing weather, and to risk presence at the rim, even when nothing seems to change.

The Symbolic as Living Medium

What enables recursive transformation is the symbolic field itself—the medium in which secrecy and surprise do their work. The symbolic is not the endpoint of analytic work, but its ongoing invitation. Every secret that becomes symbolized, every surprise that erupts in the field, generates new possibilities for relation, play, and meaning. Yet, the symbolic also preserves what cannot be known, allowing for future crossings and recursive returns.

The weather of analytic life is never settled; the rim is always in view. Both analyst and patient become, in time, more comfortable with the ambiguity, the partialness, and the movement among climates. This is the deepest gift of recursive presence: not the mastery of all secrets or the elimination of surprise, but the cultivation of a field where becoming is unending and where new forms of psychic life can take shape at the edge.

Closing Vignette: Transformation at the Rim

In the final year of analysis, Leah arrives one day with a dream: she is standing at the edge of a lake, unable to see the bottom. She does not fear the darkness below, but feels curious, even hopeful. "Maybe I don't have to know what's down there," she says. "Maybe it's enough to stand here and wonder."

The analyst smiles, recognizing the recursive weather of the field. No longer haunted by the secret, Leah is able to dwell at the rim—present to surprise, open to not-knowing, alive to the movement of the symbolic field. The transformation is not final or total; the weather will shift again. But for now, both analyst and patient can stand together at the edge, companions in a climate where secrecy, surprise, and the symbolic are not obstacles, but resources for ongoing life.

Closing Reflection—Unmastered Knowing

To dwell in psychoanalysis is to make a life at the rim of knowing. No matter how often we return, how deeply we inquire, the field remains charged by what is withheld, what erupts unexpectedly, and what can never be fully named. This chapter has traced the recursive crossings that animate analytic life—the atmospheres of secrecy and surprise, the shifting weather of the symbolic, and the endless movement among climates of knowing and not-knowing. The very tool we have used—the epistemic-affective matrix—is more map than territory, a provisional chart for moving through atmospheres that can never be fully contained.

The matrix, in its refusal of closure, stands as an emblem of unmastered knowing. Each cell is a climate, not a category; each crossing, a recursive act of presence and return. If at times the analyst or patient longs for a final articulation—a secret revealed, a meaning pinned down, a surprise made safe—the deeper ethic of psychoanalysis is to resist that longing for mastery. The "other side of knowing" is not the dark twin of insight, but the necessary climate in which symbolization, play, and transformation are perpetually reborn.

Secrecy, in this light, is not the enemy of analysis but its guardian. It marks the edge where knowledge cannot—and perhaps must not—arrive too quickly. In the climate of secrecy, what is withheld preserves the possibility of renewal, of future surprise, of psychic forms not yet imagined. The analyst's discipline is not to vanquish secrecy, but to sustain its generative atmosphere: to dwell with the unspoken, the ambiguous, the unformulated, and to honor the recursive movement that keeps the field alive.

Surprise, too, is not simply the result of analytic failure or oversight. It is the signature of an analytic field that remains open, alive to its own emergent possibilities. Surprise breaks through when the recursive weather has shifted enough—when secrecy has been tended, when the symbolic field is ready for new play, or when the climate itself invites something unplanned. Surprise is not a rupture to be repaired, but a call to humility, a sign that psychoanalytic life is never reducible to technique or interpretation.

The symbolic, throughout this chapter, has been reframed not as a stable structure but as a living medium. It is less a system of meaning than a weather system: always in motion, always holding within it the residues of secrecy and the promise of surprise. The symbolic field shelters the ambiguous, the liminal, and the emergent; it is the climate where recursive knowing and unknowing are continually negotiated. Here, meaning is never final; symbolization is a practice of ongoing return, a recursive presence at the edge.

In the end, the ethic that emerges from these crossings is an invitation rather than a conclusion. It is the invitation to analytic presence at the rim—to make a home in the atmospheres of secrecy, surprise, and the symbolic, without demanding resolution or mastery. This is an ethic of humility and of hospitality, an ongoing negotiation with the unknown and the unfinished. In a world that prizes certainty and speed, psychoanalysis offers something rarer: the discipline to wait, to return, to risk presence where knowing breaks down and new forms of life shimmer at the edge.

The future of psychoanalysis, like the weather, cannot be forecast. Its promise lies not in what is mastered but in what is kept open: the recursive movement among climates, the readiness for surprise, the dignity of secrecy, and the capacity to bear the symbolic as an ever-shifting field. In this future, the analyst and patient remain companions at the rim—bearing together the joy, sorrow, and creativity of life lived in the unmastered zone.

Chapter 13

Coda—Recursive Ethics and the Future of Unknowing

To unknow is a quiet willingness to be with what arrives before giving it a name.

This concluding chapter gathers the book's recursive threads into an open, resonant horizon. Rather than offering synthesis or closure, the coda foregrounds the ethics of not-knowing and the generativity of recursive return as the living core of psychoanalytic practice. Drawing deeply on the motifs of music, art, and poetry, it explores how these aesthetic forms model the open-ended, unfinished quality of analytic life—where silence, negative space, ambiguity, and improvisation are resources for presence rather than obstacles to understanding. Through sustained meta-commentary, this chapter reflects on its own recursive structure, inviting the reader to experience the book as a living field—a weather map, a score, a poem—meant for repeated engagement, surprise, and creative attunement. By revisiting key themes of inversion, refusal, and curved epistemology, and by situating the future of psychoanalysis in its ongoing hospitality to what cannot be mastered, the coda calls for an analytic ethos that remains porous, creative, and ethically vibrant. Ultimately, it invites the reader to dwell at the edge of the knowable, to love the questions themselves, and to imagine psychoanalysis as a field forever unfinished and open to renewal.

Introduction—Coda as Opening, Not Closure

A coda is not an ending but an aperture—an echo at the threshold of silence that refuses final cadence and leans the ear toward what returns. In psychoanalytic writing, as in art or music, the coda gestures outward—toward a horizon that cannot be circumscribed by the chapters preceding it, a future

DOI: 10.4324/9781003747109-17

that shimmers with all that has not been, and may never be, fully said. If this book has circled, doubled back, and advanced in recursive arcs, it is because the analytic field it describes resists both linearity and closure. It is not a field of certainties, but of atmospheres—spaces of opacity, surprise, refusal, and unfinished becoming.

This coda does not pretend to synthesize what has unfolded. Instead, it offers a recursive return to the book's central motifs: not as a summary, but as a movement that reframes and reanimates what has come before. To write from the edge—and to inhabit a stance of unknowing—is to relinquish mastery in favor of disciplined hospitality to what resists capture (Bion, 1962). It is to recognize that the field of psychoanalysis—and of writing itself—unfolds in atmospheres, not arguments, in recursive gestures, not conclusions. The spirit animating these pages is one of disciplined hospitality: a stance that holds open the space for the unassimilable, the ambiguous, and the yet-to-be-symbolized. It is an ethos that privileges presence over certainty, the curved movement of return over the fantasy of linear advance.

If the recursive is the signature of psychic life, it is also the rhythm of the creative act. The process of composing this book has been less an act of invention than of listening—for echoes, for atmospheric shifts, for the unthought known. It has been a writing in the register of weather: attuned to pressure changes, fronts, and unpredictable clearings. Each chapter has returned, not to the same point, but to a field transformed by repetition and difference. This is not mere reiteration but the deepening spiral of recursive presence: the curve that returns, but never identically; the refrain that gathers new resonance each time it is sounded.

To write from this stance is to be marked by humility: not only the humility to acknowledge what cannot be known, but also the willingness to remain a companion to what cannot be mastered. In this, the analyst and the writer share a discipline—the discipline to witness, to accompany, to hold open the climate where surprise is possible and closure is perpetually deferred. The coda, then, is not the place where everything comes together, but where meaning is dispersed again, scattered like seeds into a new season, or like musical notes suspended at the edge of hearing.

Meta-commentary is not a departure from the analytic or artistic field, but its deepening. To write about recursion is to write recursively; to invite unknowing is to risk the open. The book itself is a recursive object: composed of loops, returns, and atmospheric motifs, it resists being mastered by a single reading, just as analysis resists being finished by a single interpretation. Each encounter—whether on the couch, in supervision, or in these pages—enacts the ethos it proposes: the recursive discipline of return, the hospitality to surprise, the refusal to foreclose what is not yet known.

The horizon of psychoanalytic life, like the horizon of art or music or poetry, is always in motion. It recedes as we approach, inviting us into further movement, further wonder. The coda, in honoring this horizon, asks the reader not to seek closure but to linger in the unfinished, to inhabit the echo, the weather, the curve. It is an invitation to dwell at the edge of the knowable—not as exile, but as the most vital space for the generativity of psychic, analytic, and creative life.

As this coda opens, rather than closes, the field, it calls for a discipline of hospitality to what lies beyond our frames: the secrets, surprises, and atmospheric shifts that recur, transform, and sustain us. The future of psychoanalysis—like the future of any living art—resides not in what has been mastered, but in the recursive movement of unknowing: the presence, humility, and imaginative discipline to accompany the unfolding of life at the rim.

Recursion and the Ethics of Not-Knowing

Recursion is not simply a technical term, nor merely an intellectual style; it is a living principle—a way of moving through psychic, ethical, and creative life that embraces the necessity of return. In psychoanalysis, as in all creative disciplines, true knowing is never linear. It is marked by detour, return, inversion, and the capacity to revisit what cannot be grasped all at once. Recursion is not compulsion but craft: a disciplined openness to being altered by each return—new weather, new resonance, no simple repeat (Keats, 1958; Bion, 1962).

This ethic of recursion, so often misunderstood as a refusal to move forward, is in fact the very condition of movement itself. Linear mastery, the fantasy of progress without remainder, always founders on the rocks of the unconscious. There is no straight path through the psyche; every approach circles, doubles back, and reconfigures what was thought to be known. The recursive ethos acknowledges this: it enshrines not-knowing not as a deficit but as a discipline. The analyst who returns again and again to the site of uncertainty, who welcomes surprise, who resists the pull of premature synthesis, is not abdicating their responsibility. Rather, they are enacting the highest ethical calling of psychoanalytic work—the hospitality to what cannot be assimilated or resolved.

To embrace recursion is to accept that knowledge is always provisional. In the analytic hour, interpretations are offered, but never once and for all. The meanings that arise are shaped by the weather of the day, the mood of the patient, the unthought residues that hover in the room. What was true yesterday may lose its charge today; what was once a revelation may become, in time, dead knowledge, no longer alive with affect. Recursion is the willingness to return to the scene, to risk new surprise, to mourn the loss of certainty, and to honor the emergence of meaning that could not have been anticipated in advance.

This discipline of recursive not-knowing is not only a clinical technique; it is an ethical stance. The analyst who embodies it refuses the temptations of omniscience and instead cultivates presence at the rim of understanding. This stance is not passive, but rigorously attentive. It requires the analyst to be vigilant to their own impulses toward closure, to recognize when they are being pulled by the desire to explain, to integrate, to heal too quickly. The recursive ethic asks instead: can I stay with the unformulated and bear the interval where meaning has not yet condensed (Ogden, 1997)? Can I accompany the patient through ambiguity and loss, through repetition and surprise, without forcing an ending?

It is here that the motifs of inversion and refusal become central. To invert is to unsettle the expected order, to reveal the underside of what was taken for granted. In analytic life, this may mean discovering that what seemed pathological is in fact protective, or that what appeared to be failure is the site of new generativity. Refusal, in this sense, is not resistance to the analytic process, but an active stance against false resolution. The patient who refuses to be known, who withholds or obfuscates, is often protecting something vital—a remainder, a kernel of experience that cannot yet, or perhaps should not, be assimilated. The analyst's willingness to respect this refusal is itself an ethical act, an honoring of the patient's right to opacity, to secrecy, to the unmastered remainder.

Curved epistemology—one of this book's anchor motifs—describes the movement of mind and method that privileges attunement to atmosphere over linear sequence. Curved knowing is the willingness to follow the recursive path, to circle back, to notice what returns in new form. In this mode, the analyst is not a detective seeking clues, but an accompanist in the unfolding of psychic weather. Curved epistemology is musical, artistic, poetic: it is a form of being-with that recognizes the limits of direct approach, and that trusts in the generativity of return.

In practice, this recursive stance means accepting that analytic work is rarely about getting to the bottom of things, but about dwelling with what emerges at the surface—where affect shimmers, symbols condense, and the unknown exerts its gravitational pull. The analyst's responsibility is to provide a holding environment where these recursive movements can unfold. Sometimes this means waiting with the patient through long stretches of silence, or through repeated retellings of the same story, or through resistances that refuse to yield to interpretation. At other times, it means naming the weather, acknowledging the atmosphere of not-knowing, or inviting surprise into the field.

There is a humility here, one that is not weakness but ethical courage. The recursive analyst does not presume to heal, to synthesize, or to resolve, but rather to bear witness—to accompany the patient into the unknown, to share the risk of psychic transformation, to remain faithful to the movement of life beyond inherited frames. This stance is neither resignation nor nihilism. On the contrary, it is a source of hope: for in the recursive field, each return offers the chance for something new to emerge, for surprise to break through, for old meanings to be revised or relinquished.

This discipline of recursive not-knowing is not without cost. It can be uncomfortable to resist the urge for closure, to dwell in the ambiguity and messiness of psychic life. Analysts, like all humans, crave coherence, reassurance, and the mastery of the unknown. But the recursive stance asks us to hold these desires lightly, to recognize their limits, and to remain open to the possibility that what is most vital cannot be known in advance. The analyst who can model this stance for the patient, who can tolerate their own anxiety at the edge, provides a powerful invitation: to inhabit a life that is more porous, more creative, and more alive to the generative ground of unknowing.

In the context of this book, recursion is both theme and method. Each chapter, each motif, returns with a difference—reframed, expanded, unsettled by what has come before. The book itself enacts the recursive discipline it advocates, refusing linear progress in favor of atmospheric movement, curved return, and the ongoing negotiation of meaning at the rim. The coda, then, is not an ending, but a recursive crossing—a place where the ethics of not-knowing are reanimated, and where the field of psychoanalysis is opened once more to surprise, reversal, and creative possibility.

Music as Analytic Atmosphere

If psychoanalysis is, as this book proposes, an art of recursive presence and unfinished knowing, then music is perhaps its closest kin. Musical experience is itself a recursive field: melodies return, motifs recur and transform, silences shape the space as much as sound, and the unresolved becomes a vital source of affective energy. To listen musically is to inhabit a field where meaning is made and unmade—surprise and return providing the grammar, silence the punctuation (Cage, 1961).

Music teaches us about the ethics and generativity of not-knowing. In every composition, there are moments of suspended resolution—chords that refuse to settle, themes that circle back rather than conclude, silences that invite the listener to lean into what cannot be named. The recursive structure of music is not merely technical; it is existential. Each return of a motif brings both recognition and transformation: what comes back is never the same as what first appeared. In this, music models the analytic hour's looping through memory, affect, and symbolization—a movement that deepens rather than closes, that holds open the possibility of new forms.

Improvisation is one of music's most vital recursive practices. In jazz, for example, musicians return to a theme or chord progression not to repeat it, but to find new pathways, new weather, within its structure. The improviser listens, responds, dwells in uncertainty, and trusts in the emergence of form through the recursive discipline of return. So, too, the analyst: practicing a kind of deep listening—present to emergence, responsive to shift, letting silence be medium rather than lack (Oliveros, 2005).

Consider the analytic field as a kind of score—a set of motifs, affective signatures, and recurring themes that shape the "weather" of the hour. Each session is both new and not-new, echoing prior hours and anticipating future ones. The analyst and patient become, in a sense, co-composers: they play with memory, repeat and vary themes, sometimes lose their way, sometimes find themselves caught in unexpected harmonies or ruptures. There are refrains—the same story told again, the old symptom reappearing in a new key, the return of a childhood song or a half-remembered phrase. These are not failures to progress but invitations to dwell in the recursive life of the field, where meaning is not fixed but alive to change.

Silence, in both music and analysis, is generative. The rest between notes is not emptiness, but the very space in which anticipation, affect, and surprise are born. In music, a pause before the return of a theme heightens its impact, inviting the listener to inhabit the uncertainty of what comes next. In analysis, silence is the space where what cannot be said hovers—the unformulated, the secret, the withheld. The analyst's discipline is not to rush to fill these silences, but to witness their weather, to dwell with the not-yet, to let the patient's psychic music unfold at its own tempo.

The unfinished is the hallmark of both musical and analytic form. Great compositions end on open chords, unresolved cadences, or simply fade into silence, leaving the listener suspended at the rim of what might yet be. Psychoanalysis, too, refuses closure: each session ends not with a final interpretation, but with the field left open for future returns. The recursive movement is ongoing—each analytic hour is a reprise, a coda, an unfinished phrase.

A patient once described analysis as "a song I can't remember the words to, but I know when I hear it." This is the recursive memory of music: the way affective life returns as echo, as atmosphere, as half-known refrain. The analyst's role is not to supply the missing lyrics, but to accompany the patient in listening, to mark the changes in key, tempo, or theme. The music of analysis is improvised, recursive, unfinished. Its beauty lies in the courage to return, to risk surprise, to allow meaning to arise not from mastery, but from presence at the edge of knowing.

In the history of psychoanalytic thought, music has often been invoked as a metaphor, but rarely as a method. Yet the musical is more than a figure; it is a way of being-with. The analyst who works musically is attuned to repetition, variation, silence, and rupture. They hear the weather of the session, the tonal shifts, the recurring notes of desire, grief, or hope. They trust that what is played today may sound different tomorrow, that what was unresolved yesterday may return transformed. This is not passivity, but a form of creative discipline—the willingness to risk not-knowing, to dwell in ambiguity, to let the analytic field be shaped by its own recursive score.

In the coda to this book, music offers both an image and a practice: the courage to return, the willingness to dwell with the unfinished, the invitation to presence at the rim. Just as no two performances of a piece are ever the same, no two analytic hours repeat themselves precisely. Recursion, in both music and analysis, is a practice of renewal: it makes possible the emergence of the new from the material of the known.

To listen musically is to welcome surprise, to honor silence, to trust the generativity of what recurs without resolving. In this, music models the very ethics at the heart of psychoanalytic life: the discipline to remain with the unknown, to allow for the unexpected, and to receive each return as both echo and invitation. The future of psychoanalysis, if it is to remain alive, must become ever more musical—willing to improvise, to listen, to begin again, and to end, always, with the field left open for the next refrain.

Art and the Curved Gaze

If music teaches us about the recursive atmospheres of psychic life, art reveals the generative power of the unfinished, the fragmentary, and the curved gaze. In the visual field, as in the analytic, what matters most is rarely at the center; meaning accumulates in the margins, in negative space, in the subtle play of color, form, and absence. To witness is not to dominate but to be moved—to receive an unfolding image that withholds as it reveals, inviting a curved gaze rather than a totalizing one (Foucault, 1983).

The history of modern and contemporary art is a history of refusal—of frames, of perspective, of totalizing vision. The turn toward abstraction, surrealism, and fragmentation was, in part, a revolt against the fantasy of perfect representation. In analytic life, a similar refusal animates the recursive stance: the willingness to dwell with what cannot be integrated, to let meaning remain open, ambiguous, or hidden. Surrealist art, for instance, makes visible the logic of dreams, of condensation and displacement, of uncanny juxtapositions. It is not content to "explain" the world, but instead multiplies possible readings, inviting the viewer to return again and again, to circle the image, to be changed by the act of looking.

The analyst's gaze is never simply neutral or objective. Like the painter or photographer, the analyst frames the field, selects what comes into focus, and is herself implicated in the picture. There is an ethics to this gaze, a discipline of restraint and openness: to allow the patient's experience to emerge in its own time and form, to resist the urge to fill in every gap, to respect the opacity and negative capability that sustain psychic life. The curved gaze is not a matter of willful obscurity, but of hospitality to what cannot be known at once, or perhaps ever. It is a form of witness that holds space for the unassimilated, the ambiguous, the unfinished.

Consider the role of negative space in painting and drawing. In many traditions—Eastern ink painting, Western abstraction, minimalist installation—the empty or unpainted areas are not simply background, but integral to the work's meaning and affect. The eye is drawn to what is absent as much as to what is present; the composition breathes through its gaps and silences. In analysis, negative space appears as silence, as the unsaid, as the affective atmospheres that surround speech. The analyst learns to read the interval—the unpainted ground—as meaning-bearing; absence becomes a mode of presence that organizes the whole (Berger, 1972).

Surrealist art, with its recursive motifs, visual paradoxes, and fractured realities, mirrors the analytic hour's unpredictable returns and shocks of recognition. The dreamlike juxtapositions of Magritte, the metamorphoses of Ernst, the defamiliarized objects of Duchamp—all enact a refusal of closure, a delight in surprise, a recursive invitation to look again. These works do not surrender to chaos, but neither do they impose an artificial order. Instead, they invite the viewer into a liminal space, where meaning is both given and withheld, offered and deferred.

The analyst, too, is called to such creative hospitality. To hold the field as an artist does is to risk being surprised by what appears, to welcome the unexpected, to remain available to what emerges at the edge of comprehension. The analytic hour becomes a kind of studio, a place where both participants are co-creators, shaping and being shaped by the weather of affect, symbol, and relation. There is no final painting, no perfect portrait of the patient or the self—only a series of attempts, sketches, and reworkings, each deepening the atmosphere, each returning the gaze in a new form.

Art also teaches us the value of ambiguity, of works that "hold open" multiple interpretations. A painting by Rothko is both color and emotion, surface and depth; a collage by Hannah Höch is both critique and celebration, fragmentation and connection. These works refuse the binary of explanation and nonsense; they thrive in the middle space, the borderlands, the weather systems of the in-between. So too does analysis, which lives at the intersection of symbol and symptom, of speech and silence, of presence and absence. The analyst's discipline is to remain at this threshold, to allow meaning to accumulate through recursive returns, through patient attention to the unfinished and the unspoken.

Art's history is also a history of rupture—of sudden breaks, shocks, and estrangements. The emergence of Cubism, the violence of Dada, the quiet radicalism of minimalism—each represents a recursive refusal to be contained by inherited forms. In analysis, similar ruptures may appear: moments when the old frame no longer fits, when a symptom reappears in a new guise, when the field is shaken by loss or surprise. These are not failures, but opportunities for creative transformation. The analyst's task is not to restore the old order, but to hold the space in which new images, new relations, and new forms of life might take shape.

To gaze with a curved eye is to resist both mastery and retreat. It is to acknowledge that seeing is always partial, always shaped by what is not visible, always open to revision. The curved gaze is recursive: it bends, it returns, it changes with each movement. The analyst who adopts this stance is not an outsider looking in, but a participant in the unfolding of the field. They are attuned to the play of presence and absence, to the weather of affect and symbol, to the generative possibilities that arise when meaning is left unfinished.

As this coda unfolds, let art be a companion and a guide. Let the analytic field be understood as a canvas in motion, always returning, always opening to surprise and revision. Let the curved gaze invite both humility and creative engagement, a willingness to dwell at the threshold of the known and the unknown. In this way, the future of psychoanalysis might be envisioned not as a science of closure, but as an art of recursive presence—a living field where the unfinished is not a failure, but the very condition for life.

Poetry, Negative Capability, and Analytic Presence

If music offers psychoanalysis the lesson of return and improvisation, and art reveals the generative force of ambiguity and negative space, then poetry teaches the discipline of inhabiting the unformulated—of living within, rather than resolving, the liminal weather of experience. Poetry's affinity with analysis is not just in its use of metaphor or symbol, but in its recursive capacity to hold open what cannot be finalized, to dwell with multiplicity, resonance, and creative uncertainty. The poetic is not merely a mode of speaking, but a way of being: receptive to ambiguity, sensitive to atmospheric shift, and attuned to what shimmers at the edge of language.

Keats's "negative capability"—remaining "in uncertainties, mysteries, doubts, without any irritable reaching after fact and reason" (1958)—is foundational here. For Keats, the greatest writers and thinkers possess "negative capability." This is not indifference or passivity; it is a courageous receptivity to the ambiguous, the unfinished, the yet-to-be-named. In the analytic field, negative capability becomes the analyst's willingness to sit with uncertainty, to resist the pull toward rapid interpretation, to accompany the patient through silences, fragments, and recursive returns. It is an ethical stance: a refusal to foreclose meaning, a discipline of waiting, an invitation to what is not yet known.

Poetry, at its most vital, is recursive. The return of words, images, and forms is never simple repetition; each recurrence resonates differently, colored by new weather, altered by what has intervened. The poetic refrain is both anchor and opening, a place to land and a site for launching into new meaning. In analysis, this is mirrored by the return of themes, symptoms, and affects—never quite the same, always shaped by context and relation. The analyst who can hear these recursions as poetry—who can attend to the rhythm, the echo, the surprise—offers a space for psychic life to unfold in its own tempo.

Consider Emily Dickinson, whose elliptical lines make weather of meaning—condensing and dispersing sense, refusing closure. "Tell all the truth but tell it slant— / Success in Circuit lies" (Dickinson, 1958, Poem 1263). Dickinson's lines are weather systems—condensing and dispersing meaning, refusing closure, inviting the reader into a field of atmospheric possibility. "Tell all the truth but tell it slant," she writes; "Success in circuit lies." The poetic "slant" is the curved epistemology of analysis: not a straight line to revelation, but a recursive circling, a willingness to let meaning come obliquely, unexpectedly, as a surprise. For Dickinson, as for the analyst, truth is not a commodity to be delivered, but an event that emerges, fleetingly, in the weather of relation.

Rainer Maria Rilke, another poet of recursive atmosphere, urges us to "live the questions now." He invites us to be "patient toward all that is unsolved in your heart and try to love the questions themselves, like locked rooms and like books that are now written in a very foreign tongue." This patient, poetic stance is not a renunciation of knowledge, but a discipline of remaining with what is unfinished, of loving the generative force of uncertainty. In analysis, this means welcoming the unknown not as a threat but as the very space in which new psychic forms may arise.

Poetry's ambiguity is not confusion but creative multiplicity. The best poems hold open multiple readings, shifting with each return, inviting new interpretations without ever settling into a single meaning. Psychoanalytic presence, similarly, thrives in the refusal to collapse ambiguity into explanation. The analytic hour becomes a poem: rhythms of speech and silence, image and gap, repetition and transformation. The analyst's voice, like the poet's, may be spare, elliptical, suggestive—making room for the patient's imagination, affect, and surprise.

The practice of writing and reading poetry is itself a recursive discipline. The poet revises, returns, listens for what does not yet fit. The reader, too, is called to return, to let the poem work over time, to hear new meanings in the same lines as life changes. The analyst's discipline is much the same: a recursive willingness to revisit what has been said, to hear old material in new weather, to trust that understanding will arrive not as sudden mastery, but as the slow work of attunement, resonance, and presence.

Clinical life is full of moments that call for poetic, not propositional, knowing. A patient brings a dream fragment—unsettling, beautiful, incomplete. The analyst listens, resists the urge to explain, allows the image to linger in the room. The silence between them becomes charged with possibility; meaning accumulates in the pause, in what is not spoken. Or a patient returns again and again to a word, a gesture, a half-remembered story. Each recurrence is an opportunity—not to close the loop, but to deepen the spiral, to allow affect, memory, and symbol to reverberate through new climates of relation.

The poetic discipline of negative capability is also an ethic of humility. It acknowledges that not all can be known, that the psyche is full of weather that escapes capture. The analyst who can dwell in this humility models for the patient a form of psychic hospitality: an openness to the unfinished, the ambiguous, the surprising. This is not the abdication of meaning, but its very source—the climate in which new forms, new stories, and new selves may take shape.

In the context of this book, poetry stands as both method and companion. The recursive structure of chapters, the atmospheric style, the motifs that return with difference—all are efforts to write analysis as poetry, to live psychoanalysis as weather, as refrain, as open form. The future of analytic presence may well depend on our capacity for negative capability, for poetic humility, for recursive attunement to what cannot be finalized. To read and write, to speak and listen, as a poet is to dwell at the rim—to live in the weather of unknowing, where surprise and renewal remain possible.

Meta-Reflections—The Book as Recursive Object

To write a book about recursion, unknowing, and the atmospheric ethics of psychoanalytic life is inevitably to find oneself drawn into the form one is describing. This book was never imagined as a straightforward treatise, nor as a manual for technique. Its aspiration has been to model, in style and structure, the very recursive, curved, and atmospheric epistemology it proposes. It is a book shaped by weather—returning, looping, echoing, and opening rather than marching toward definitive closure. In this way, the text becomes a recursive object, inviting the reader not only to learn but also to experience, to read and reread, to move through motifs and climates that are themselves in motion.

From its opening pages, the book's compositional rhythm has been one of return. Each chapter orbits a core set of motifs—inversion, refusal, remainder, secrecy, surprise, curved epistemology, recursive presence—yet each return is different, refracted through new clinical scenes, theoretical lenses, or aesthetic atmospheres. This is not an accident of style but a deliberate stance: a refusal of linear progress and final synthesis in favor of recursive movement and ongoing negotiation. The hope has been that the reader will feel, as much as understand, the lived rhythms of psychic life—the circling, the doubling back, the dwelling at the rim of the knowable.

In the process of writing, the recursive ethic has repeatedly intervened. Drafts have been revised, sentences rewritten, chapters reordered, not in pursuit of seamlessness but in the spirit of hospitality to surprise, ambiguity, and unfinishedness. Each attempt to "get it right" has instead revealed new atmospheres, unexpected connections, and the inevitable remainder that cannot be integrated. The writing itself has been an analytic process: improvisational, iterative, open to rupture and renewal. There has been no single path, but a series of returns, detours, and discoveries—sometimes frustrating, often generative, always marked by the limits of mastery.

This meta-reflection is not mere self-commentary; it is an ethical and epistemological gesture. In the recursive method, self-reflexivity is not a turn away from the subject but a deepening of engagement—a willingness to look again, to question one's assumptions, to allow the work to undo and remake itself. The recursive book is not finished when the final chapter is written; it is a field that remains open to the weather of new readings, future contexts, and the unpredictable shifts of meaning that time and relation will bring.

To read recursively is also an act of discipline and generosity. The reader is invited not to extract "takeaways" or to master the text, but to linger in its atmospheres, to allow motifs to return and gather new resonance, to risk surprise in the act of engagement. The book is not a map to a destination, but a weather map—a score for improvisation, a gallery of images always in flux. It asks to be read not in a single, linear sweep, but in multiple passes, with pauses for reflection, with openness to being unsettled, with patience for what remains ambiguous or in suspension.

The hope is that the book's recursive form will model for the reader the very stance it advocates: a discipline of return, an ethics of not-knowing, a hospitality to the unfinished. Each chapter, each section, is an invitation to dwell with what is not resolved, to accompany the unfolding of meaning without the demand for mastery. The analytic field, as the book understands it, is not a place for final answers, but a horizon for ongoing life, relation, and transformation.

This meta-reflective stance is also an acknowledgment of the reader's agency and subjectivity. Every encounter with the book will be different, shaped by mood, context, personal history, and the weather of the day. The book is written in anticipation of these recursive readings, these unpredictable crossings, these private returns. It is a living object, always incomplete, always open to the next engagement.

In the tradition of psychoanalytic writing, much has been made of the "case," the interpretation, the insight. This book aspires, instead, to become a kind of companion—a recursive presence at the reader's side, offering not solutions but atmosphere, not certainty but the invitation to return. The analyst who reads may find echoes of their own clinical hours, the patient their own psychic weather, the supervisor their own recursive anxieties. The book hopes to serve as a weather map, score, and poem—a resource to which one might return, again and again, finding something different each time.

If the recursive method has a future in psychoanalysis, it will be not as a doctrine, but as a discipline of presence. The recursive book is only one instance, one attempt, among many possible. It is both an artifact and an experiment—a weather system in print, designed to keep the field of analytic life open, alive, and unfinished.

A Future for Psychoanalysis—Invitation and Unfinishedness

To conclude with a vision of the future for psychoanalysis is itself a paradox. The very ethos of this book resists finality, resists the horizon as destination. Instead, it invites a living relationship to the future: one in which the field remains porous, creative, and radically unfinished. The analytic future is not a path already paved, but an expanse of possible weather—full of storms and calms, echoes and ruptures, recurring motifs and unprecedented events. To stand at the edge of this horizon is not to predict, but to attune oneself to what emerges, to the movement and recurrence of meaning, affect, and surprise.

The recursive discipline at the heart of this work demands that psychoanalysis continue to return, not to a static tradition, but to its own capacity for reinvention and surprise. The "recursion" of analytic life is not simple repetition, but a spiraling engagement with what remains unassimilated: the secrets, refusals, ruptures, and reversals that have animated the analytic encounter since Freud and beyond. Each new generation of analysts, patients, and readers stands at the edge of a weather system both familiar and new. The field's vitality depends not on the mastery of its past, but on its willingness to circle back, to revisit its own ground with humility and wonder, to let the unfinished be a source of life rather than a sign of failure.

If psychoanalysis is to remain alive, it must become ever more attuned to the recursive atmospheres of art, music, and poetry. These fields do not offer models of closure, but practices of return, improvisation, and dwelling in ambiguity. The analytic hour as a musical refrain, the clinical encounter as a canvas always in progress, the patient's narrative as a poem that refuses easy sense—these are not metaphors but kinships, signals of a shared ethic of openness and creative risk.

The future analyst will be less master interpreter than companion at the edge—witness to psychic weather, curator of atmospheres, co-traveler in recursive return (Ogden, 2005). Their presence will be marked not by authority, but by hospitality—an openness to surprise, a patience for what emerges slowly, an ethics of care for the secret, the remainder, the ambiguous. In this future, supervision will become an even more recursive field, a space where not-knowing is not shameful but honored as generative. The analyst's own process—full of uncertainty, error, and revision—will be seen not as failure but as the discipline of hospitality to psychic life.

This vision also requires the analytic field to become more porous to other forms of knowledge, other disciplines, and other arts. To read psychoanalysis musically, to paint it with the brush of abstraction, to inhabit it as a poem—these are invitations to make the field more plural, more creative, more responsive to the complexity of psychic and social life. It means giving up the fantasy of a single frame or final interpretation, and instead cultivating a practice of recursive attention: a willingness to see, hear, and speak anew, even as old motifs return.

To stand at the threshold of the future is to remain a companion to the unfinished. In the analytic hour, this may mean waiting through long silences, welcoming the patient's resistance, or allowing meaning to arrive in its own time. In the broader field, it means holding space for new voices, dissenting perspectives, and emergent forms. The discipline of not-knowing, so often maligned as indecisive or weak, is revealed as a source of strength: the ground on which surprise, change, and renewal can take root.

This unfinishedness is not only a limitation but also a resource. It is the "negative capability" that makes the analytic field creative, the ambiguity that gives rise to new forms of relation and thought. The recursive return to what cannot be resolved is not a circling in vain, but the spiraling movement by which the psyche grows, the analytic relationship deepens, and the field itself becomes more capacious. The future of psychoanalysis, if it is to be worthy of its object, must remain unfinished, recursive, and open to weather.

As the book comes to its own threshold, it offers not a set of answers, but an invitation: to dwell at the edge, to risk hospitality to surprise, to welcome the unknown as both limit and generative ground. The analyst, patient, supervisor, and reader are all called to be companions in this field—to listen, to wait, to return, to create anew from the materials of the past. To read this book is to join a recursive conversation, to become part of the unfinishedness that animates all analytic life.

A future psychoanalysis—curved, recursive, poetic, and porous—awaits those willing to accompany what cannot be mastered. The horizon is never reached, but always returns: a weather system of possibility, an atmosphere of hope, a field forever opening to what comes next.

Let the future be a refrain, not a finale; a canvas ever in process, not a finished work. Let the recursive discipline of unknowing be our common ground. And let the field remain alive, open, and unfinished—for this, above all, is the true horizon of psychoanalytic life.

Afterthinking at the Edge

Recursive Hospitality, Tögal, and the Weather of Analytic Life

This chapter is written as an afterthinking—a recursive gesture at the rim of psychoanalytic knowing, where field, weather, and luminous presence converge. Drawing from analytic field theory, recursive epistemology, and the visionary tradition of Tögal within Dzogchen and Bön, this chapter weaves together motifs of not-knowing, paradox, and the subtle body as a living field. Clinical and contemplative invitations are offered as "weather practices" for inhabiting analytic life at the edge, emphasizing direct presence, humility, and hospitality to difference and the unformulated. Rather than seeking closure or mastery, the text invites readers to dwell in recursive hospitality: a discipline of staying with the climate of the moment, letting light, surprise, and the unspeakable become analytic partners. This chapter closes with a coda—welcoming the reader back to the unfinished horizon where knowing and not-knowing shimmer together. This is psychoanalysis as living weather: luminous, recursive, and always arriving at the rim.

Opening: At the Edge of Knowability

As John Wheeler argues, the observer is implicated in the very phenomena that appear—our participation helps bring what happens into being (Wheeler, 1983). To write—and to read—at the edge of knowability is to enter a weather, not just a text. The field of analytic life, like the wider field of consciousness, is not made of certainties, but of atmosphere, pressure, and recurring fronts: the recursive conditions by which knowing and not-knowing become weather events, inverting, coalescing, and dissolving at the horizon of experience. If this book offers anything new, it is not only in its attention to paradox but also in its devotion to the ongoing movement of **epistemological inversion**—the way in which each act of knowing brings its own shadow, each attempt at mastery returns us to the rim, and every answer becomes the soil for new, generative doubt.

The edge of knowability is not a line, nor a void, but a living rim—weathered by longing, by difference, by history, by the press of what remains unformulated. It is the site where the self is not a fixed entity, but a pattern in a shifting field, where the analyst's effort to know, to witness, to contain, always meets its own recursive undoing. The analytic field is not neutral; it is dense with affect, culture, memory, and the always-excessive presence of the Other. As Levinas reminds us, the encounter with the Other is irreducibly ethical, always exceeding what can be grasped or assimilated (Levinas, 1969). To linger at this edge is not a failure, but a stance: a discipline of recursive hospitality, of holding open the space where knowledge and unknowing fold into one another.

This book, then, is written as an **invitation to weather**—not just to read about, but to co-create the atmospheric conditions of analytic knowing. You, the reader, are not outside this process; your own presence, attention, and mood shape the field as much as any idea or interpretation. As Donnel Stern argues, thinking is fundamentally intersubjective, emerging in the field between people (D. B. Stern, 2010). The self that reads, like the self that analyzes or dreams, is always already plural, porous, composed by an ensemble of moods, echoes, and half-remembered dialogues.

To approach psychoanalytic life in this spirit is to turn away from static binaries of knowing and not-knowing, presence and absence, self and other. Instead, it is to dwell in the recursive movement of the field—a weather that is never just cognitive, but always affective, bodily, and relational. Every interpretation, every silence, every sigh or glance is a shift in atmospheric pressure, a microclimate in the larger weather system of the analytic encounter. Sullivan (1953) recasts personality as an enduring pattern of recurrent interpersonal situations—a processual rhythm rather than a fixed essence. What we call "insight" or "resistance" is, from this angle, simply the crest and trough of a larger pattern of inversion and return.

Epistemological inversion is the event by which background becomes foreground, certainty gives way to surprise, and the familiar is suddenly strange. It is not merely paradox—though paradox is the air it breathes—but the dynamic, lived reversal by which the field of knowing is constantly reconstituted at its edge. In this sense, analytic work is never just about integrating what is split, or resolving what is paradoxical, but about learning to inhabit the recursive horizon where every figure invites a new ground, and every weather a new forecast.

The field is always more than two: shaped by culture, by the unspoken, by the ghosts of history, and by the insistent presence of difference. No weather is neutral. Levinas (1969) would insist that the edge of knowability is always an ethical zone: the place where the I is called by the face of the Other, and the Other's presence exceeds grasp and leaves an inexhaustible remainder that renders any knowledge and relation incomplete (Levinas, 1969, p. 194). To stay at the edge, to refuse premature closure, is to remain open to the possibility that something unthinkable, something truly new, might arrive—not as a solution, but as a shift in the weather of the field.

As you read, notice the ways in which your own attunement changes—the microclimates of certainty and confusion, openness and resistance, invitation and withdrawal. You are not just reading; you are **weathering** the field. The edge of knowability is not a boundary to be crossed, but a rim to be inhabited, recursively, with presence, patience, and the discipline of not-knowing.

If there is an ethics to this work, it is this: to dwell at the edge, to host the recursive arrival of new weather, to remain faithful to the field's unmastered horizon. The analytic field, after all, is not made once and for all but remade in every act of presence, every act of witness, every act of thought. In this sense, as Wheeler (1983) suggests, we are always co-creating the world that appears—not as masters, but as weather-makers, partners in thought, participants in the recursive weather of analytic life.

Field Weather and Inversion at the Horizon

To speak of the analytic field as "weather" is not simply to borrow a metaphor, but to risk a more radical epistemology. Weather is neither fully knowable nor wholly unpredictable; it is the recursive, lived backdrop of all experience, shaping and shaped by every presence within it. The field, in this sense, is not a neutral container, but a dynamic system of currents, temperatures, and fronts—a participatory climate where knowing and not-knowing are always in flux, always on the move.

In analytic work, the "weather" of the field is not only a backdrop for meaning but also the very substance of what is known and felt. There are hours when the room is clear, the air bright with the possibility of connection, words coming easily, and insights blooming. There are other times when a chill descends, when silence presses inward, and every interpretation falls flat, disintegrating in the fog of affect and ambiguity. This is not simply the analyst's mood or the patient's resistance; it is the field itself "weathering"—the product of countless visible and invisible forces, including culture, history, transference, and the plural presence of every participant (Sullivan, 1953).

At the horizon of analytic weather lies the phenomenon of **epistemological inversion**: the lived event in which what is background becomes foreground, what is known is suddenly unmoored, and the presumed "object" of analysis reveals itself as participant, even as weather-maker. The field, in these moments, is not passively received but recursively produced; it inverts, turns, and remakes itself at the edge of knowability. This is never a simple movement from ignorance to insight, or from confusion to clarity, but a recursive oscillation—an ongoing series of reversals that keep the analytic process alive, creative, and unfinished.

Such inversion is not only cognitive but also deeply affective: it is the sense, in the middle of an hour, that what one felt certain of is now strange, that a mood has shifted, that something unnameable is now at the center. One might recall the way a sudden summer storm remakes the entire atmosphere of a city; what was only background haze becomes the main event, and everyone finds themselves pausing, reorienting, recalibrating. In the analytic setting, these shifts can be subtle—a patient's laughter turns to tears with no apparent cause, or the analyst, usually so attuned, suddenly feels "out of phase," unable to track the undercurrents. The "meaning" of such events is not always clear, but their weather is unmistakable. Here, affect is epistemology: the field's mood is not a barrier to knowing, but its very texture and method (Bollas, 1987).

This is the recursive logic of the field: knowing and not-knowing are not endpoints or opposites, but recurring positions in an ongoing atmospheric drama. Each new insight is provisional, each clarity haunted by the possibility of inversion. As the philosopher Emmanuel Levinas (1969) suggests, the edge of encounter is always a site of excess—an Otherness that resists containment, continually destabilizing the apparent order of the field. In analytic weather, the Other is not just the patient or analyst, but the unassimilable remainder—the unsymbolized, the unspeakable, the remaindered affect that returns in new forms. At the rim of knowability, the field itself is Other: a horizon that cannot be possessed, only inhabited, moment by recursive moment.

Consider a vignette. In the middle of a session, a patient who has been speaking in careful, rehearsed language suddenly falls silent. The room thickens; both participants sense a shift, a front moving in. The analyst offers an interpretation, but it falls flat—meaning is no longer where it was. What was background—an undercurrent of grief or anger—now swells, taking center stage. The weather has turned. Words, for a time, are useless; what matters is the shared affective field, the willingness to dwell in opacity, to let the storm pass, or to reconfigure what can be said. Eventually, something new arises—not necessarily insight, but a new pattern, a clearing in the weather, an opening to a different mode of presence. Here, inversion is not a disruption, but a necessary event—the recursive movement by which the field remains alive.

This weather logic is not unique to analysis. In music, as in art, the shift of background and foreground is a primary tool of composition. A melody may fade into harmony, and the accompaniment, once mere support, becomes the main line. In painting, what was once the shadow or negative space can claim the eye, transforming the whole. These are not simple reversals, but recursive processes—each new configuration is temporary, held open by the play of inversion and return. In analytic life, such moments are invitations: to hear what is not yet audible, to see what has not yet come to form, to remain receptive to the field's next weather.

Paradox, in this context, is not a static tension to be resolved but the very atmosphere that sustains the analytic field. It is the sense that knowing and not-knowing, form and emptiness, presence and absence are not opposites but recursive partners in the making of experience. Inversion is the weather event—the moment when the paradox becomes lived, when the "logic" of analysis is revealed to be a practice of recursive attunement at the edge. To be an analyst, or a participant in any field of meaning, is to become a forecaster of sorts: not predicting outcomes, but staying attuned to the subtle shifts that mark the rim of the knowable.

This is why, as readers and practitioners, we are always already in the weather, never outside it. Our efforts to know are themselves atmospheric disturbances, contributing to the patterns that emerge. The edge of knowability is not a stable threshold, but a moving front—one that requires recursive humility and a willingness to be surprised. As the analytic field turns, so too does our sense of self, of Other, of what might be possible.

If there is an ethics to analytic weather, it is to linger at the edge, to attend to the recursive movements of inversion and return, to refuse the comforts of mastery for the generative discomfort of not-knowing. Here, knowing is less a possession than a weather pattern—something to be noticed, tracked, and participated in, but never fully owned. The field, in its weather, invites us to relinquish control, to host the unpredictable, to receive the arrival of the Other not as a threat, but as the very condition for new meaning.

As you continue through these pages, notice how your own inner weather shifts—the changes in mood, in attention, in openness, or in resistance. Each reading is a new field; each encounter with the text is a chance for inversion, for the background to become foreground, for a new weather to announce itself. You are not simply a reader of analytic weather; as Wheeler (1983) reminds us, the observer is inescapably involved in bringing about what appears to be happening. The field is yours as much as it is mine. We inhabit its recursive horizon together.

The Participatory Self—Partners in Thought at the Edge

To inhabit the field at the edge of knowability is, inevitably, to encounter the dissolution of "I"—to sense the self not as a bounded substance, but as a rhythmic, weathered phenomenon of relation and participation. Sullivan (1953) long ago proposed that personality consists of relatively enduring patterns of recurrent interpersonal situations, shifting the locus of selfhood from inner substance to patterned field. In this view, the self is not a private core but a mutable, recursive climate—always being remade by the currents of relationship, language, and affect that move through the analytic encounter.

This weathered self is never solitary. The field of analytic life is always plural, always intersubjective, always porous to the presence of another. Even our most private experiences, our deepest moments of knowing and not-knowing, are shaped by the imagined or actual presence of another mind. The analyst's thought, the patient's symptom, even the act of reading these words—none emerge in a vacuum, but in the participatory weather of the field.

At the edge, the "I" loosens. The solid sense of agency—"I am thinking, I am interpreting, I am analyzing"—dissolves into something more recursive, more atmospheric. Stern (2010) reminds us that we are *partners* in the generation of meaning, not its masters. The subject is not an island, but a node in a web, a swirl in the weather. The field is always more than the sum of its parts. This is especially evident in analytic moments of intense contact, rupture, or creativity: when self and other are mutually implicated in an atmosphere of surprise, or when what had felt most private suddenly finds resonance in the relational field.

A vignette: A patient comes into session gripped by a mood that she cannot name. The analyst, too, feels a heaviness, a quiet anxiety whose origin is unclear. For a time, both are adrift; interpretations falter, and neither can locate the source of the weather. Gradually, through shared silence and the analyst's gentle witnessing, a memory surfaces—not just for the patient, but in the shared field itself. It is not spoken as a declaration, but as a joint emergence, a weather event that belongs to both and neither. The room feels lighter, the mood shifts, and both are left with the sense that something important has happened—something that could not have come into being without the recursive attunement, the willingness to let "I" become "we," and to linger at the rim of the knowable.

Such moments are not rare—they are the heartbeat of analytic work at its most vital. They show us that knowing is never only "mine" or "yours," but always relational, always emerging in the participatory field between. Even the act of not-knowing—the analyst's hesitation, the patient's confusion—takes on new meaning in the field. The refusal to foreclose, the discipline of shared uncertainty, becomes a resource: Stern argues that unformulated experience—and the capacity to symbolize it—emerges between people, within the field (2010).

Affect, here, is the key epistemological vector. The weather of the field is not just cognitive, but emotional—joy, anxiety, strangeness, resonance, rupture. At the edge, these affects are not simply owned by one or the other, but circulate in the atmosphere. The analyst's shame at not knowing, the patient's terror of recognition, the shared moment of delight or sorrow—all are weather events that shape what is possible to know and to become. Affect is not an obstacle to understanding, but the very climate in which knowing unfolds.

Levinas (1969) gives ethical gravity to this field logic. The encounter with the Other, he writes, is not an act of possession or comprehension, but a site of infinite responsibility and exposure. The face of the Other calls the self into being, not as a master, but as a host—responsible for making space, for lingering at the edge, for receiving what cannot be assimilated or explained. In analytic life, to become a partner in thought is to accept this ethical demand: to witness what is strange or unwelcome, to hold presence for what cannot yet be named, to remain hospitable to the "unformulated" and the "unforeseeable" (D. B. Stern, 2010).

To say that the field is always plural is also to acknowledge that it is shaped by difference—by race, gender, sexuality, culture, history, and the unspoken "weather" of the social world. No analytic atmosphere is ever neutral; the room is always crowded with ghosts and absences, with the excess of the world beyond its walls. Each partner brings their own weather, and together they generate a climate that is never entirely predictable, never fully owned. The edge of knowability is thus also an edge of difference: a horizon where the limits of empathy, understanding, and shared meaning are continually redrawn.

The reader, too, enters this participatory weather. As you move through these words, notice how your own sense of self shifts—how you may feel called into the field, implicated in its moods, responsible for its atmosphere. This is not accidental; the book itself is written as a recursive invitation, a weather system in which every act of attention, resistance, or curiosity generates new patterns. You, too, are a partner in thought, a participant at the edge. What emerges in your own mind as you read—the hesitations, the recognitions, the refusals—is not private, but part of the recursive field we inhabit together.

The "I" that writes and the "you" that reads are both weathered by this encounter. At the edge, the boundary is always moving; agency, knowing, and affect pass between us like clouds or currents. To dwell here is not to lose the self, but to feel its recursive pluralization—to become field, to become weather, to become a partner in the ongoing generation of meaning. Stern (2010) emphasizes that psychoanalysis is most vital when it does not foreclose the field but keeps it open to the arrival of new thought, feeling, and being (p. 18).

The analytic field, then, is a discipline of recursive hospitality—a stance of ongoing readiness to be moved, to be undone, to receive the unexpected. It is a commitment to linger at the rim of the knowable, to stay with the weather of unknowing, and to make presence available for what might yet emerge. Here, as everywhere in this book, the self is always a plural event, and the field is the unfinished weather of our shared attunement.

Unformulated Emptiness, Psychedelic States, and Recursive Emergence

The analytic field is, at its most generative, a climate of unformulated possibility—a weather thick with unsymbolized affect, half-formed images, and the shimmers of meaning that have not yet taken shape. Ogden (1994) called this "the analytic third": a space of co-creation where neither analyst nor patient is fully in control, and where experience emerges in the space between, often surprising both partners. Bollas (1987) named the "unthought known" as the residue of experience not yet thinkable, the background weather that nonetheless shapes the present; Bion (1962) differently tracks how raw (beta) elements require transformation to become thinkable.

Psychoanalytic process, in this view, is not the progressive conquest of ignorance, but the recursive discipline of returning to the edge of what can be known. The most creative moments are often those in which symbolization fails—where language breaks down, concepts dissolve, and the field is saturated with a kind of fertile emptiness. It is here, in the liminal zone of unformulated experience, that something new may arise: a feeling, a memory, a dream, a piece of music or art that opens the field to fresh weather.

Psychedelic states, dream states, and moments of extreme affect can all bring us to this rim. In the midst of a psychedelic session, the usual coordinates of self and world may vanish; boundaries blur, time thickens, and meaning becomes atmospheric, no longer tied to narrative or explanation. The analytic weather in such moments is unpredictable—a storm, a shimmer, a hush. There is often a sense of being suspended on the threshold of symbolization, with experience felt as intensity, color, or sensation before it coalesces into thought. This is not the absence of knowing, but its precondition—the field as unformulated emptiness, a weather waiting to be named.

Consider a clinical moment: a patient returns from a week-long psychedelic retreat. He tries to describe what he experienced, but words fail. "It was like being inside a painting," he says, "or maybe a song. There was no me, just colors, feelings, waves." In the analytic hour, he sits in silence, and the room fills with a palpable charge. The analyst resists the urge to interpret, instead leaning into the affective weather. Slowly, something shifts: tears come, then laughter, then a story, half-formed and elliptical. The meaning is not in the narrative but in the shared willingness to stay with the field as it is—in all its unformulated, recursive possibility.

What is background becomes figure. The weather of the session—at first chaotic, then coherent, then open again—models the recursive process by which new knowing emerges from the unthought known. Affect is epistemology: the analytic field teaches us to trust the mood, the silence, the tension in the air. These are not obstacles to meaning, but its generative soil. Recursive emergence is the method—returning again and again to the edge, letting the weather shift, letting the unformulated become thinkable in its own time.

Difference is always present in this weather. Every field is shaped by the cultural, historical, and relational currents that move through it. The analytic space is haunted by ghosts: the histories of race, gender, sexuality, trauma, migration, and class that inflect every silence, every breath. Some weather patterns are personal, others collective; some are fleeting, others ancient and persistent. To attend to the field is to attune to these differences, to let the weather teach us what can and cannot be known, what is allowed to emerge, and what remains unformulated, perhaps for generations.

Levinas (1969) reminds us that the edge of knowing is always an encounter with Otherness—with that which cannot be fully grasped or contained. The patient's unformulated experience, the analyst's bewilderment, the cultural ghosts in the room—all are faces of the Other, inviting us to linger at the edge, to remain hospitable to what exceeds our categories. In analytic life, this is not simply a matter of method but of ethics: to bear witness to the unthought, to refuse to collapse the weather into explanation, to honor the recursive rhythms by which new forms of knowing may eventually arise.

Even outside the analytic dyad, these patterns hold. In the weather of culture, new meanings emerge from zones of unformulated emptiness—art forms that erupt from the margins, social movements that break through the silence, poetry that names what was previously unspeakable. The recursive field is always alive, always returning to its edge, always welcoming the next front, the next storm, the next clearing. The weather is never finished.

As you reflect on your own experience, you may notice how certain memories, moods, or images hover at the edge of articulation—neither present nor absent, but shimmering in the background. These, too, are part of the recursive field. To attend to them is to enter the weather, to let the unformulated speak in its own time. The process is never linear; it moves in cycles, reversals, and unpredictable turns. Each reading, each analytic hour, is a new chance for recursive emergence, for the background to become figure, for the weather to teach us what is possible.

To practice psychoanalysis—or to live deeply in any field of meaning—is to surrender to this recursive logic, to let the weather do its work, to host the ongoing dance of figure and ground, form and emptiness, knowing and not-knowing. The discipline is not to master the weather, but to learn to dwell within it—to stay with the moods, the silences, the storms, and the moments of sudden, unspeakable clarity that only arise at the edge.

The Symbolic and Subtle Body—Sensing at the Edge

The field of analytic knowing is not just linguistic, not just cognitive—it is vibrantly somatic, a living weather that courses through and as the body. To attend to the edge of knowability is to sense, quite literally, the borderlands where thought, affect, and sensation become indistinguishable. Gendlin (1978) called this the **felt sense**: that subtle, bodily resonance which signals meaning before words, the raw, unformulated weather that precedes and undergirds all symbolization. The analyst who listens at this edge learns to recognize knowing as an embodied event, an atmospheric pulse rather than a propositional content.

Here, the body is not simply the patient's or the analyst's; it is a shared field, an interpenetrating atmosphere where affect circulates and shifts, where the line between "mine" and "yours" is as porous as a summer sky. Eigen (2004) explores the **mysticism of the body**—its capacity to register contact, trauma, joy, and mystery at the most granular levels of sensation. In analytic work, this means that knowing is never purely mental; it is always mediated by the body's capacity to feel, to bear, to resonate with what cannot yet be said.

This is not a new insight. Traditional yoga, before its Western translation as fitness or stress reduction, was a discipline of subtle body practice—a way of listening to the currents and channels that move beneath the surface of ordinary awareness (White, 2012). In Tibetan traditions, **Tummo** (inner fire) and **Chandali** practices cultivate sensitivity to energy, heat, and space as epistemological events: not metaphysical oddities, but recursive invitations to feel the world as a field, the self as weather, the edge as a living rim (Longchenpa, 2014). The symbolic body is not merely a metaphor; it is the site where the analytic field becomes incarnate, where weather is felt as heat, shiver, constriction, or release.

Consider an analytic vignette. A patient, reflecting on a recurring dream, grows suddenly quiet. "I can feel it here," she says, hand on her chest, "like a knot. I can't name it, but it's there." The analyst, noticing his own breath catch, becomes aware of a tingling in his arms. For a moment, neither speaks. The room hums with a kind of charged silence—the weather thick, almost tactile. In this shared atmosphere, meaning hovers at the edge; the knot is not yet a narrative, not yet a memory, but a climate in the body, awaiting its time.

Slowly, as the hour unfolds, words begin to surface. The patient speaks of longing, of fear, of the way her body "holds onto" what her mind cannot express. The analyst, now more attuned, finds language for his own sensations—a sense of pressure, a fleeting sadness, a desire to comfort and to wait. The weather shifts: what was once a mute presence in the chest becomes an image, a phrase, a new understanding. The subtle body, here, is the analytic field itself—felt, shared, weathered together.

Such moments are not reducible to technique. They arise from the recursive discipline of staying at the edge, of trusting the body's knowing as a form of analytic hospitality. The "felt sense" is not a thing, but a weather event—a signal that something is forming, that the edge is alive. Gendlin (1978) emphasizes that bodily experience carries forward more than has yet taken conceptual form. To listen for this "more" is to welcome the weather as a teacher, to recognize that not-knowing is always lived, not just thought.

In some analytic traditions, these somatic shifts are dismissed as "noise"—artifacts to be bracketed in the pursuit of insight. But in recursive, field-based work, the noise is the music; the body's weather is the analytic weather. What cannot be articulated in speech is often expressed in posture, in tone, in the subtle choreography of presence and absence. Affect, here, is epistemology: what the body feels, what the field knows, and what the field knows is always on the move.

Levinas (1969) offers a further deepening: the body is not merely "mine," but always already a site of encounter with the Other. The face-to-face meeting, he insists, is irreducibly ethical—a summons to responsibility that exceeds knowledge or mastery. In the analytic field, this means that bodily sensation is never just an internal event; it is an invitation, a call, a weathering by difference and relation. The edge of knowability is thus always a horizon shaped by otherness, by the mystery of what cannot be absorbed into the self.

Cultural and relational differences saturate this weather. The meanings the body carries—its heat, its silence, its vulnerabilities—are never universal. They are shaped by histories of gender, race, trauma, migration, and desire. To listen for the symbolic body is to listen for the weather of difference, to attend to the ways the field is marked by what is absent as much as what is present. Each encounter brings new weather; each body signals new conditions at the rim.

Analytic practice at this edge is not about "decoding" symptoms or making the implicit explicit. It is a discipline of field-listening, a willingness to trust the weather, to let the subtle body's knowledge unfold on its own terms. Some sessions are thunderous, others quiet as dawn; some are charged with tension, others lull with calm. The analyst's task is not to master this weather, but to attune—to feel, to wait, to recognize the recursive patterns by which knowing and not-knowing alternate, coalesce, and dissolve.

The body's wisdom, in this sense, is recursive: it returns again and again to the edge, signaling with shivers, aches, and pulses what cannot be said but must be lived. To dwell at this rim is to become a partner in the field's ongoing generation of meaning—a participant in the weather, a witness to the subtle turnings of the symbolic body as it leans into its next horizon.

As you read, notice the weather of your own body—the tension in your jaw, the warmth in your hands, the flutter of anxiety or curiosity as ideas land and recede. This, too, is field knowledge: the subtle body as participant, as weather-maker, as the site where meaning takes shape and dissolves, only to return again in new forms. The edge of knowability is not elsewhere; it is here, in the flesh, in the weather of sensation, at the rim of every analytic and lived encounter.

Tögal as Epistemology—Things as They Are, Light at the Edge

To speak of Tögal here is, for me, a first—an extension and intensification of the nondual thread woven through earlier works, but now named and inhabited as an epistemology of the field itself. Tögal (*thod rgal*), meaning "leap over" or "direct crossing," is a visionary contemplative practice rooted in the **Dzogchen tradition** of Tibetan Buddhism, itself with antecedents in the ancient Tibetan Bön religion (Reynolds, 2005; Klein, 2006; Longchenpa, 2014). Within these lineages, Tögal is not simply a metaphorical gesture but a sophisticated, embodied discipline for encountering the nature of reality through direct vision and the radiance of awareness. Light, in this tradition, is not an abstraction; it is both phenomenon and method—a recursive meeting of self, world, and experience at their most luminous edge.

What matters for analytic life is not the esoteric ritual or doctrinal precision of Tögal, but the stance it models: the radical willingness to meet experience as it is—luminous, unresolved, unpossessed—at the living rim of knowability. While Tögal is traditionally practiced in mountain hermitages, with intricate supports and lineages of transmission, its fundamental invitation—to turn toward the "light" of awareness, to participate in the weather of experience without grasping or turning away—is available wherever there is openness to the edge. My use of Tögal here is not an attempt to reproduce its ritual or doctrinal form, but to learn from its epistemological stance: a discipline of participatory presence at the threshold of knowing, of meeting what arises without the compulsion to resolve or assimilate.

In analytic life, we are accustomed to seeking—tracking meaning, decoding symptoms, laboring to bind what is split or heal what has ruptured. Yet there are moments when the very structure of seeking itself becomes the site of transformation: the light of attention turns back on itself, revealing that what is sought is already present, if only forgotten. This is the recursive logic at the heart of Tögal. The field becomes luminous not through conquest or mastery, but by allowing what arises to shine in its own time. The task is not to render all weather transparent, but to honor the atmosphere's ability to illuminate itself.

Things are as they are, and your seeking is the light that already knows what it seeks but has forgotten so.

Let this phrase resonate—poetic, recursive, an invitation rather than a doctrine. In Tögal, the "light" is not simply a visual metaphor, but the living atmosphere of awareness—a participatory field that includes both seer and seen, knower and unknown, rim and center. The discipline is to let appearances come and go, to allow the field's weather to unfold without grasping, without turning every shimmer into a sign or every surprise into a problem to be solved.

A clinical vignette: a patient, in the midst of complicated grief, begins to describe moments of seeing "light" at the edges of things—"as if the world is outlined in something I can't quite touch." The analyst, who in other moments might have interpreted this as a defensive formation or a wishful regression, instead chooses to pause. Together, they dwell in this luminous edge of the field—a silence charged with expectancy, humility, and the unmistakable sense that something real, and rare, is happening. There is no rush to interpretation, no attempt to "resolve" the light. Instead, both linger in its presence, letting the weather of the field become its own form of knowing. In the days that follow, both analyst and patient notice the world appearing differently—colors sharper, time slowed, grief and hope fused in a shared shimmer.

Tögal's invitation is not to escape the analytic field, but to dwell in it more deeply—to meet its weather as luminous, recursive, always more than the sum of its interpretations. In the contemplative practice, the meditator is instructed to "look directly into the light"—not to find answers, but to rest in the knowing that is already present. So too in analytic life: the analyst who can meet the field without fleeing from opacity, without demanding closure, is practicing Tögal in spirit if not in form. This is not spiritual bypass, not an avoidance of suffering, but a willingness to let the edge of knowability shine as it is—a horizon always unfinished, always inviting.

Meta-commentary is crucial here: as you read, notice the moments when something in you "lights up," when the weather of attention changes, when you sense a shimmer at the rim of meaning. These are not accidents; they are recursive invitations, field-events that cannot be owned or explained away. You are not outside this weather, but a participant—your seeking, your hesitation, your surprise are all part of the field's light.

Levinas (1969) offers a sobering complement: the light of the field is never total, never a conquest. The Other—whether the patient, the analyst, the text, or the world—always exceeds the frame, always escapes full illumination. The face, according to Levinas, brings an infinity beyond comprehension. Tögal, then, is not the mastery of experience but the discipline of allowing what is inexhaustible, what cannot be fully known, to shine in its own time, at its own edge.

Sometimes this light arrives as silence. In analytic work, there are sessions when nothing seems to happen—no new insight, no catharsis, no breakthrough. Yet, in the quiet, something shimmers: a glance, a phrase, a tear, a shared breath. These are field-events, weathered moments of Tögal, where the light of knowing is not a floodlight but a candle at dusk—enough to see by, but never enough to end the night.

Tögal as epistemology is not a method to be mastered, but a field to be inhabited—a recursive practice of letting the weather of experience be as it is, knowing that the seeking itself is already participation, already light. In this, psychoanalysis and contemplative life are not so far apart: both rest on the discipline of staying with the edge, of honoring what cannot be named, of welcoming the field's shimmer as a presence in its own right.

To live this is to risk a new kind of humility—not the humility of ignorance, but the humility of participation. The analyst, the patient, the reader, the thinker—all become weather-makers, witnesses to the recursive light that moves through the field. The edge of knowability is thus not a barrier, but a living invitation—a call to dwell, to wait, to see what shines, and to let the light teach us what it knows.

Synthesis: Paradox, Inversion, and Recursion at the Horizon

To draw together the weather patterns traced in these pages is not to bring closure, but to reveal their recursive logic, their never-ending hospitality to what remains unresolved. Here, at the edge of knowability, every motif—the shifting patterns of knowing and not-knowing, the plural field of partners in thought, the recursive return of affect, the shimmer of light at the rim—finds itself doubled, echoed, turned inside out. The field is both familiar and strange; what we thought was a conclusion is only another change in the weather.

Paradox, in this project, is not a static condition to be "solved," but an atmosphere that sustains the analytic field. It is the mood of the recursive horizon: the knowledge that knowing and not-knowing, presence and absence, self and other, are not opposites, but forms of attunement—always in movement, always prone to inversion. Every figure emerges on a shifting ground; every certainty contains the seed of its own reversal. In this sense, paradox is not a defect in the field, but its method, its weather—what makes new meaning, and new being, possible.

Epistemological inversion is the weather event—the lived moment when background becomes foreground, when the logic of analysis is shown to be recursive, never final. The analytic hour is rarely a linear march from ignorance to insight; it is a looping, wandering, folding of experience, in which the old returns in new forms, and the most important knowing often appears as surprise, reversal, or the eruption of difference. To dwell at this rim is not to possess knowledge, but to be possessed by it—to be moved by the field, to let oneself be undone and remade in the weather of encounter.

This is the work of recursive hospitality. The analytic field, like the weather, is never finished, never entirely "ours." It calls for an ethics not of mastery, but of presence—an ongoing willingness to host what arrives, to welcome the unformulated, to bear witness to what cannot be resolved or explained. As Levinas (1969) reminds us, the encounter with the Other is always an invitation to responsibility, a summons to receive what exceeds our categories, to make room for the stranger, the unspoken, the irreducibly plural.

Art, poetry, and music offer analogies for this field. In a symphony, a theme is introduced, varied, returned to, inverted, echoed across instruments, never quite the same twice. In a poem, a phrase recurs—sometimes identical, sometimes changed by context, always alive to the weather of the line. In a painting, background and foreground continually trade places; a color or shape that seemed unimportant suddenly becomes the heart of the scene. Analytic life is much the same: it is the play of motifs, the return of themes, the recursive shimmer of meaning at the edge.

Affect is epistemology. The weather of the field—its joy, its anxiety, its confusion and wonder—is not just background noise, but the very stuff of knowing. To attend to affect is to attend to the weather; to be moved by mood, by silence, by the pressure in the air, is to be in the field. The analyst's task, and the reader's, is not to stand apart but to join in—to recognize that every act of knowing is already a participation, a weather event, a form of hospitality.

The field is always plural, always shaped by difference. Every encounter is a meeting of histories, cultures, desires, absences. No weather is neutral; no field is without its ghosts. The analytic hour is a weather system in which every partner brings their own storm, their own calm, their own atmospheric pressure. The edge of knowability is always the edge of difference—an invitation to stay with what cannot be integrated, to listen for what is missing, to honor the ways the field is haunted by what will not be assimilated.

Recursive sincerity is the discipline that emerges here. It is the willingness to be sincere about not-knowing, to name the recursive returns, to let the weather of the field be what it is, rather than what we wish it to be. It is a kind of faithfulness—not to answers, but to the process, to the endless horizon of the field. To practice recursive sincerity is to become a partner in the unfinished, a witness to the ever-returning invitation of the edge.

As you read, you may notice certain phrases returning: weather, edge, recursion, hospitality, difference, light. These are not mere repetitions, but invitations—ways the text, and the field, beckon you to dwell, to return, to notice the new in what seems familiar. You are not outside this weather; you are part of the field's ongoing horizon. Every act of reading, every breath of attention, is a shift in the atmosphere, a recursive participation in the open field.

The work of psychoanalysis—and, perhaps, of living—is not to resolve paradox or conquer the edge of knowability, but to dwell within its recursive weather. The field's horizon is always ahead, always arriving, always inviting the next act of hospitality, the next surprise, the next echo. In this, analytic life becomes an ongoing discipline: to keep the field open, to make room for what returns, to live at the edge, where knowing is always new, always unfinished.

Closing: Afterthinking as Unfinished Weather

If you have lingered with these pages, you have already felt the weather change—the slow thickening of clouds, the sudden shaft of light, the restless movement of wind at the horizon of the knowable. This is the atmosphere of afterthinking: not an ending, but an open sky. The recursive field of analytic and contemplative life does not resolve; it returns, refracts, hovers, and invites.

What you seek is the light already present, weathering the edge of the knowable.

This is the paradox and the promise of the field: that every act of seeking, every gesture of thought or presence, is already participation in the recursive shimmer of knowing. The analyst and the analysand, the writer and the reader, are weather-makers—partners in the unfinished hospitality of the field. What arises between us, in silence and in word, is a mood, a climate, a subtle radiance that cannot be contained by concept or closed by explanation.

Afterthinking is not an act of mastery. It is a willingness to remain in motion, to let motifs recur, to allow the weather to unsettle certainty and open new routes of sense and surprise. In this, the discipline is humility—what Levinas (1969) might call the ethical demand of the Other, the call to hospitality that keeps the field plural, open, incomplete. The edge of knowability is not a barrier to cross, but a place to dwell—a horizon that will always move as we approach it, a weather that will always return in new forms.

There is no neutral field. Every climate is colored by difference, by history, by the unspoken and the unspeakable. The analytic hour, like the world itself, is full of absences and presences, storms and calms, inheritances and losses. To dwell at the edge is to honor these conditions, to make space for the ghosts, the ungrievable, the not-yet-known. Recursive hospitality is the ongoing stance: not to finish the work, but to witness its unfolding, to welcome the weather's return.

Perhaps, as you read, you have noticed how certain lines or images circle back—how weather, recursion, edge, light, and hospitality have become more than words, but fields you have inhabited, climates you have co-created. This is not an accident. The recursive field is participatory: your attention, your affect, your resistance, and your wonder, have weathered these pages as much as any concept. What you seek here has always also been seeking you.

Afterthinking, then, is an unfinished invitation. It is the practice of dwelling at the rim—where what is unformulated can arrive, where knowing is always alive to difference, and where the light of the field is always both gift and mystery. As every weather does, this writing passes, leaves traces, echoes, a changed horizon. But it does not close the field; it opens it again.

Return, if you wish. Orbit back. Let the recursive weather of analytic and contemplative life teach you again what it means to stay at the edge, to welcome what returns, to host what remains unsaid and unsayable. The horizon is not behind us, but ahead, shimmering with every act of presence, every refusal of closure, every recursive hospitality to the unmastered field.

Afterthinking is only weather on the way to something else.

Coda: Weathering the Edge—Clinical Invitations for Recursive Hospitality

Yet as with all weather, the practice is lived—embodied in presence, not only conceived in thought. What follows is a coda: a series of invitations for analytic life at the edge, drawn from the recursive field and inflected by luminous, Tögal-like presence. May these gestures accompany you as you return to your own weather.

1 Begin with the Weather
   Before each session, pause to sense your field. Notice the climate of your own mood, body, and attention. Is the air bright or heavy? What old fronts linger, what new atmospheres want to break in? Let this moment of attunement be the threshold into analytic presence.
2 Let the Field Shine
   When a patient brings an unnameable sensation, a half-articulated image, or even a flicker of light in their dream or memory, pause with them. Instead of interpreting or moving quickly to meaning, let the shared field shimmer. Practice "looking into the light" of the experience, trusting the weather to reveal what is needed, or nothing at all. Sometimes, sitting quietly in this edge is the deepest analytic work.

3 Name Not-Knowing—Together
If understanding falters or the analytic space grows foggy, try naming not-knowing aloud. "I'm not sure what this is yet, but let's stay with it." Notice how the field responds—does something shift, clarify, or deepen? Make room for the generative presence of unformulated experience.
4 Partner in the Weather
Remind yourself: the field is never yours alone. At moments of clinical impasse or surprise, wonder, "Who else is in this weather?" The patient's parents, culture, history; your own unseen teachers or moods—each may be shaping the climate. In supervision, make explicit the mood or front you both sense. "There's a chill in the room today," or "It feels luminous, even if we don't know why."
5 Stay with the Shimmer at the Rim
Encourage both yourself and your patient to notice the moments that resist articulation—a heat in the chest, a pause before tears, a strange lightness after silence. Name these as weather, not symptoms. "Something's hovering here, just at the edge." Tögal teaches that what appears at the rim is already meaningful, even if we never find its name.
6 Journal the Weather
After sessions, write down a brief account of the climate you noticed—oppressive, buoyant, flickering, charged. Return to these entries to track how your own presence, and the field's mood, shape the work over time. Let this recursive awareness become part of your clinical discipline.
7 Practice Recursive Return
If a motif, phrase, or emotional pattern returns in the work—week after week or across cases—pause to sense the weather conditions that surround its arrival. Does the return signal a new front, or the persistence of something ungrievable? Each recurrence is an opportunity for new knowing, not a failure of resolution.
8 Welcome Silence as Light
When nothing seems to happen in a session, trust the silence as field-event. Tögal invites us to rest in the luminous stillness that is neither absence nor avoidance, but the light at the edge of experience. Some of the deepest transformations occur in these unscripted pauses.

9 Honor Difference, Host the Other
Notice how the weather of the field is shaped by cultural, historical, and personal differences. Welcome these "fronts" not as problems but as creative conditions. Levinas reminds us: the Other always exceeds our frame. Make hospitality to difference a central analytic stance.

10 Trust the Weather
Most of all, trust the recursive field—the discipline of presence at the edge. Let not-knowing, surprise, light, and storm become analytic teachers. What you seek is already arriving, weathering the horizon, shimmering at the rim.

Appendix A—Listening as Knowing

A Mikrokosmos Study Guide

On Mikrokosmos and the Curvature of Listening

In psychoanalysis, as in music, form is not a vessel for meaning but the movement of meaning itself. Béla Bartók's *Mikrokosmos*—153 pieces across six books—functions as both pedagogy and revelation: a topology of form learning to hear itself. Unison bends toward counterpoint, pattern curves into rhythm, and equal temperament is bent into curvature. Each miniature enacts a principle of psychic structure. Like the analytic hour, the cycle proceeds not by linear development but by recursive listening—returning to what has already sounded in order to hear it differently.

Composed for his son yet addressed to anyone who listens, *Mikrokosmos* also reads as a study in how consciousness learns to listen: how the known folds back into the unformulated, how order bears dissonance without repair. Within the tempered grid, Bartók lets natural harmonics, folk modes, and asymmetrical rhythms press against the system without breaking it. Psychoanalysis performs a parallel operation within language: bending symbolization to the edge of its grid, revealing the residue of experience the symbolic cannot fully absorb.

Listening psychoanalytically means hearing remainder as rhythm. Every phrase in *Mikrokosmos* trains the ear to notice what repeats, what distorts, and what persists as difference. The analyst, like the pianist, works within a tempered instrument—language—and yet reaches toward what exceeds it. The recursive structures here model an ethic of tension sustained without repair: to stay inside modulation and honor the stayed note that does not resolve.

What follows are 12 brief "studies" that pair analytic capacities—contact, differentiation, holding, translation, remainder, opacity, recursion, threshold, repetition, polyphony, reverie, release—with selected *Mikrokosmos* pieces. Each entry offers a one-sentence gloss and a concise practice cue. Hear theory as sound; hear sound as thought.

I. Contact—Unison and Primary Process
(Nos. 1–6, Book I): Parallel motion as first communication—sameness quickening in resonance until difference stirs.
Instruction: Listen for the instant two lines become just distinct.

II. Differentiation—Dialogue and Otherness
Dialogue (No. 65, Book II); *Question and Answer* (No. 14, Book I): Call-and-response marks recognition—the self hears itself as other and replies.
Instruction: Attend to the moment imitation turns to speech.

III. Holding—Accompaniment and Ground
(Nos. 79, 86, Book III): A melody wanders while its ground keeps faith; containment is timing, not control—the analyst's breath sustaining the patient's phrase.
Instruction: Hear the patience beneath movement—the tempo of reverie.

IV. Translation—Crossing Voices
Canon at the Octave (No. 28, Book I); *Imitation and Inversion* (No. 25, Book I): A voice returns altered yet recognizably itself; transference as imitation that re-means by re-entry.
Instruction: Follow the voice that comes second; it knows what the first forgot.

V. Remainder—Dissonance and Delay
(Nos. 100, 102, Book IV): The unresolved interval vibrates like thought still forming—dissonance keeps time with what cannot yet be symbolized.
Instruction: Let the tone hang and notice how the body waits.

VI. Opacity—Modes within Constraint
(Nos. 126, 130, Book V): Inside equal temperament, modal turns and irregular meters bend the system until it shimmers; law contains its own curvature.
Instruction: Hear how form strains against itself yet does not break.

VII. Recursion—Return and Transformation
(Nos. 148, 151, Book VI): Themes re-enter altered; recognition parts company with memory as the same figure returns as its own echo.
Instruction: Compare the beginning and the end—find identity reappearing as evolution.

VIII. Threshold—Silence Between Notes
Diminished Fifth (No. 101, Book IV); *Whole-Tone Scale* (No. 136, Book V): Between fixed tones lies audible latency; the diminished fifth hinges open a pause that feels like sound.
Instruction: Attend to rests and decays—treat silence as event.

IX. Repetition—Compulsion and Freedom
Ostinato (No. 146, Book VI); *In Hungarian Style* (No. 43, Book II); *Chromatic Inventions* (No. 91-92, Book III): Small loops repeat until they transform; pattern both binds and releases.
Instruction: Listen until the loop becomes trance, and then catch the first breath of change.

X. Integration—Polyphony and Layering
From the Island of Bali (No. 109, Book IV); *Intermezzo* (No. 111, Book IV); *In Dorian Mode* (No. 32, Book I): Independent lines interlace without loss—self-states in conversation across distinct time senses.
Instruction: Move your ear among lines and refuse the comfort of a single melody.

XI. Reverie—Nocturnal Atmosphere
Notturno (No. 97, Book IV): Thinking-in-the-dark; form relaxes into weather and the psyche breathes through night air.
Instruction: Listen softly—do not disturb your own hearing.

XII. Release—Cadence Without Closure
(Nos. 148–153, Book VI): Resolution suspends rather than erases tension; ending returns quiet as continuation.
Instruction: When the last note fades, keep listening inwardly for the echo.

Coda

To listen this way is to practice analysis. The ear replaces interpretation; form replaces explanation. Each interval, each remainder, becomes an act of ethical attention. *Mikrokosmos* teaches what the analytic hour repeats: that knowing and unknowing are not opposites but two voices of the same phrase. Curved, recursive listening is the method—keeping form open, letting cadence suspend, and hearing remainder as rhythm.

This listening, curved and recursive, is what this book has tried to do in another register.

Bibliography

Abraham, N., & Torok, M. (1978/1994). *The shell and the kernel: Renewals of psychoanalysis.* (N. T. Rand, Ed. & Trans.). University of Chicago Press. (Original work published 1978).

Akhtar, S. (2009). *Comprehensive dictionary of psychoanalysis*. Karnac.

Anderson, T. (2025). Post-mutuality ethic: Presence, witnessing, and the ethics of non-relation in relational psychoanalysis. *Psychoanalysis, Self, and Context.* Advance online publication.

Anzaldúa, G. (1987). *Borderlands/La Frontera: The new mestiza.* Aunt Lute Books.

Atlas, G., & Aron, L. (2018). *Dramatic dialogue: Contemporary clinical practice.* (1st Ed.). Routledge.

Atwood, G. E., & Stolorow, R. D. (2014). *Structures of subjectivity: Explorations in psychoanalytic phenomenology and contextualism* (2nd Ed.). Routledge.

Bach, S. (1994). *The language of perversion and the language of love.* Jason Aronson.

Bachelard, G. (1969). *The poetics of space.* (M. Jolas, Trans.). Beacon Press.

Balint, M. (1968). *The basic fault: Therapeutic aspects of regression.* Northwestern University Press.

Baranger, M., & Baranger, W. (2008). The analytic situation as a dynamic field. *International Journal of Psychoanalysis, 89*(4), 795–826.

Baranger, M., & Baranger, W. (2009). *The work of confluence: Listening and interpreting in the psychoanalytic field.* (L. G. Fiorini, Ed.). Karnac. (Original work published 1961).

Bartók, B. (1940/1987). *Mikrokosmos: 153 progressive piano pieces in six volumes.* (Definitive Edition). Boosey & Hawkes.

Beckett, S. (1983). *Worstward ho.* Grove Press.

Benjamin, J. (1988). *The bonds of love: Psychoanalysis, feminism, and the problem of domination.* Pantheon.

Benjamin, J. (1990). An outline of intersubjectivity: The development of recognition. *Psychoanalytic Psychology, 7*(suppl), 33–46. https://doi.org/10.1037/h0085258

Benjamin, J. (1995). *Like subjects, love objects: Essays on recognition and sexual difference*. Yale University Press.

Benjamin, J. (2004/2017). Beyond doer and done to: An intersubjective view of thirdness. In L. Aron & A. Harris (Eds.), *Relational psychoanalysis* (Vol. 2, pp. 5–46). Routledge. (Original work published 2004).

Benjamin, J. (2018). *Beyond doer and done to: Recognition theory, intersubjectivity, and the third*. Routledge.

Benjamin, W. (1999). *The arcades project*. (H. Eiland & K. McLaughlin, Trans.). Belknap Press. (Original work written 1927–1940).

Benvenuto, S. (2016). *What are perversions? Sexuality, ethics, psychoanalysis*. Routledge.

Benvenuto, S. (2020). *Conversations with Lacan: Seven lectures for understanding Lacan*. Routledge.

Berger, J. (1972). *Ways of seeing*. BBC/Penguin.

Bersani, L. (1986). *The Freudian body: Psychoanalysis and art*. Columbia University Press.

Bersani, L. (2010). *Is the rectum a grave? and other essays*. University of Chicago Press.

Bion, W. R. (1959). Attacks on linking. *International Journal of Psychoanalysis, 40,* 308–315.

Bion, W. R. (1962). *Learning from experience*. Heinemann.

Bion, W. R. (1965). *Transformations*. Heinemann.

Bion, W. R. (1970a). *Attention and interpretation*. Tavistock.

Bion, W. R. (1970b). Notes on memory and desire. *Psychoanalytic Forum, 4,* 279–282.

Bollas, C. (1987). *The shadow of the object: Psychoanalysis of the unthought known*. Columbia University Press.

Bollas, C. (1992). *Being a character: Psychoanalysis and self experience*. Routledge.

Bollas, C. (2018). *Meaning and melancholia: Life in the age of bewilderment*. Routledge.

Boulanger, G. (2007). *Wounded by reality: Understanding and treating adult onset trauma*. Analytic Press.

Bromberg, P. M. (1998). *Standing in the spaces: Essays on clinical process, trauma, and dissociation*. Analytic Press.

Bromberg, P. M. (2006). *Awakening the dreamer: Clinical journeys*. Analytic Press.

Bromberg, P. M. (2011). *The shadow of the tsunami and the growth of the relational mind*. Routledge.

Bronfen, E. (1992). *Over her dead body: Death, femininity and the aesthetic*. Manchester University Press.

Bronfen, E. (1998). *The knotted subject: Hysteria and its discontents*. Princeton University Press.

Buchholz, M. B. (2014). Temporal patterns in therapeutic interaction. *Research on Language and Social Interaction, 47*(2), 105–129.

Buchholz, M. B. (2022). Doing we—Working alliance as a building process: A recursive model. In A. Hepburn, G. Raymond & J. Heritage (Eds.), *Talk in social interaction: Basic points and tenacious misconceptions* (pp. 71–95). John Benjamins.

Buchholz, M. B., & Kächele, H. (2013). Conversation analysis—A powerful tool for psychoanalytic practice and psychotherapy research. *Language and Psychoanalysis, 2*(2), 4–30.

Buñuel, L. (Director). (1962). *El Angel Exterminador [The Exterminating Angel]* [Film]. Producciones Gustavo Alatriste.

Butler, J. (2000). *Antigone's claim: Kinship between life and death.* Columbia University Press.

Cage, J. (1961). *Silence: Lectures and writings.* Wesleyan University Press.

Campbell, J. (1949). *The hero with a thousand faces.* Princeton University Press.

Chasseguet-Smirgel, J. (1985). *The ego ideal: A psychoanalytic essay on the malady of the ideal.* W. W. Norton.

Chodorow, N. (1994). *Femininities, masculinities, sexualities: Freud and beyond.* University Press of Kentucky.

Chodorow, N. (1999). *The power of feelings: Personal meaning in psychoanalysis, gender, and culture.* Yale University Press.

Civitarese, G. (2010). *The intimate room: Theory and technique of the analytic field.* Routledge.

Civitarese, G. (2016). *Truth and the unconscious in psychoanalysis.* Routledge.

Civitarese, G. (2019). *An apocryphal dictionary of psychoanalysis.* Routledge.

Civitarese, G. (2024). *On arrogance: A psychoanalytic essay.* Routledge.

Cooper, S. H. (2016). *The analyst's experience of the depressive position: The melancholic errand of psychoanalysis.* Routledge.

Corbett, K. (2009). *Boyhoods: Rethinking masculinities.* Yale University Press.

Csikszentmihalyi, M. (1990). *Flow: The psychology of optimal experience.* Harper & Row.

Dalí, S. (1929). *The great masturbator* [Painting]. Museo Nacional Centro de Arte Reina Sofía.

Dalí, S. (1931). *The persistence of memory* [Painting]. The Museum of Modern Art.

Damasio, A. (1999). *The feeling of what happens: Body and emotion in the making of consciousness.* Harcourt Brace.

Davies, J. M. (1994). Love in the afternoon: A relational reconsideration of desire and dread in the countertransference. *Psychoanalytic Dialogues, 4*(2), 153–170. https://doi.org/10.1080/10481889409539005.

Davies, J. M., & Frawley, M. G. (1994). *Treating the adult survivor of childhood sexual abuse: A psychoanalytic perspective.* Basic Books.

Dean, T. (2000). *Beyond sexuality.* University of Chicago Press.

Derrida, J. (1972/1982). *Margins of philosophy.* (A. Bass, Trans.). University of Chicago Press.

Derrida, J. (1978). *Writing and difference.* (A. Bass, Trans.). University of Chicago Press. (Original work published 1967).

Derrida, J. (1994). *Specters of Marx: The state of the debt, the work of mourning, and the New International.* (P. Kamuf, Trans.). Routledge.

Derrida, J. (1997). *Of grammatology.* (G. C. Spivak, Trans., corrected ed.). Johns Hopkins University Press. (Original work published 1967).

Derrida, J. (2000). *Of hospitality.* (A. Dufourmantelle, Trans.). Stanford University Press.

Dickinson, E. (1958). *The complete poems of Emily Dickinson.* (T. H. Johnson, Ed.). Little, Brown. (Poem 1263.)

Dimen, M. (2003). *Sexuality, intimacy, power.* Routledge.

Duchamp, M. (1917). *Fountain* [Readymade sculpture]. Photograph by Alfred Stieglitz. Public domain.

Eigen, M. (1993a). *The electrified tightrope.* Karnac.

Eigen, M. (1993b). *The psychoanalytic mystic.* Free Association Books.

Eigen, M. (1996). *Psychic deadness.* Harvard University Press.

Eigen, M. (1999). *Damaged bonds.* Continuum.

Eigen, M. (2004). *The sensitive self.* Wesleyan University Press.

Eigen, M. (2005). *Emotional storm.* Wesleyan University Press.

Eigen, M. (2006). *Flames from the unconscious.* Karnac.

Eigen, M. (2009). *Contact with the depths.* Karnac.

Eigen, M. (2014). *Faith.* Routledge.

Eigen, M. (2015). *The challenge of being human.* Karnac.

Erikson, E. H. (1950). *Childhood and society.* W. W. Norton.

Ernst, M. (1921–1938). *Collages and paintings* [Various works]. Various collections.

Escher, M. C. (1953). *Relativity* [Lithograph]. The M.C. Escher Company.

Fairbairn, W. R. D. (1952). *Psychoanalytic studies of the personality.* Routledge & Kegan Paul.

Ferenczi, S. (1988a). Confusion of tongues between adults and the child. (M. Balint, Trans.). In M. Balint (Ed.), *Final contributions to the problems and methods of psycho-analysis* (pp. 156–167). Karnac. (Original work published 1932).

Ferenczi, S. (1988b). *The clinical diary of Sándor Ferenczi.* (J. Dupont, Ed. M. R. Rudnytsky, Trans.). Harvard University Press. (Original work written 1932).

Ferenczi, S. (1994). Introjection and transference (E. Mosbacher, Trans.). In J. Rickman (Ed.), *First contributions to psycho-analysis* (pp. 35–93). Karnac. (Original work published 1909).

Ferro, A., & Civitarese, G. (2016). *The analytic field and its transformations.* Routledge.

Fink, B. (2007). *Fundamentals of psychoanalytic technique: A Lacanian approach for practitioners.* W. W. Norton.

Foucault, M. (1975/1995). *Discipline and punish: The birth of the prison.* (A. Sheridan, Trans.). Vintage Books.

Foucault, M. (1976/1990). *The history of sexuality, volume 1: An introduction.* (R. Hurley, Trans.). Vintage Books.

Foucault, M. (1980). *Power/knowledge: Selected interviews and other writings, 1972–1977.* (C. Gordon, Ed.). Pantheon.

Foucault, M. (1983). *This is not a pipe.* (J. Harkness, Trans.). University of California Press.

Foucault, M. (1986). *The care of the self: The history of sexuality, Vol. 3.* (R. Hurley, Trans.). Pantheon.

Foucault, M. (1997). *Ethics: Subjectivity and truth.* (P. Rabinow, Ed. R. Hurley et al., Trans.). The New Press.

Freud, S. (1900/1953). The interpretation of dreams. In J. Strachey (Ed. & Trans.), The standard edition of the complete psychological works of Sigmund Freud (Vols. 4–5, pp. ix–627). Hogarth Press. (Original work published 1900).

Freud, S. (1901/1953). The psychopathology of everyday life. In J. Strachey (Ed. & Trans.), *The standard edition of the complete psychological works of Sigmund Freud* (Vol. 6, pp. 1–279). Hogarth Press. (Original work published 1901).

Freud, S. (1905/1953). Three essays on the theory of sexuality. (J. Strachey, Trans.). In J. Strachey (Ed. & Trans.), *The standard edition of the complete psychological works of Sigmund Freud* (Vol. 7, pp. 123–246). Hogarth Press. (Original work published 1905).

Freud, S. (1910/1957). Wild psycho-analysis. In J. Strachey (Ed. & Trans.), *The standard edition of the complete psychological works of Sigmund Freud* (Vol. 11, pp. 219–227). Hogarth Press. (Original work published 1910).

Freud, S. (1911/1958). Psycho-analytic notes upon an autobiographical account of a case of paranoia (Dementia paranoides). In J. Strachey (Ed. & Trans.), *The standard edition of the complete psychological works of Sigmund Freud* (Vol. 12, pp. 1–82). Hogarth Press. (Original work published 1911).

Freud, S. (1911/1958). Formulations on the two principles of mental functioning. In J. Strachey (Ed. & Trans.), *The standard edition of the complete psychological works of Sigmund Freud* (Vol. 12, pp. 213–226). Hogarth Press.

Freud, S. (1912/1958). The dynamics of transference. In J. Strachey (Ed. & Trans.), *The standard edition of the complete psychological works of Sigmund Freud* (Vol. 12, pp. 97–108). Hogarth Press. (Original work published 1912).

Freud, S. (1915/1957). Instincts and their vicissitudes. (J. Strachey, Trans.). In J. Strachey (Ed. & Trans.), *The standard edition of the complete psychological works of Sigmund Freud* (Vol. 14, pp. 117–140). Hogarth Press. (Original work published 1915).

Freud, S. (1915/1957). The unconscious. In J. Strachey (Ed. & Trans.), *The standard edition of the complete psychological works of Sigmund Freud* (Vol. 14, pp. 159–215). Hogarth Press. (Original work published 1915).

Freud, S. (1917/1957). Mourning and melancholia. In J. Strachey (Ed. & Trans.), *The standard edition of the complete psychological works of Sigmund Freud* (Vol. 14, pp. 243–258). Hogarth Press.

Freud, S. (1918/1955). From the history of an infantile neurosis. In J. Strachey (Ed. & Trans.), *The standard edition of the complete psychological works of Sigmund Freud* (Vol. 17, pp. 1–122). Hogarth Press.

Freud, S. (1919/1955). A child is being beaten: A contribution to the study of the origin of sexual perversions. In J. Strachey (Ed. & Trans.), *The standard edition of the complete psychological works of Sigmund Freud* (Vol. 17, pp. 175–204). Hogarth Press.

Freud, S. (1919/1955). The uncanny. In J. Strachey (Ed. & Trans.), *The standard edition of the complete psychological works of Sigmund Freud* (Vol. 17, pp. 217–256). Hogarth Press. (Original work published 1919).

Freud, S. (1920/1961). *Beyond the pleasure principle.* (J. Strachey, Trans.). W. W. Norton. (Original work published 1920).

Freud, S. (1923/1961). The ego and the id. In J. Strachey (Ed. & Trans.), *The standard edition of the complete psychological works of Sigmund Freud* (Vol. 19, pp. 12–66). Hogarth Press.

Freud, S. (1924/1961). The loss of reality in neurosis and psychosis. In J. Strachey (Ed. & Trans.), *The standard edition of the complete psychological works of Sigmund Freud* (Vol. 19, pp. 183–187). Hogarth Press. (Original work published 1924).

Freud, S. (1925/1961). Negation. In J. Strachey (Ed. & Trans.), *The standard edition of the complete psychological works of Sigmund Freud* (Vol. 19, pp. 235–239). Hogarth Press. (Original work published 1925).

Freud, S. (1930/1961). Civilization and its discontents. In J. Strachey (Ed. & Trans.), *The standard edition of the complete psychological works of Sigmund Freud* (Vol. 21, pp. 57–145). Hogarth Press.

Freud, S. (1937/1964). Analysis terminable and interminable. In J. Strachey (Ed. & Trans.), *The standard edition of the complete psychological works of Sigmund Freud* (Vol. 23, pp. 209–254). Hogarth Press.

Freud, S. (1937/1964). Constructions in analysis. In J. Strachey (Ed. & Trans.), *The standard edition of the complete psychological works of Sigmund Freud* (Vol. 23, pp. 255–270). Hogarth Press. (Original work published 1937).

Freud, S. (1960). *The psychopathology of everyday life.* (A. A. Brill, Trans.). W. W. Norton. (Original work published 1901).

Fromm, E. (1941). *Escape from freedom*. Farrar & Rinehart.

Gendlin, E. T. (1978). *Focusing*. Everest House.

Glissant, É. (1997). *Poetics of relation.* (B. Wing, Trans.). University of Michigan Press.

Green, A. (1975). The analyst, symbolization, and absence in the analytic setting (On changes in analytic practice and analytic experience). *International Journal of Psycho-Analysis, 56*(1), 1–22.

Green, A. (1986). *On private madness.* (A. Weller, Trans.). Hogarth Press.

Green, A. (1986). The dead mother. In *On private madness.* (A. Weller, Trans., pp. 142–173). Hogarth Press. (Original work published 1983).

Green, A. (1999). *The work of the negative.* Free Association Books.

Green, A. (2001). *Life narcissism, death narcissism.* (A. Weller, Trans.). Free Association Books. (Original work published 1983).

Gödel, K. (1931/1986). On formally undecidable propositions of *Principia Mathematica* and related systems I. (B. Meltzer, Trans.). In S. Feferman et al. (Eds.), *Collected works* (Vol. 1, pp. 144–195). Oxford University Press. (Original work published 1931).

Guntrip, H. (1968). *Schizoid phenomena, object relations and the self.* International Universities Press.

Harris, A. (2009). *Gender as soft assembly.* Routledge.

Harris, A. (2021). Discussion: "synchronicity, acausal connection, and the fractal dynamics of clinical practice." *Psychoanalytic Dialogues, 31(*4), 487–492.

Heidegger, M. (1962). *Being and time.* (J. Macquarrie & E. Robinson, Trans.). Harper & Row. (Original work published 1927).

Hirshfield, J. (1994). The weighing. In J. Hirshfield (Ed.), *The October palace* (p. 79). HarperCollins.

Höch, H. (1919–1920). *Cut with the kitchen knife dada through the last weimar beer-belly cultural epoch of Germany* [Collage]. Staatliche Museen zu Berlin.

Hofstadter, D. R. (1979). *Gödel, Escher, Bach: An eternal golden braid.* Basic Books.

Horney, K. (1937). *The neurotic personality of our time.* W. W. Norton.

Isaacs, S. (1948). The nature and function of phantasy. *International Journal of Psycho-Analysis, 29*, 73–97.

Joseph, B. (1985). *Psychic equilibrium and psychic change: Selected papers of Betty Joseph.* Routledge.

Keats, J. (1817/1958). Letter to George and Thomas Keats, 21 December 1817. In H. E. Rollins (Ed.), *The letters of John Keats, 1814–1821* (Vol. 1 pp. 193–195). Harvard University Press.

Keats, J. (1958). *Selected letters of John Keats.* (L. B. Adams, Ed.). Harvard University Press. (Letter of Dec. 21/27, 1817 for "negative capability.")

Kernberg, O. F. (1975). *Borderline conditions and pathological narcissism.* Jason Aronson.

Kernberg, O. F. (1992). *Aggression in personality disorders and perversions.* Yale University Press.

Klein, M. (1937). Love, guilt and reparation. In M. Klein & J. Riviere (Eds.), *Love, guilt and reparation and other works 1921–1945* (pp. 306–343). Hogarth Press.

Klein, M. (1940/1975). Mourning and its relation to manic-depressive states. In M. Klein & J. Riviere (Eds.), *Love, guilt and reparation and other works 1921–1945* (pp. 344–369). Hogarth Press. (Original work published 1940).

Klein, M. (1946/1975). Notes on some schizoid mechanisms. In M. Klein & J. Riviere (Eds.), *Envy and gratitude and other works 1946–1963* (pp. 1–24). Hogarth Press. (Original work published 1946).

Klein, M. (1959). *Our adult world and its roots in infancy*. Tavistock.

Klein, M. (1975). *The psycho-analysis of children.* (A. Strachey, Trans.). The Hogarth Press. (Original work published 1932).

Klein, A. C., & Wangyal, T. (2006). *Unbounded wholeness: Dzogchen, Bon, and the logic of the nonconceptual*. Oxford University Press.

Knoblauch, S. H. (2000). *The musical edge of therapeutic dialogue.* The Analytic Press.

Knoblauch, S. H. (2020). *Bodies and social rhythms: Navigating unconscious vulnerability and emotional fluidity*. Routledge.

Kristeva, J. (1982). *Powers of horror: An essay on abjection.* (L. S. Roudiez, Trans.). Columbia University Press.

Lacan, J. (1966/2006). The function and field of speech and language in psychoanalysis (B. Fink, Trans.). In *Écrits: The first complete edition in English* (pp. 197–268). W. W. Norton. (Original work published 1953).

Lacan, J. (1977). *The four fundamental concepts of psycho-analysis.* (A. Sheridan, Trans.). W. W. Norton. (Original work published 1973).

Lacan, J. (1977). *Écrits: A selection.* (A. Sheridan, Trans.). W. W. Norton.

Lacan, J. (1992). *The ethics of psychoanalysis, 1959–1960.* (D. Porter, Trans.). W. W. Norton.

Laplanche, J. (1999). *Essays on otherness.* (J. Fletcher, Trans.). Routledge.

Laplanche, J., & Pontalis, J.-B. (1974). *The language of psycho-analysis.* (D. Nicholson-Smith, Trans.). W. W. Norton. (Original work published 1973).

Laub, D., & Auerhahn, N. C. (1993). Knowing and not knowing massive psychic trauma: Forms of traumatic memory. *International Journal of Psycho-Analysis, 74*(2), 287–302.

Lee, L.-Y. (1986). From blossoms. In G. Stern (Ed.), *Rose* (p. 24). BOA Editions.

Levertov, D. (1987). Making peace. In *Breathing the water* (p. 34). New Directions.

Levinas, E. (1969). *Totality and infinity: An essay on exteriority.* (A. Lingis, Trans.). Duquesne University Press.

Loewald, H. W. (1960). On the therapeutic action of psycho-analysis. *International Journal of Psycho-Analysis, 41*, 16–33.

Loewald, H. W. (1978). Primary process, secondary process, and language. *Psychoanalytic Quarterly, 47*(4), 430–451.

Loewald, H. W. (1980). *Papers on psychoanalysis.* Yale University Press.

Lombardi, R. (2017). *Body–mind dissociation in psychoanalysis: Development after Bion.* Routledge.

Longchenpa. (2014). *The practice of Dzogchen: Longchen Rabjam's writings on the great perfection.* (Tulku Thondup, Trans. & Ed., & Harold Talbott, Ed.). Snow Lion. (Original work written in the 14th century).

Magritte, R. (1928). *The lovers* [Painting]. Museum of Modern Art.

Magritte, R. (1937). *Not to be reproduced* [Painting]. Museum Boijmans Van Beuningen.

Main, R. (2004). *The rupture of time: Synchronicity and Jung's critique of modern western culture*. Routledge.

Man Ray. (c. 1958, replica of 1921 original). *The gift* [Readymade]. The Museum of Modern Art.

McWilliams, N. (1999). *Psychoanalytic case formulation*. The Guilford Press.

McWilliams, N. (2004). *Psychoanalytic psychotherapy: A practitioner's guide*. The Guilford Press.

McWilliams, N. (2011). *Psychoanalytic diagnosis: Understanding personality structure in the clinical process*. (2nd Ed.). Guilford Press.

McWilliams, N. (2021). *Psychoanalytic supervision*. The Guilford Press.

Mitchell, J. (1974). *Psychoanalysis and feminism: Freud, Reich, Laing and women*. Pantheon Books.

Mitchell, S. A. (1988). *Relational concepts in psychoanalysis: An integration*. Harvard University Press.

Mitchell, S. A. (1993). *Hope and dread in psychoanalysis*. Basic Books.

Mitchell, S. A., & Aron, L. (Eds.). (1999). *Relational psychoanalysis: The emergence of a tradition*. The Analytic Press.

Muñoz, J. E. (1999). *Disidentifications: Queers of color and the performance of politics*. University of Minnesota Press.

Ogden, T. H. (1994). *Subjects of analysis*. Jason Aronson.

Ogden, T. H. (1994). The analytic third: Working with intersubjective clinical facts. *International Journal of Psycho-Analysis, 75*(1), 3–19.

Ogden, T. H. (1997). Reverie and interpretation. *Psychoanalytic Quarterly, 66*(4), 567–595.

Ogden, T. H. (1997). *Reverie and interpretation: Sensing something human*. Karnac.

Ogden, T. H. (2004). The analytic third: Implications for psychoanalytic theory and technique. *Psychoanalytic Quarterly, 73*(1), 167–195.

Ogden, T. H. (2005). *This art of psychoanalysis: Dreaming undreamt dreams and interrupted cries*. Routledge.

Ogden, T. H. (2009). *Rediscovering psychoanalysis: Thinking and dreaming, learning and forgetting*. Routledge.

Ogden, T. H. (2016). *Reclaiming unlived life: Experiences in psychoanalysis*. Routledge.

Oliveros, P. (2005). *Deep listening: A composer's sound practice*. iUniverse.

Orange, D. M. (1995). *Emotional understanding: Studies in psychoanalytic epistemology*. Guilford Press.

Orange, D. M. (2011). *The suffering stranger: Hermeneutics for everyday clinical practice*. Routledge.

Parsons, M. (2000). *The dove that returns, the dove that vanishes: Paradox and creativity in psychoanalysis*. Routledge.

Parsons, M. (2014). *Living psychoanalysis: From theory to experience.* Routledge.

Phillips, A. (1993). *On kissing, tickling, and being bored: Psychoanalytic essays on the unexamined life.* Harvard University Press.

Phillips, A. (1995). *Terrors and experts.* Harvard University Press.

Rabaté, J.-M. (2003). Lacan's turn to Freud. In J.- M. Rabaté (Ed.), *The Cambridge companion to Lacan* (pp. 1–24). Cambridge University Press.

Rabaté, J.-M. (2014). *The Cambridge introduction to literature and psychoanalysis.* Cambridge University Press.

Racker, H. (1968). *Transference and countertransference.* International Universities Press.

Rank, O. (1929/1989). *Will therapy and truth and reality.* (J. Taft, Trans.). W. W. Norton.

Reik, T. (1962). *The haunting melody: Psychoanalytic experiences in life and music.* Farrar, Straus & Giroux. (Original work published 1948).

Reynolds, J. M. (2005). *The oral tradition from Zhang Zhung: An introduction to the Bonpo Dzogchen teachings of the oral tradition from Zhang Zhung and instructions on the practice of the four bonpo Dzogchen yogas of contemplation.* Vajra Publications.

Rilke, R. M. (1934). *Letters to a young poet.* (M. D. Herter Norton, Trans.). W. W. Norton & Company.

Rilke, R. M. (1992). *The Duino Elegies.* (S. Mitchell, Trans.). Shambhala.

Rilke, R. M. (1996). *Rilke's Book of Hours: Love Poems to God* (A. Barrows & J. Macy, Trans.). Riverhead Books. (Original work published 1905).

Ringstrom, P. A. (2014). *A relational psychoanalytic approach to couples psychotherapy.* Routledge.

Ringstrom, P. A. (2025a). On play in psychoanalysis. *Psychoanalytic Inquiry.* (In press).

Ringstrom, P. A. (2025b). Psychedelics and clinical uses of play. *Psychoanalytic Inquiry.* (In press).

Rothko, M. (1960). *No. 14* [Painting]. San Francisco Museum of Modern Art.

Roudinesco, É. (1999). *Jacques Lacan & Co.: A history of psychoanalysis in France, 1925–1985.* University of Chicago Press.

Roudinesco, É., & Plon, M. (1997). *A dictionary of psychoanalysis.* Columbia University Press.

Russell, B. (1903). *The principles of mathematics.* Cambridge University Press.

Sedgwick, E. K. (1990). *Epistemology of the closet.* University of California Press.

Segal, H. (1957). Notes on symbol formation. *International Journal of Psycho-Analysis, 38*, 391–397.

Slochower, J. (1991). *Holding and psychoanalysis: A relational perspective.* The Analytic Press.

Slochower, J. (1996). *Psychoanalytic collisions.* The Analytic Press.

Slochower, J. (2020). *Holding and psychoanalysis: A relational perspective.* (2nd ed.). Routledge.

Slochower, J. (2024). *Psychoanalysis and the unspoken.* Routledge.

Sophocles. (1984). *Antigone.* (R. Fagles, Trans.). In *The three Theban plays.* Penguin Classics. (Original work ca. 441 BCE).

Stern, D. B. (1997). *Unformulated experience: From dissociation to imagination in psychoanalysis.* Analytic Press.

Stern, D. B. (2010). *Partners in thought: Working with unformulated experience, dissociation, and enactment.* Routledge.

Stern, D. B. (2015). *Relational freedom: Emergent properties of the interpersonal field.* Routledge.

Stern, D. B. (2018). *The infinity of the unsaid: Unformulated experience, language, and the nonverbal.* Routledge.

Stern, D. B. (2024). *On coming into possession of oneself: Transformations of the interpersonal field.* (1st Ed.). Routledge.

Stern, D. N. (1985). *The interpersonal world of the infant: A view from psychoanalysis and developmental psychology.* Basic Books.

Stern, D. N. (2010). *Forms of vitality: Exploring dynamic experience in psychology, the arts, psychotherapy, and development.* Oxford University Press.

Stevens, W. (1990). The poems of our climate. In W. Stevens (Ed.), *The collected poems of Wallace Stevens* (p. 193). Vintage.

Stolorow, R. D., & Atwood, G. E. (1992). *Contexts of being: The intersubjective foundations of psychological life.* Analytic Press.

Stolorow, R. D., Atwood, G. E., & Orange, D. M. (2002). *Worlds of experience: Interweaving philosophical and clinical dimensions in psychoanalysis.* Basic Books.

Sullivan, H. S. (1953). *The interpersonal theory of psychiatry.* W. W. Norton.

Tanguy, Y. (1942). *Indefinite divisibility* [Painting]. Albright-Knox Art Gallery.

Taylor, D. (1997). Disappearing acts: Spectacles of gender and nationalism in Argentina's "dirty war." *Theatre Journal, 49*(2), 174–188.

Tomkins, S. (1962). *Affect imagery consciousness, Vol. 1: The positive affects.* Springer.

Tomkins, S. (1963). *Affect imagery consciousness, Vol. 2: The negative affects.* Springer.

Wheeler, J. A. (1983). Law without law. In J. A. Wheeler & W. H. Zurek (Eds.), *Quantum theory and measurement* (pp. 182–213). Princeton University Press.

White, D. G. (Ed.). (2012). *Yoga in practice.* Princeton University Press.

Winnicott, D. W. (1958/1965). The capacity to be alone. In D. W. Winnicott (Ed.), *The maturational processes and the facilitating environment* (pp. 29–36). Hogarth Press. (Original work published 1958).

Winnicott, D. W. (1963/1965). Communicating and not communicating leading to a study of certain opposites. In D. W. Winnicott (Ed.), *The maturational processes and the facilitating environment: Studies in the theory of emotional development* (pp. 179–192). International Universities Press. (Original work published 1963).

Winnicott, D. W. (1965). *The maturational processes and the facilitating environment*. International Universities Press.

Winnicott, D. W. (1969/1971). The use of an object and relating through identifications. In *Playing and reality* (pp. 86–94). Tavistock.

Winnicott, D. W. (1971). *Playing and reality*. Tavistock.

Wittgenstein, L. (1953). *Philosophical investigations*. (G. E. M. Anscombe, Trans.). Blackwell.

Wolfson, E. R. (1995). *Along the path: Studies in Kabbalistic hermeneutics, myth, and symbolism*. State University of New York Press.

Wolfson, E. R. (1995). *Circle in the square: Studies in the use of gender in Kabbalistic symbolism*. State University of New York Press.

Žižek, S. (1991). *For they know not what they do: Enjoyment as a political factor*. Verso.

Index

For Product Safety Concerns and Information please contact our EU representative GPSR@taylorandfrancis.com
Taylor & Francis Verlag GmbH, Kaufingerstraße 24, 80331 München, Germany

www.ingramcontent.com/pod-product-compliance
Lightning Source LLC
LaVergne TN
LVHW010852110826
845149LV00005B/1392

* 9 7 8 1 0 4 1 2 5 0 8 4 5 *